_k_

CULTURE CARE
DIVERSITY AND
UNIVERSALITY

A Worldwide Nursing Theory

SECOND EDITION

Madeleine M. Leininger,
PhD, LHD, DS, CTN, RN, FAAN, FRCN,

Professor Emeritus
College of Nursing
Wayne State University
Detroit, Michigan

Adjunct Faculty Memeber
College of Nursing
University of Omaha
Omaha, Nebraska

Marilyn R. McFarland, PhD, RN, CTN

Family Nurse Practitioner Student
Adjunct Faculty
Crystal M. Lange College
of Nursing and Health Sciences
Saginaw Valley State University
University Center, Michigan

JONES AND BARTLETT PUBLISHERS
Sudbury, Massachusetts
BOSTON   TORONTO   LONDON   SINGAPORE

World Headquarters

Jones and Bartlett
Publishers
40 Tall Pine Drive
Sudbury, MA 01776
978-443-5000
info@jbpub.com
www.jbpub.com

Jones and Bartlett
Publishers Canada
6339 Ormindale Way
Mississauga, ON
L5V 1J2
CANADA

Jones and Bartlett
Publishers International
Barb House, Barb Mews
London W6 7PA
UK

Jones and Bartlett's books and products are available through most bookstores and online booksellers. To contact Jones and Bartlett Publishers directly, call 800-832-0034, fax 978-443-8000, or visit our website, www.jbpub.com.

Substantial discounts on bulk quantities of Jones and Bartlett's publications are available to corporations, professional associations, and other qualified organizations. For details and specific discount information, contact the special sales department at Jones and Bartlett via the above contact information or send an email to specialsales@jbpub.com.

Production Credits

Acquisitions Editor: Kevin Sullivan
Production Director: Amy Rose
Associate Editor: Amy Sibley
Associate Production Editor:
    Carolyn F. Rogers
Marketing Manager: Emily Ekle
Manufacturing and Inventory
    Coordinator: Amy Bacus

Composition: Jason Miranda, Spoke & Wheel
Cover Design: Anne Spencer
Cover Image: Courtesy of Dr. Madeleine M. Leininger
Interior Design: Paw Print Media
Printing and Binding: Malloy, Inc.
Cover Printing: Malloy, Inc.

Library of Congress Cataloging-in-Publication Data
Culture care diversity and universality : a worldwide nursing theory / [edited by] Madeleine M. Leininger, Marilyn R. McFarland.-- 2nd ed.
    p. ; cm.
Includes bibliographical references and index.
ISBN 0-7637-3437-3 (pbk. : alk. paper)
1. Transcultural nursing. 2. Nursing--Cross-cultural studies. 3. Nursing--Philosophy.
    [DNLM: 1. Transcultural Nursing. 2. Nursing Theory. WY 107 C9678 2006]
I. Leininger, Madeleine M. II. McFarland, Marilyn R.
    RT86.54.C85 2006
    610.73'01--dc22

                                                            2005023891

Printed in the United States of America
09 08 07 06 05   10 9 8 7 6 5 4 3 2 1

Contents

The goal of transcultural nursing is to discover and creatively use culturally based research knowledge in order to provide culturally congruent care to people of diverse cultures.

—M. M. Leininger, 1978, 1991, 2004

Foreword

Since the publication of *Culture Care Diversity and Universality: A Theory of Nursing* (1991) by Dr. Madeleine Leininger, the entire world has been undergoing unprecedented rapid and often volatile change. Social, political, and economic issues in the 21st century are radically different from what they were in the 20th century producing forces that create uncertainty as well as opportunities for individuals, families, communities, and nations. Globalization has become a fact of life. Various migrations have brought unparalleled numbers of immigrants into nations that once consisted of a single ethnic group or religion. Large numbers of refugees have left their countries of origin because of war, persecution, or economic reasons. Some refugees have been forced to roam from place to place or from continent to continent. In addition, the technology revolution has changed the way we interact in the world and the way information is disseminated.

The impact of these changes on nursing and health care has also been unprecedented. As persons from diverse cultures encounter one another, cultural shock, ethnocentrism, prejudicial beliefs and behaviors, and cultural conflict are common. At this time, caring in nursing and other health care professions and the delivery system must assume strong leadership for effective and culturally congruent health care to occur. Benner and Wrubel, in *The Primacy of Caring* (1989, xi), stated, "Nursing is viewed as a caring practice whose science is guided by the moral art of ethics and responsibility." Leininger has stated since the early 1960s that *care is the essence of nursing*. Caring is viewed as a moral art and a primary need for health practices (Leininger, 1984, 1988). Leininger's theory of Culture Care Diversity and Universality was the first seminal work to demonstrate through research, practice, and education that cultural caring is essential in nursing and health care. This book and Leininger's other publications give nurses and other healthcare providers a most current and relevant knowledge base for understanding culturally based caring.

In the *Theory of Culture Care Diversity and Universality*, Dr. Leininger has combined her broad and extensive background in nursing and anthropology to thoughtfully create a new field called Transcultural Nursing. Her first book, *Nursing and Anthropology: Two Worlds to Blend* (1970) showed the potential for this new field of nursing. This potential has been presented further in many additional publications and is again clearly evident in this edition.

I was extremely fortunate to be one of Dr. Leininger's first students in the field of transcultural nursing in the early 1970s at the University of Washington in Seattle, Washington, USA. My interdisciplinary doctoral program included nursing, anthropology, and sociology. As my academic advisor and mentor, Dr. Leininger guided my study and dissertation, which were focused on phenomena in maternal and child nursing among women on a small Native American reservation of the Northwestern United States (Horn, 1975). In this early study, cultural caring was discovered to be central and essential to nursing care. I was also fortunate to observe how Leininger developed the caring constructs and further refined the theory and the ethnonursing method over these several years.

For the last half of the 20th century and now into the 21st century, Dr. Leininger has studied caring in many cultures. She has disseminated her findings in numerous publications and through teaching many undergraduate and graduate students. During this time she worked with many students around the world as well as in the United States. Under Dr. Leininger's mentorship and tutelage, students learned the culture care theory and ethnonursing method firsthand. These students were also coparticipants in the elucidation and explication of the theory and research method. Numerous theses, dissertations, and publications have their theoretical and conceptual underpinnings in the Culture Care Theory and have used the ethnonursing research method. In addition, the theory has been extensively used in practice settings in the United States and worldwide for cultural care assessments. This text gives many excellent examples of practice applications of the theory and research method. Developing the method to fit the theory was a unique and major contribution by Leininger.

Dr. Leininger has worked relentlessly to perfect the components of the theory and the ethnonursing research method over these past decades. Clearly, holistic health care is in great demand today, which necessitates indepth understanding of cultural and care phenomena to provide culturally congruent and effective nursing care. A superficial approach to these areas can be more harmful than helpful. Leininger's philosophy is that indepth reading and study of the subject matter are essential; her many publications and those of others have provided this indepth knowledge base. The theory of Culture Care with the ethnonursing research method has led to a substantial body of knowledge for nursing and for other health care providers. Knowledge obtained using the theory and ethnonursing method has earned professional confidence as a result of the high degree of rigor used in data collection and analysis. Research findings from the use of the method with the theory have brought new approaches and knowledge to the care of diverse cultures (Leininger & McFarland, 2002).

This book is a unique, outstanding, and rich resource for nurses and healthcare providers. A full explication of the theory and ethnonursing method provides a comprehensive approach to the study of caring with a focus on universal and diverse aspects. The multiple clinical examples based on the theory and research method are especially useful because they provide a clear explanation of how theory and research are critical in nursing practice.

This book has multiple applications and uses for nurses and health care personnel. Nurse educators will find the book invaluable and practitioners will find that it has immediate application to varied health care situations and settings, and all health care providers will find information essential to holistic and culturally based care. I am very pleased to have the opportunity to recommend this excellent text to all in health care today. It is a significant landmark in the advancement of health care to diverse cultures.

Beverly Horn, RN, CHN, CTN, PhD
Professor Emeritus
University of Washington
Seattle, WA

References

Benner, P., & Wrubel, P. (1989). *The primacy of caring: Stress and coping in health and illness*. Menlo Park, CA: Addison-Wesley.

Horn, B. M. (1975). *An ethnoscientific study to determine social and cultural factors affecting Native American women during pregnancy*. Unpublished doctoral dissertation, University of Washington, Seattle, Washington.

Leininger, M. (1970). *Nursing and anthropology: Two worlds to blend*. New York: John Wiley & Sons.

Leininger, M. (1984). *Caring: The essence of nursing and health*. Detroit, MI: Wayne State University Press.

Leininger, M. (1988). *Care: The essence of nursing and health*. Detroit, MI: Wayne State University Press.

Leininger, M., & McFarland, M. (2002). *Transcultural nursing: Concepts, theories, research and practices* (3rd ed.). New York: McGraw-Hill, Inc.

Preface

Madeleine M. Leininger

The purpose of a book preface is to alert readers to what they might anticipate in this publication. In the preface, the authors share the purpose of the book and some of the major features. The purpose of this book is to update the reader about the theory of Culture Care Diversity and Universality and recent developments with the ethnonursing research method. Since the first edition was published in 1991, there have been several refinements to clarify the theory and make it meaningful for use in different contexts. In the past decade many nurses have discovered the theory and are using it to study diverse cultures, subcultures, and different phenomena of interest to them. The theory has become popular and very important in gaining indepth knowledge about a particular domain of inquiry of interest to a researcher. It has been encouraging to see undergraduate and graduate nursing students use the theory and discover remarkable insights about its use in relation to health, care, illness, and wellness contexts. The students often relate how exceedingly pleased they have been to use the theory and method. They tell about discoveries and new insights not known before in their profession.

Through the years, the authors have mentored many of these students and have helped them become skilled in theory and method uses. They find the theory is relevant to nursing and 'makes sense.' The theory and method have become well known as 'user friendly,' rewarding, and exciting to use. Thus, several suggestions from the users of the theory have been included in this revised edition. Readers can benefit from these suggestions and from the many authors who have made chapter contributions.

This book contains many new and original chapters and a few classic chapters from the 1991 book which have been preserved and present the use of the theory with the ethnonursing method in different cultures in clinical and community environments. There are new chapters about people from different cultures and ideas for using the theory in nursing practice, administration, and research. The classic chapters were included because they have been so essential and meaningful to transcultural nurses over time. Brief synopses of other classic chapters have been included to inform readers that these cultures have been studied with the theory and method and can be useful to health professionals. These brief summaries include the Philippine and Anglo American cultures and research on dying and hospice clients in institutional contexts. Most importantly the ethnonursing research enablers have been included from the original 1991 book because they remain in great demand in transcultural nursing as well as in other disciplines.

As many researchers know, the authors value the importance of indepth *emic* and *etic* knowledge to fully grasp the phenomena under study. Qualitative research methods have at last taken hold in nursing and have slowly been introduced to other health care fields. Indeed, transcultural nurse researchers have taken the lead with qualitative methods and have been 'ahead of their time' in their use. The ethnonursing qualitative research method was developed by me in the 1950s. This method and other qualitative methods are being valued to discover largely invisible, covert knowledge about care, wellbeing, health, and wellness phenomena. This shift to the recognition of the importance of qualitative research and the use of the ethnonursing method designed to fit the theory has been a major breakthrough for nursing and other health disciplines. The ethnonursing research method was different from the quantitative approach with traditional measurement of a few specific variables and reductionistic data analyses. The ethnonursing method with newly developed enablers was designed to systematically study the major tenets of the Culture Care Theory. These points are reinforced in this revised edition with new researchers presenting their discoveries.

The Culture Care Theory remains one of the most holistic and comprehensive theories in nursing and in most health disciplines. It is the only theory focused explicitly on discovering the relationships of care (caring) and health phenomena of specific and diverse cultures related to wellness or illness, and the only one to address death and dying among diverse cultures. In the past five decades, the discovery of specific care and health meanings, expressions, and symbols have been noteworthy contributions of transcultural nurse researchers. The use of culture specific care knowledge about wellness, health, and wellbeing related to people care has been a major breakthrough to help cultures attain, regain, or maintain health within their familiar contexts. It has been a powerful experience to study and to promote respect of cultural values, beliefs, and practices of diverse cultures. Nearly 50 years have passed since this largely unknown body of culture care knowledge, so needed in nursing and health care services, began to be slowly discovered. It is this knowledge base that is also viewed by many health personnel as the new and major breakthrough in health care. The use of this knowledge has led to new ways to prevent illnesses and to maintain health by relying on research data related to cultural values, beliefs, and practices.

The comparative knowledge has been valuable to discover and appreciate cultural diversities and commonalities in health care. Most importantly, the reader will discover ways the theory and method are used together to obtain culture care knowledge which includes both therapeutic generic and professional care. The reader will gain many new culturally based insights into how cultures have promoted care, health, and wellbeing that are meaningful and acceptable to them. More and more, the Culture Care Theory is being recognized and appreciated as a guide to gain new knowledge and for holistic health care assessments. The well-known Sunrise Enabler and several other enablers are presented to guide researchers to discover actual and potential factors that can influence care and wellbeing. Thus the close relationship between the use of the Culture Care Theory and the ethnonursing research method originally envisioned with the theory has become valuable, especially to provide culturally congruent and appropriate care practices.

The goal to provide culturally congruent care is being sought and taught worldwide in order to prevent negative care practices and other unfavorable or inappropriate care and healing practices. It is the Culture Care Theory with the ethnonursing method that is currently recognized as beneficial to provide congruent and appropriate care outcomes. Furthermore, many cultures are now expecting—and some demanding—culturally congruent care. This book addresses this critical need and a wealth of culturally based care knowledge with therapeutic practices.

In the first part of the book the chapters are broad and open to capture the reader's interest. Basic and substantive ideas on the relevance of the theory and the method are presented as foundational ideas. In subsequent chapters, the focus is directed toward linking the theory with the specific domains of inquiry or the interest areas of the researchers and providers. The reader of this book is, therefore, encouraged to focus on seeking culturally congruent findings, and to think broadly and holistically to grasp the multiple factors influencing care and health. Researchers, however, should remain focused on the theory tenets and their specific domain of inquiry under investigation. The researcher will find that the use of enablers is a most helpful means to tease out or probe for covert knowledge. These enablers help one to discover indepth knowledge about culture, care, and health related to specific values and beliefs of past or current practices. The reader will find the contents of this book greatly expand one's ways of understanding cultures and their unique or common culture care practices and beliefs. One will realize the new insights into cultures are very different from traditional nursing and traditional medicine with their largely biophysical approaches. The findings will change health care myths and misunderstandings of cultures. As the culture and care factors become understood, the practices will, out of necessity, change. Grasping and providing holistic care and using multiple cultural factors influencing health and caring in different environments, contexts, and geographic areas over time will be new challenges. The reader will value this new world of transcultural research knowledge, along with the theory and research method with therapeutic care practices. The authors, therefore, hope this second edition will lead to new pathways to discover and provide cultural specific care, and to value the uniqueness and commonalities among cultures.

Discovering that cultures have differences and similarities is essential to being a culturally competent professional practitioner. One will realize the benefits of the theory and the method and the critical need for transcultural nursing research to provide quality care to diverse cultures. We contend this book is a major step toward this goal as one lives and works in a rapidly growing multicultural world.

Dedication and Acknowledgments

This book is dedicated to our beloved family members and to the many nursing students, faculty, and multidisciplinary colleagues who have been with us in the process of writing this book. For several decades we have worked with, taught, and mentored many students in transcultural nursing. These special friends have been genuinely interested in establishing and advancing transcultural nursing knowledge and care practices. We are, indeed, most grateful to those undergraduate and graduate students and other scholars who have recognized the great importance of the theory of Culture Care Diversity and Universality. Many students have been quick to recognize the need for transcultural nursing knowledge and for discovering a theory to explicate humanistic care and health of diverse cultures. To these perceptive and enthusiastic learners and practitioners, we dedicate this book. We know their interest, enthusiasm, and commitment to the theory and the ethnonursing method has been remarkable. They will continue to use and sustain the theory and the method well into the future.

This book reflects the work of two committed transcultural nurse authors, leaders, teachers, practitioners, and researchers who have dedicated many teaching and mentoring hours to help others learn the theory and method. The authors have taught hundreds of nursing students from diverse cultures. We dedicate this book to these students, and to all others over time, who have shared their research findings and experiences with us.

Many of the contributors to this book are doctorally prepared transcultural nurses who continue to forge ahead with their teaching, research, consultation, and practice in creative ways. The theory and the method have been viewed as invaluable to them. This book, therefore, is also dedicated to these pioneers and persistent users of the theory and the method. These nurses have been courageous leaders by showing 'newcomers' the importance of and ways to use the theory and the method. Their persistent and enthusiastic efforts are known to many nursing students and to interdisciplinary colleagues who have recently become knowledgeable about the theory and method.

Teaching and conducting holistic transcultural nursing with theory based research in diverse and often high risk environments has often been difficult and challenging, but most rewarding. It has also been difficult to move from being a cultural stranger to a 'research friend' while remaining patient and understanding of complex cultural explanations in the research learning process. Many transcultural nurse leaders and students have been exemplars in discovering new research insights and by providing culturally congruent care. We appreciate the persistent efforts of these nurses and their enthusiastic transcultural nursing research endeavors and discoveries. They have been invaluable in leading the way to new approaches in health care and in establishing the new body of transcultural nursing knowledge we use today. Therefore, we also dedicate this book to these leaders in grateful appreciation of their creative endeavors and persistent efforts.

The authors would be remiss if we did not fully and gratefully acknowledge the faithful and competent secretaries and assistants who helped with this book, namely Arlene Mayberger, Angela LeFevre Welke, Marilyn Eipperle, Adebola Grillo, and Evison Kalulu. These dedicated persons and others have been most helpful and competent in seeing this book become a reality. We also appreciate that several transcultural nurse leaders have shared their ideas with us in the process of writing and reflecting on the content of these chapters. We are grateful to Penny Glynn of Jones & Bartlett for her encouragement and openness in working with us. Her help and that of others from the book company have been greatly appreciated.

Most of all, we dedicate this book to our families for their patience and their 'never-ending' understanding of our not being available while writing this book over many months. Their attitude and understanding have been deeply appreciated, and so this book is dedicated to them with our love and gratitude.

The contributing authors have provided their fresh insights and creative ways for studying culture care and health phenomena using the theory and the method. Their contributions to this second edition are deeply appreciated. Many of these contributions are unique and original. They are most important for advancing the body of transcultural nursing knowledge and for demonstrating the use of the theory and the ethnonursing research method. To all those who have been loyal and dedicated supporters over the past years in establishing and promoting the new discipline of transcultural nursing and for promoting the teaching and importance of transcultural research, we are most grateful. Accordingly, we dedicate this book to these many leaders and followers who have often faced difficult struggles in teaching and performing this new kind of research using a holistic theory. They have also struggled to obtain transcultural nursing courses and implement these practices into professional curricula and to conduct transcultural nursing research using qualitative methods. Indeed, these leaders have all been significant contributors in carving out the new pathway of transcultural nursing knowledge for the growing and important discipline of transcultural nursing. So our most grateful thanks goes to all these committed and persistent leaders and followers of this new movement in nursing and health care.

Finally, I (Leininger) have been most grateful to God that my health was maintained allowing me to complete this major book, for it reflects many years of my career in transcultural nursing as well as my contributions to other health disciplines. This book and my many publications are essential for the continuity of the discipline of transcultural nursing and health care services to often neglected cultures. It has been a pleasure to work with my coauthor, Dr. Marilyn McFarland, for we have learned and grown together in this sustained endeavor.

If we have missed giving acknowledgments to others who have in some way contributed to or assisted with this publication, please accept our sincere apologies and sincere thanks.

Madeleine M. Leininger
Marilyn R. McFarland

Contributors

Margaret Andrews, RN, PhD, CTN, FAAN
Faculty
University of Northern Colorado
Greeley, Colorado

Debra A. Curren, RN, MS, CTN
Curren Culture Care Consulting
Greeley, Colorado

Cheryl Easley, PhD, RN
Dean of College of Health and
  Social Welfare
University of Alaska–Anchorage
Anchorage, Alaska

Linda S. Farrell, PhD, RN
Michigan, USA

Ann O. Hubbert, PhD, RN, CTN
Assistant Professor of Nursing
University of Nevada–Reno
Reno, Nevada

Madeleine M. Leininger, PhD, LHD, DS, CTN, RN, FAAN, FRCNA
Professor Emeritus
College of Nursing
Wayne State University
Detroit, Michigan
and
Adjunct Faculty Member
College of Nursing
University of Omaha
Omaha, Nebraska

Averetta E. Lewis, RN, PhD, APRN-BC
Family Nurse Practitioner
Saginaw, Michigan
and
Professor of Nursing
Crystal M. Lange College of Nursing
  and Health Sciences
Saginaw Valley State University
University Center, Michigan

Marilyn R. McFarland, PhD, RN, CTN
Family Nurse Practitioner Student
and
Adjunct Faculty
Crystal M. Lange College of Nursing
  and Health Sciences
Saginaw Valley State University
University Center, Michigan

Sandra Mixer, MSN, RN
Doctoral Student
University of Northern Colorado
Greeley, Colorado
and
Assistant Professor of Nursing
Middle Tennessee State University
Murfreesboro, Tennessee

Hiba Wehbe-Alamah, APRN-BC, MSN
Doctoral Student, Duquesne University
Pittsburgh, Pennsylvania
and
Adjunct Faculty
Crystal M. Lange College of Nursing and Health Sciences
Saginaw Valley State University
University Center, Michigan USA
and
Nurse Practitioner
Saginaw County Health Department
Saginaw, Michigan

Anna Frances Z. Wenger, PhD, RN, CTN, FAAN
Senior Scholar, Interfaith Health Program
Rollins School of Public Health
Emory University
Atlanta, Georgia
and
Faculty/Consultant, Ethiopia Public Health Initiative
The Carter Center
Atlanta, Georgia

Norma Zehnder, RN, PhD, APRN-BC
Adjunct Faculty
Crystal M. Lange College of Nursing and Health Sciences
Saginaw Valley State University
University Center, Michigan

CHAPTER ONE

Culture Care Diversity and Universality Theory and Evolution of the Ethnonursing Method

Madeleine M. Leininger, PhD, LHD, DS, CTN, RN, FAAN, FRCNA

The Culture Care Theory

Leininger's (1991a/b) theory of Culture Care Diversity and Universality is the creative outcome of independent thinking, a keen awareness of a rapidly changing world, and more than five decades of using and refining the theory. It is not a borrowed theory but has been independently developed as a theory highly relevant to discover the care and health needs of diverse cultures. The theory draws upon the theorist's experiences and creative thinking to construct a theory useful to nursing and other health fields. The roots of the theory reflect the theorist's early and current nursing practice in hospitals, clinics, community settings, and her study of many cultures worldwide. In the late 1940s patients often expressed their appreciation to the theorist for healing them through her <u>caring actions</u>. Many direct observations and experiences with clients of diverse cultures with a variety of health conditions led the theorist to realize that the human care mode was important for recovery from illnesses and maintaining health and wellbeing. Most importantly, a caring nurse who understood and could provide therapeutic care to people of diverse cultures was a critical and longstanding need in nursing and all health practices (Leininger, 1977, 1988a/b/c, 1991a/b; Leininger & McFarland, 2002).

In the early 1950s, the theorist worked as a clinical mental health specialist in a child guidance center with mildly disturbed children of diverse cultural backgrounds. It was during this time she saw differences in the care of children and realized that only limited research had been conducted in relation to care within specific cultures and in health institutions. It was evident that nurses and other health professionals failed to recognize and appreciate the important role of culture in healing, caring processes, and in medical treatment practices. Culture and care were identified by Leininger as major dimensions missing in nursing and health care services (Leininger, 1978, 1995). The theorist tried to use psychoanalytic and other mental health ideas popular after World War II to help clients, but these practices were woefully inadequate to explain or help children and adults of different cultural backgrounds. The theorist's interest continued to grow along with many questions about the interface of culture and care. Understanding and responding appropriately and therapeutically to clients of different cultures was a critical need that merited theoretical explanations and research investigation for beneficial outcomes.

Given that the theorist had no substantive knowledge about cultures and care in her basic and advanced nursing education, and no preparation in cultural anthropology, she decided to pursue an academic doctoral program in anthropology at the University of Washington in Seattle in the early 1960s. Her goal was to become knowledgeable about different cultures and the theories with research findings related to diverse cultures and caring. During this educational process the theory of Culture Care Diversity and Universality was developed with a specific focus on nursing and health outcomes. Her goal was to provide a sound theory in nursing but also one that could be used in other health-related disciplines. She envisioned a new field of transcultural nursing as an important discipline for study and practice in the mid 1950s. Through creative thinking and the discovery of the close relationship between culture and care phenomena, Leininger began to envision the theory. Bringing culture and care together into a new conceptual and theoretical relationship was a major challenge. It was a difficult endeavor due to the lack of studies and limited interest by nurses in the idea. However, the need became more and more apparent in Leininger's clinical observations and studies. Gradually the theorist envisioned a theory of Culture Care Diversity and Universality as a new way to discover and help people. Both culture and care needed to be studied in depth and worldwide with a comparative focus. The theorist envisioned that such knowledge could greatly transform nursing and health in both education and practice worldwide. But extensive research and systematic study were needed in the two major domains of culture and care and the interrelationships between them. Care research with a theoretical base was definitely needed. Care meanings and actions were vague and limitedly understood. In the period following World War II, many immigrants and refugees from diverse cultures were moving to the United States and to other places worldwide. There was also the need to bring this knowledge into nursing as a sound basis for the new discipline of transcultural nursing.

After five decades of study and research, the Theory of Culture Care Diversity and Universality has been established as a major, relevant, and dominant theory in nursing. It is also used by other health-related disciplines to provide transcultural care to people of diverse cultures. Most importantly, transcultural nursing has become a recognized field of study and practice. Knowledge of cultures with their care needs using the Culture Care Theory has become a major and unique emphasis in nursing as a means to know and help cultures (Leininger, 1988a/b/c, 1991a/b, 1995a; Leininger & McFarland, 2002). Culturally based care factors were being recognized as influences upon human expressions related to health, illness, wellbeing or to face death and disabilities. The theory became meaningful and a guide to nurses' thinking, practices, and research. The process of envisioning and reconceptualizing care as the essence of nursing from a holistic care perspective was an exciting and new way of knowing and understanding people.

Epistemically and ontologically, the theorist held that *care* was the essence of nursing or what made nursing what it is or could be in healing, wellbeing, and to help people face disabilities and dying. The theorist held that *care is nursing, care is health, care is curing, and care is wellbeing* (Leininger 1988a/b/c, 1991a/b; Leininger & McFarland, 2002). The theorist also postulated that human care is what makes people human, gives dignity to humans, and inspires people to get well and to help others (Leininger, 1977, 1984; Leininger & McFarland, 2002). Leininger further held and predicted that there could be no curing without caring, but caring could exist without curing (Leininger, 1984, 1988a; Leininger & McFarland, 2002). This was a profound theoretical hunch predicting that care was a powerful and central dominant force for healing and wellbeing. Indeed, this statement continues to be studied with a transcultural focus (Leininger & McFarland, 2002). Research focused on culture care as an interrelated phenomenon was crucial to identify and advance nursing and health care. Care needed to become meaningful, explicit, and beneficial; it had to be conceptualized showing the interrelationships of care to culture and to different cultures—the transcultural nursing focus. Care was a powerful and dynamic force to understand the totality of human behavior in health and illness worldwide. Action modes related to care that were culturally based and maintained beneficial health outcomes were needed. Care needed to be understood and actualized in diverse and specific cultural contexts.

Leininger (1988) held that culture was the broadest, most comprehensive, holistic, and universal feature of human beings and care was predicted to be embedded in culture. Both had to be understood to discover clients' care needs. Caring was held as the action mode to help people of diverse cultures while care was the phenomenon to be understood and to guide actions. Culture care together was predicted to be a powerful theoretical construct believed essential to human health, well-being, and survival. Knowledge of the specific culture care values, beliefs, and lifeways of human beings within life's experiences was held as important to unlock a wealth of new knowledge for nursing and health practices. These ideas had not been studied indepth or from a transcultural comparative perspective. In fact, culturally based care was held by Leininger (1994b) as essential and long overdue to help people of diverse cultures in healing, recovery, and to face death and disabilities.

The theorist predicted that culture and care were embedded in each other and needed to be teased out and understood within a cultural context. Most importantly, this knowledge would contribute to transcultural nursing as a discipline and practice field. The Culture Care Theory and transcultural nursing were closely related modes as bases for being human, but also for health and wellbeing. The embedded phenomenon of culturally based care was new and significant and needed to be discovered and the research findings creatively used to provide transcultural nursing care. Such care could be culturally meaningful, therapeutic, congruent, and safe for people of diverse and similar cultures. Using culturally based research about care was a significant challenge to promote healing, recovery, wellbeing, and healthy lifeways. This goal remains a major challenge for health care professionals. These ideas and predictions were very exciting to the theorist. However, they needed to be rigorously studied transculturally for explicit knowledge in order to guide nurses and other health professionals in their caring actions and decisions. Both culture and care were of equal importance and neither could be neglected. The idea of culture care as a synthesized dominant and central construct within the theory of Culture Care Diversity and Universality was the new focus. Culturally based care needed to be studied in a unique way to discover fresh and different ways to serve people, especially those of diverse cultures. Most importantly, the theorist challenged nurses to discover both cultural diversity and universality about care worldwide.

The purpose of the theory of Culture Care was to discover, document, know, and explain the interdependence of care and culture phenomena with differences and similarities between and among cultures. Such knowledge was believed to be essential for current and future professional nursing care practice and for that of other health care providers. A new body of research based culture care knowledge was envisioned as opening new ways to practice nursing and provide health care services. This body of knowledge could revolutionize and transform nursing and health care with benefits to people of similar and different cultures. Most importantly, this would support the new discipline of transcultural nursing envisioned by the theorist and lead to therapeutic outcomes.

From the beginning, the goal of the Culture Care Theory has been to use culture care research findings to provide specific and-or general care that would be culturally congruent, safe, and beneficial to people of diverse or similar cultures for their health, wellbeing, and healing, and to help people face disabilities and death (Leininger, 1963, 1991a/b, 1994a, 1995; Leininger & McFarland, 2002).

Basic Theoretical Differences

Philosophically and professionally many questions about culture, care, and nursing were raised but few nursing research studies were available. Many nurses viewed *care* as an important word to use in teaching and practice, but few possessed substantive care knowledge or could explain care within a culture. Care knowledge that had scientific and accurate data about cultures with care meanings, expressions, and beneficial outcomes was missing. Indeed, many nurses in the 1950s and 1960s were absorbed in studying medical diseases, symptoms, and regimens of treatment for many diseases.

While working on the theory, it became apparent that the Theory of Culture Care would be very different from other existing ideas or emerging nursing theories in several respects. *First*, the central domain of the theory was focused on culture and care relationships. This theory was directed mainly toward discovering largely unknown or vaguely known ideas about care and culture. For Leininger, care should not be taken for granted or remain as an invisible, covert, and unknown dimension (Leininger, 1988b). It was time that care became explicit, confirmed, and documented within and among cultures. *Second*, some theorists used the terms *theories* and *models* in the same way. But as one studied the constructs of theory and models, they were different. Theories should predict and lead to discovery of unknown or vaguely known *truths* about some phenomena. Such theoretical knowledge should explain and guide nurses' thinking, actions, and decisions. Models are mainly pictorial diagrams of some idea, but they are not theories as they usually fail to show predictive relationships. There are different kinds of theories used by different disciplines to generate knowledge. However, all theories have as their primary goal to discover new phenomena or explicate vaguely known knowledge (Leininger 1991a/b). *Third*, theorists have hunches and predictions about the interrelationships of the major phenomena or variables under study. The Culture Care Theory was open to the discovery of new ideas that were vague or largely unknown but influenced people's culture care outcomes related to their health and wellbeing. No other theorist had focused explicitly on synthesized culture care using an open discovery process. Some researchers focused on a few specific variables to be measured. However, Leininger's theory focused on <u>culture care as a broad yet holistic phenomenon and the central domain of care inquiry with multiple factors or influencers on care and culture</u>. *Fourth*, the theorist valued an open discovery and naturalistic process to explore different aspects of care and culture in natural or familiar living contexts and in unknown environments. *Fifth*, Leininger developed a specific research method, namely the ethnonursing method, to systematically and rigorously discover the domain of inquiry (DOI) concerning culture care. This method was new and unknown in nursing and was different from other qualitative methods including ethnography. The ethnonursing method was designed as an open, natural, and qualitative inquiry mode seeking informants' ideas, perspectives, and knowledge about care and culture. The theorist did not want a method that controlled, reduced, or manipulated culture and care as with the quantitative methods. Studying only a few variables selected by the researcher was not acceptable. To discover entirely new or different phenomena it was necessary for the researcher to hear informants tell stories about their health and cultural lifeways. Indeed, narrow hypotheses with reductionistic goals could greatly limit obtaining holistic and unknown culture and care knowledge, and would curtail the discovery of complex, covert, and embedded phenomena about culture and care (Leininger, 1985, 1991a/b, 1995; Leininger & McFarland, 2002).

Furthermore, the new Culture Care Theory was focused on obtaining <u>indepth knowledge of care and culture constructs</u> from key and general informants related to health or wellbeing, dying or disabilities. Again, nurse theorists in the 1950s and 1960s were very few and most focused on a few concepts to be measured. They followed the quantitative paradigm and philosophy. In contrast, Leininger's theory and method followed the qualitative paradigm and was used to tease out largely unknown or vaguely known data about culture care.

Most importantly, Leininger's theory differed considerably from other nurses' work or thinking in the mid 1980s as the few nurse leaders concerned with theory development relied on the four metaparadigm concepts of <u>person</u>, <u>environment</u>, <u>health</u> and <u>nursing</u> to explain nursing. These concepts were proclaimed as <u>the definitive metaparadigm of nursing</u> (Faucett, 1984; Fitzpatrick & Whall, 1989). However, Leininger (1991a/b; 1994b) found these four concepts were very questionable, limited, inappropriate, and inadequate to explain or fully discover nursing and especially ideas bearing on transcultural nursing. Of great concern, <u>care</u> and <u>culture</u> were unfortunately *excluded* from the metaparadigm. In critiquing these four metaparadigm concepts, several problems prevailed from viewpoints within transcultural nursing and general logic. First, it is not logical to use <u>nursing</u> to *explain* <u>nursing</u>. It is a theoretical and logical contradiction to use the <u>same term to explain or predict the same phenomenon</u>. Such illogical and inappropriate reasoning violates scholarly research and discovery principles. Most importantly, Leininger's early definition of nursing had become known and was desired by many nurses. Nurses were beginning to study human care as an area of interest to them. The absence of <u>care</u> in the metaparadigm demonstrated limited nurses' interest or value in studying care as a nursing phenomenon needing to be explained. The theorist [Leininger] had defended nursing as a "...*learned humanistic and scientific profession and discipline which is focused on human care phenomena and activities in order to assist, support, facilitate, or enable individuals or groups to maintain or regain their wellbeing (or health), in culturally meaningful and beneficial ways or to help people face handicaps or death*" (Leininger, 1991a, p. 47). This definition was held by academically prepared and perceptive nurses as giving credence to the true nature of nursing. However, only a few nurses identified care and culture as worthy of study. Why were care and culture excluded from nursing? Did it reflect a lack of knowledge and interest in these two major phenomena? Was it a failure to envision the great relevance and potential for nursing?

The Culture Care Theory explicitly focused on care and culture because they were the missing phenomena that had been long neglected and needed to be discovered in order to grasp the full nature of nursing or to explain nursing. Indeed, the Culture Care Theory was the only theory focused on developing a new knowledge for the discipline of transcultural nursing. There was evidence that nurses needed to provide care to diverse cultures worldwide but were unable to do so without a base of culture care research knowledge (Leininger, 1970, 1988b, 1994b). Culture and care were new to most nurses in the 1950s. Leininger (1988a/b/c) saw culture and care knowledge as critical societal and global needs for sustaining and maintaining nursing as a profession. Culturally congruent care for the health or wellbeing of humans was largely undiscovered. The theory with its focus on culture and care was in its infancy and long overdue for study by nursing. Care and culture were held by Leininger as the heart and soul of nursing, and essential for developing new transcultural nursing knowledge and practices and to move nursing into a predicted multicultural and global world (Leininger, 1980, 1988b, 1991a/b).

Yet another major difference in Leininger's theory in comparison with other nursing ideas was that this theory predicted three action modalities or decision modes for providing culturally congruent nursing care. The three modes were highly innovative and unique in nursing and health care. Leininger (1994b) held that nurses needed creative and different approaches to make care and culture needs meaningful and helpful to clients. These three theoretically predicted action and decision modes of the culture care theory were defined as follows (Leininger, 1991a/b; Leininger & McFarland, 2002).

1. Culture care preservation and-or maintenance referred to those assistive, supportive, facilitative, or enabling professional acts or decisions that help cultures to retain, preserve, or maintain beneficial care beliefs and values or to face handicaps and death.
2. Culture care accommodation and-or negotiation referred to those assistive, accommodating, facilitative, or enabling creative provider care actions or decisions that help cultures adapt to or negotiate with others for culturally congruent, safe, and effective care for their health, wellbeing, or to deal with illness or dying.
3. Culture care repatterning and-or restructuring referred to those assistive, supportive, facilitative, or enabling professional actions and mutual decisions that would help people to reorder, change, modify, or restructure their lifeways and institutions for better (or beneficial) health care patterns, practices, or outcomes. (Leininger, 1991a/b, 1995; Leininger & McFarland, 2002).

These three action-decision care modes were unique and were not found in other theories or in current nursing and health practices. Furthermore, the three modes based on research data were held to be essential for caring and to be used with specific research care data discovered from the theory. The theory challenged nurses to discover specific and holistic care as known and used by the cultures over time in different contexts. Both care and culture were held to be central and critical nursing constructs for any nursing metaparadigm. Leininger's theory was the first theory directed toward discovering and using culturally based or derived research care knowledge in nursing obtained from culture informants. To achieve this goal, both *emic* [insider] and *etic* [outsider] knowledge were two new and important constructs in the theory introduced by the theorist to differentiate the informants' inside knowledge in contrast with the researcher's outsider or professional knowledge. This was another unique difference from other theorists' or nurses' work. The cultural informants' *emic* knowledge about care was deeply valued. Both *emic* and *etic* data were studied as integral parts of the theory to obtain comparative and contrasting care knowledge. Such insider [*emic*] and outsider [*etic*] knowledge gave valuable insights to nurses caring for cultures, and to date have led to many new ideas about culture care that nurses need to know and understand.

The reader will find that the frequently used phrase *nursing interventions* is seldom used in the Culture Care Theory or in transcultural nursing. This term has often been used inappropriately and is viewed by several cultures as too controlling or all knowing. When used by nurses, this term may lead to interferences through words or actions with the cultural lifeways, values, and practices of others. This is because it often refers to or represents <u>cultural imposition</u> nursing practices used when providing care to clients which may be offensive or in conflict with their lifeways.

Returning to the metaparadigm, the second concern with the four metaparadigm concepts (Faucett, 1989) was the use of *person*. From transcultural knowledge, *person* may not be used and may not be the central, meaningful, or dominant term in some cultures (Leininger, 1991a/b, 1995; Leininger & McFarland, 2002). Instead, the linguistic terms of *human beings, families, clans,* and *collective groups* are frequently used transculturally because these terms have cultural meanings and are often used by the people. These terms in many cultures are spiritually derived. Moreover, in nonWestern cultures *person* or *individual* may be culturally taboo and not used as these terms are too egocentric and do not fit the philosophy of people. This practice sharply contrasts with American, Canadian, European, and other Western cultures where <u>person</u> and <u>individualism</u> tend to dominate Western thoughts and communication modes. The use of *person* in the metaparadigm is highly questionable. Using *person* may lead to cultural clashes, cultural biases, and cultural imposition practices or to serious ethical–moral conflicts. The use of the term *human beings* has a more universal transcultural meaning, carries dignity and respect for people, and is generally more acceptable transculturally. In cultures that acknowledge God as a supreme being who created human beings, this term or the use of a similar term known to the culture should be used and respected. Most human beings believe they are endowed with rights to live, were created by a supreme being, and need to be cared for by other human beings including nurses. Certain human care rights, obligations, and privileges are known in many cultures even though they vary in actions, interpretation, and practices. In general, human beings are valued and respected and often viewed as sacred. The Culture Care theorist holds that respecting human beings from a spiritual, cultural, and holistic perspective while caring for them is essential for human care and caring.

It was important for nurses to discover humanistic *culture care differences* and *similarities*. The theorist believed that dominant specific culture care constructs could be discovered from a holistic viewpoint.

The lifeways and care patterns of human beings or groups were important to be discovered. Such <u>comparative</u> data about culture care phenomena was unique and another way to know and help people.

Third, the concept of <u>environment</u> was a complex and multifaceted dimension in all cultures. It varied transculturally and required very broad geophysical and social knowledge. Understanding ecologies and different environments in which people live and survive or die is important. Leininger (1991a/b) valued the phenomenon of environment, and it was included in the theory as depicted in the Sunrise Enabler. *Environment* as a major construct of the theory had to be systematically examined. As an influencer of health and caring, *environment* refers to the <u>totality of geophysical situation(s), or about the lived-in geographic and ecological settings of cultures</u>. Special environmental meanings, symbols, and commonly shared views and values exist as part of the environmental context. The environmental context included multiple factors such as the physical, ecological, spiritual, sociopolitical, kinship, or technological dimensions that influenced culture care, health, and wellbeing. The environmental context gives clues about care expressions, meanings, and patterns of living for individuals, groups, and families. Holistic cultural context knowledge provides for different environments as care settings for self or others living in culturally specific ways, such as woodlands, plains, wet lands, or arid areas. Such holistic dimensions of environment go beyond commonly focused biophysical and emotional foci used by nurses, and to broad areas of grasping living and caring settings. The environmental context also provides information about birthing and dying rituals in one's environmental context (Leininger, 1988b).

Fourth and finally, the concept of <u>health</u> used by Fawcett (1984) in the nursing metaparadigm has remained important in the Culture Care Theory but was predicted as an <u>outcome of using and knowing culturally based care</u>, rather than biophysical or medical procedures and treatments. The theorist has defined health as "...*a state of well-being that is culturally defined and constituted. Health is a state of being to maintain and the ability to help individuals or groups to perform their daily role activities in culturally expressed beneficial care and patterned lifeways*" (Leininger, 1991a/b; 1995). All cultures have both different and similar patterns and ways to maintain health. Observing and following cultural rules for wellness is culturally known. By using the Culture Care Theory, the nurse researcher discovers what constitutes health with its meanings and symbols, and ways cultures know, transmit, and practice health care including intergenerational practices including differences and similarities. The focus on <u>human care</u> rather than health alone has challenged nurses to discover <u>health</u> *and* <u>care together and how this</u>

knowledge has been preserved, maintained and restored for health out-comes through use of Culture Care Theory. Many nurse theorists have focused only on health as the outcome without knowledge of cultural care influences. Leininger holds that it is care and caring knowledge and actions that can explain and lead to the health or wellbeing of people in different or similar cultures (Leininger, 1984, 1988a, 1991a/b; Leininger & McFarland, 2002). The theorist predicted one can explain health in diverse contexts and also discover the commonalities or universalities transculturally. Thus, the Culture Care Theory was significantly differ-ent from other nursing theories that focused on health or a few, specific physical illnesses or conditions to arrive at nursing activities. These the-orists failed to study the importance, power, or major influence of care to explain health or wellbeing. For Leininger, care beliefs, values, and prac-tices were predicted to be the powerful explanatory means to discover and understand health as well as to explain nonhealth or predict illness conditions. To date, transcultural nursing studies have found that the terms health *and* wellbeing are often used interchangeably when explaining health and care. Such terms often explained health promoting and maintenance attributes in many cultures (Leininger, 1991a/b; Leininger & McFarland, 2002). Most importantly, *health* was discovered as an often restorative attribute, whereas wellbeing implied a quality of life or a desired state of existence in most cultures studied (Leininger, 1993a/b; Leininger & McFarland, 2002).

Thus, the four metaparadigm concepts were found to be highly ques-tionable and neglected culture and care to explain nursing. This seemed ironic and a gross oversight because of the frequent linguistic uses of *care* in nurses' daily language. The Culture Care Theory has given primary emphasis to care as the essence and central dominant construct of nurs-ing since 1960. Since the 1980s, other nurses such as Gaut (1984), Ray (1987), Watson (1985), and others have studied, valued, and stressed care as important to nursing (Leininger, 1984, 1988a/b/c, 1997d). In fact, sev-eral nurse researchers are now actively explicating care phenomena. Unfortunately, some will fail to study and link culture with care to gain new insights about nursing. Since the 1990s, *culture* has become a popu-lar public word to describe behaviors or values different from one's own and especially to understand immigrants.

Other Central Constructs in the Culture Care Theory

There are several additional constructs used in the Culture Care Theory that need to be briefly identified. Many of these constructs can be stud-ied further in Leininger's first and primary theory book as examples for reflective study (Leininger, 1991a/b). These constructs and their definitions have also been presented in several published research studies with their domains of inquiry (Leininger, 1991a/b, 1995; Luna, 1998; McFarland, 1997). Thus theory definitions are <u>orientational</u> (not <u>operational</u>) to encourage the researcher to discover new qualitative knowledge and to avoid being focused solely on the researcher's quantitative definitions or Western ideas. Cultures usually have their own definitions and uses of their terms. This is another major difference between this theory and other nursing theories that have prescribed definitions which usually reflect the researcher's interests or ethnocentric views. Due to space limitations only a few key and essential constructs are briefly defined and discussed below; others can be studied in the transcultural nursing literature. They are the following:

1. <u>Care</u> refers to both an abstract and-or a concrete phenomenon. Leininger has defined <u>care as those assistive, supportive, and enabling experiences or ideas towards others with evident or anticipated needs to ameliorate or improve a human condition or lifeway</u> (Leininger, 1988a/b/c, 1991a/b, 1995a; Leininger & McFarland, 2002). <u>Caring</u> refers to <u>actions, attitudes, and practices to assist or help others toward healing and wellbeing</u> (Leininger, 1988a/b/c, 1991a/b, 1995a; Leininger & McFarland, 2002). Care as a major construct of the theory includes both <u>folk</u> and <u>professional</u> care, which are a major part of the theory and have been predicted to influence and explain the health or wellbeing of diverse cultures. From current research, care is largely an embedded, invisible, and often *taken for granted* phenomenon that is difficult for nurses to quickly identify or grasp with indepth meaning. However, over the past five decades many books, articles, and research studies have become available enabling nurses to discover and know differential care meanings of diverse cultures (Leininger, 1976, 1984, 1988a/b/c, 1991a/b; Leininger & McFarland, 2002). Nurses are also learning that care is more than *doing* or performing physical action tasks. <u>Care</u> has <u>cultural</u> and <u>symbolic meanings</u> such as <u>care as protection</u>, <u>care as respect</u>, and <u>care as presence</u>. These care linkages are essential to provide culture specific care and are often gender linked. Several master's and doctoral research studies have discovered transcultural care meanings within and between cultures. (See Appendix.) Most of these studies are by doctorally prepared transcultural nurse researchers who have teased out covert and indepth meanings of care in scientific and authentic ways for clinical care practices. They also know how to use the Culture Care Theory and the ethnonursing method very well.

2. Culture as the other major construct central to the theory of Culture Care has been equally as important as care and is therefore not an adverb or adjective modifier *to care*. The theorist conceptualized *culture care* as synthesized and closely linked phenomena with interrelated ideas. Both culture and care require rigorous and full study with attention to their embedded and constituted relationship to each other as a human care phenomenon. Leininger has defined *culture* as "...the learned, shared, and transmitted values, beliefs, norms, and lifeways of a particular culture that guides thinking, decisions, and actions in patterned ways and often intergenerationally" (Leininger, 1991a/b; 1997a). From an anthropological perspective, culture is usually viewed as a broad and most comprehensive means to know, explain, and predict people's lifeways over time and in different geographic locations. Moreover, culture is more than social interaction and symbols. Culture can be viewed as the blueprint for guiding human actions and decisions and includes material and nonmaterial features of any group or individual. It has been a major construct in anthropology for nearly a century. Culture is more than ethnicity or social relationships. Culture phenomena distinguish human beings from nonhumans. Unfortunately, and until transcultural nursing began, these phenomena had not been studied and valued explicitly in nursing (Leininger, 1988a/b/c). Today, transculturally prepared nurses are advancing culture knowledge in many ways by uniting culture and care together conceptually and for research purposes. This new approach in nursing is encouraging. Social scientists are also learning the importance of transcultural nurse research. The powerfulness of the culture care dual construct to discover and understand illness, wellness, and other human health expressions remains a new thrust in nursing. The theorist has held that culture care phenomena conceived and linked together have great power to explain health and-or illness. To date, research studies focused on culture care phenomena have led to the discovery of important outcomes using the Culture Care Theory and the ethnonursing method. The findings are beginning to transform nursing education and practices (Leininger, 1991a/b, 1997b; Leininger & McFarland, 2002).

3. The constructs *emic* and *etic* care were another major part of the theory. The theorist wanted to identify differences and similarities among and between cultures. It was believed desirable to know what is universal [or common] and what is different [or diverse] among cultures with respect to care. The term *emic* refers to the local, indigenous, or insider's cultural knowledge

and view of specific phenomena; whereas *etic* refers to the outsider's or stranger's views and often health professional views and institutional knowledge of phenomena (Leininger, 1991a/b). *Emic* and *etic* terms were derived from linguistics but were reconceptualized by the theorist within her theoretical perspectives to discover contrasting culture care phenomena. These two dual constructs, emic and etic, have been invaluable in explicating the differences and interdependencies among cultural informants' and professional nurses' knowledge and practices over the past several decades (Leininger & McFarland, 2002).

There are two other major related constructs coined by the theorist and used in the theory:

a. Generic (*emic*) care refers to the *learned and transmitted lay, indigenous, traditional, or local folk (emic) knowledge and practices to provide assistive, supportive, enabling, and facilitative acts for or towards others with evident or anticipated health needs in order to improve wellbeing or to help with dying or other human conditions* (Leininger & McFarland, 2002).

b. Professional (*etic*) nursing care refers to *formal and explicit cognitively learned professional care knowledge and practices obtained generally through educational institutions* [usually nongeneric]. They are taught to nurses and others to provide assistive, supportive, enabling, or facilitative acts for or to another individual or group in order to improve their health, prevent illnesses, or to help with dying or other human conditions (Leininger, 1991a/b, 1995, 1997a; Leininger & McFarland, 2002).

4. Cultural and Social Structure Factors are another major feature of the theory. Social structure phenomena provide broad, comprehensive, and special factors influencing care expressions and meanings. Social structure factors of clients include religion (spirituality); kinship (social ties); politics; legal issues; education; economics; technology; political factors; philosophy of life; and cultural beliefs and values with gender and class differences. The theorist has predicted that these diverse factors must be understood as they directly or indirectly influence health and wellbeing. In the past, social structure factors were not explicitly studied in nursing nor in reference to *care* until the advent of transcultural nursing. The use of Leininger's theory has helped nurses to study these dimensions for a holistic or total view of clients. The study of these factors is providing a wealth of new

and invaluable insights about culturally based care leading to health, wellness, or illness. Culturally congruent care is indeed the desired goal of the theory (Leininger, 1991a/b, 1995, 1997a; Leininger & McFarland, 2002).

5. Ethnohistory is another construct of the theory. Ethnohistory comes from anthropology but the theorist reconceptualized it within a nursing perspective. The theorist defines ethnohistory as the *past facts, events, instances, and experiences of human beings, groups, cultures, and institutions that occur over time in particular contexts that help explain past and current lifeways about culture care influencers of health and wellbeing or the death of people* (Leininger 1991a/b; Leininger & McFarland, 2002). Ethnohistory is another guide to attain culturally congruent care. Special past and current events and conditions within the historical context of cultures and caring modalities over time are important data for transcultural nursing knowledge and caring practices especially when studied within the lifecycle of care and wellbeing.

6. Environmental context refers to the *totality of an event, situation, or particular experience that gives meaning to people's expressions, interpretations, and social interactions within particular geophysical, ecological, spiritual, sociopolitical, and technologic factors in specific cultural settings* (Leininger 1989, 1991a/b; Leininger & McFarland, 2002).

7. Worldview refers to the *way people tend to look out upon their world or their universe to form a picture or value stance about life or the world around them* (Leininger 1991a/b; Leininger & McFarland, 2002). Worldview provides a broad perspective of one's orientation to life, people, or groups that influence care or caring responses and decisions. Worldview guides one's decisions and actions, especially related to health and wellbeing as well as care actions.

8. Culture Care Preservation and-or Maintenance, Culture Care Accommodation and-or Negotiation, and Culture Care Repatterning and-or Restructuring have been defined earlier in this chapter and in Leininger & McFarland (2002, p. 84). Many examples are given in the subsequent chapters of this book within specific cultures.

9. Culturally Congruent Care refers to *culturally based care knowledge, acts, and decisions used in sensitive and knowledgeable ways to appropriately and meaningfully fit the cultural values, beliefs, and lifeways of clients for their health and wellbeing, or to prevent illness, disabilities, or death* (Leininger,

1963, 1973b, 1991a/b, 1995; Leininger & McFarland, 2002). To provide culturally congruent and safe care has been the major goal of the Culture Care Theory.

10. Care Diversity refers to the *differences or variabilities among human beings with respect to culture care meanings, patterns, values, lifeways, symbols, or other features related to providing beneficial care to clients of a designated culture* (Leininger, 1995, 1997a; Leininger & McFarland, 2002). Recently the term *cultural disparities* is being used by people with limited transcultural insights. It is not an acceptable term to use in transcultural nursing because of its negative connotations and narrow viewpoints.

11. Culture Care Universality refers to the *commonly shared or similar culture care phenomena features of human beings or a group with recurrent meanings, patterns, values, lifeways, or symbols that serve as a guide for caregivers to provide assistive, supportive, facilitative, or enabling people care for healthy outcomes* (Leininger, 1995).

For several decades, *transcultural nursing* has been defined as a discipline of study and practice focused on comparative culture care differences and similarities among and between cultures in order to assist human beings to attain and maintain meaningful and therapeutic health care practices that are culturally based (Leininger, 1963, 1991a/b, 1994b, 1995; Leininger & McFarland, 2002). Transcultural nursing continues to identify and use comparative care discoveries, skills, and standards to help human beings of diverse or similar cultures in beneficial ways. As stated earlier, transcultural nursing came into being as an essential and imperative field of study and practice to meet societal and global needs of people of diverse and similar cultures. The theory of Culture Care Diversity and Universality has been a major breakthrough for research based knowledge based on direct field experiences to support the discipline of transcultural nursing over the past many decades. This leads to offering some brief statements about the philosophical basis, theoretical tenets, and major assumptions of the theory of Culture Care Diversity and Universality.

Philosophical and Theoretical Roots

Given that the theory was developed independently without any particular persons or schools of thought, the theorist's philosophy of life, her extensive professional nursing experiences, anthropological and other relevant knowledge, diverse intellectual scholarly interests, and spiritual insights and beliefs were used. As a spiritual person, the theorist believes that God created all human beings with His caring interest and love, and that He wanted human beings to be healthy and contribute love and help to other human beings. Nursing was viewed as a unique caring profession to serve others worldwide. It is influenced by ethno-history, culture, social structure, and environmental factors in different geographic areas and by the different needs of people. Nursing is a dynamic field of study and practice that takes into account culture, religion, social change, and multiple factors that influence health and well-being. It is a profession with discipline knowledge to help people, whether ill or well, with their diverse care needs.

The theorist's intellectual and educational interest in religious beliefs and in the humanities and diverse philosophies of life were all important in developing the theory. The theorist's preparation in the biological sciences, philosophy, mental health, nursing, anthropology, psychology, and many diverse and broad life experiences of 80 years all influence ongoing development of the theory. Her 50 years as a professional nurse clinician and educator, as well as her extensive experience in nursing administration, education, and research were reflected upon in developing the theory. She was interested in developing new practices for nursing to meet diverse cultural needs and to provide therapeutic care practices. The complexity of human beings and diverse cultural lifeways challenged her thinking to provide comprehensive and holistic care practices. Thus, she contended that the medical model of focusing on diseases, symptom relief, and pathological conditions was far too narrow for a caring discipline. Holistic and broad worldviews respecting the sacredness and uniqueness of humans and their culturally based values were imperative to surpass traditionally narrow medical and past nursing perspectives. The Culture Care Theory thus had to be broad, holistic, and yet culture specific with research based knowledge to transform nursing and traditional medicine (Leininger, 1997b). The new discipline of transcultural nursing needed to be developed as an essential and long overdue field of study and practice and especially to serve neglected cultures (Leininger, 1997c).

Theoretical Tenets and Predictions

Tenets are the positions one holds or are givens that the theorist uses with a theory. In developing the theory, four major tenets were conceptualized and formulated with the Culture Care Theory:

1. Culture care expressions, meaning, patterns, and practices are diverse and yet there are shared commonalities and some universal attributes.

2. The worldview, multiple social structure factors, ethnohistory, environmental context, language, and generic and professional care are critical influencers of cultural care patterns to predict health, well-being, illness, healing, and ways people face disabilities and death.
3. Generic *emic* [folk] and *etic* [professional] health factors in different environmental contexts greatly influence health and illness outcomes.
4. From an analysis of the above influencers, three major actions and decision guides were predicted to provide ways to give <u>culturally congruent, safe, and meaningful health care to cultures</u>. The three culturally based action and decision modes were: (a) <u>culture care preservation and-or maintenance</u>; (b) <u>culture care accommodation and-or negotiation</u>; and, (c) <u>culture care repatterning and-or restructuring</u>. Decision and action modes based on culture care were key factors predicted for congruent and meaningful care. Individual, family, group, or community factors are assessed and responded to in dynamic and participatory nurse–client relationships (Leininger 1991a/b, 1993b, 2002; Leininger & McFarland, 2002).

Theoretical Assumptions

The above major theoretical tenets and predictions of the theory led to the formation of specific theoretical hunches or assumptions that the researcher could use in Western and nonWestern cultures over time and in different geographic locations. Some of the theoretical assumptions (assumed givens) were the following (Leininger & McFarland, 2002):

1. Care is the essence and the central dominant, distinct, and unifying focus of nursing.
2. Humanistic and scientific care is essential for human growth, wellbeing, health, survival, and to face death and disabilities.
3. Care (caring) is essential to curing or healing for there can be no curing without caring. (This assumption was held to have profound relevance worldwide.)
4. Culture care is the synthesis of two major constructs that guide the researcher to discover, explain, and account for health, wellbeing, care expressions, and other human conditions.
5. Culture care expressions, meanings, patterns, processes, and structural forms are diverse but some commonalities (universalities) exist among and between cultures.

6. Culture care values, beliefs, and practices are influenced by and embedded in the worldview, social structure factors (e.g., religion, philosophy of life, kinship, politics, economics, education, technology, and cultural values) and the ethnohistorical and environmental contexts.
7. Every culture has generic [lay, folk, naturalistic; mainly emic] and usually some professional [etic] care to be discovered and used for culturally congruent care practices.
8. Culturally congruent and therapeutic care occurs when culture care values, beliefs, expressions, and patterns are explicitly known and used appropriately, sensitively, and meaningfully with people of diverse or similar cultures.
9. Leininger's three theoretical modes of care offer new, creative, and different therapeutic ways to help people of diverse cultures.
10. Qualitative research paradigmatic methods offer important means to discover largely embedded, covert, epistemic, and ontological culture care knowledge and practices.
11. Transcultural nursing is a discipline with a body of knowledge and practices to attain and maintain the goal of culturally congruent care for health and wellbeing.

Culture care is the broadest, most comprehensive holistic and universal theory for the discovery of new knowledge to help people of diverse cultures. Cultural lifeways, beliefs, values, and practices are powerful means to know and assist people of diverse cultures. The above tenets and assumptions of the theory are essential to guide transcultural care research knowledge and practices. The Culture Care Theory is a fresh and bold new theory, different from existing nursing theories, which can greatly transform nursing and health practices. The purpose and the goal of the theory must always be kept foremost in researchers' minds. The ethnonursing research method was thoughtfully designed to fit the theory tenets and purpose of the theory. The six enablers were designed to tease out indepth care and culture knowledge from informants living in different cultural contexts. They will be discussed later and are also presented in the chapters on specific cultures using the theory and ethnonursing method.

An Overview of the Ethnonursing Research Method

The ethnonursing research method was explicitly designed by Leininger (1985) to fit the Theory of Culture Care Diversity and Universality and to fit the purposes of qualitative research methods. It was developed as an important means to tap vague, largely complex, covert, and unknown care and cultural phenomena in order to generate fresh data as a basis for culturally congruent care. Findings from use of the theory and the method are analyzed in detail to improve care to clients of diverse cultures (Leininger, 1985, 1993a/b, 1991a/b). Ethnonursing is a rigorous, systematic, and indepth method for studying multiple cultures and care factors within familiar environments of people and to focus on the interrelationships of care and culture to arrive at the goal of culturally congruent care services. The Sunrise Enabler and other enablers were developed by the theorist as research guides to obtain broad, yet specific, indepth knowledge bearing on the goal of the theory and researchers' domains of inquiry. The six enablers cover multiple factors influencing care patterns and expressions. The Sunrise Enabler has been widely used and valued to expand nurses' views and discoveries. The Sunrise Enabler is not the theory per se, but depicts multiple factors predicted to influence culture care expressions and their meanings (Leininger, 1988c, 1991a/b, 1994b, 1995, 1997a; Leininger & McFarland, 2002). The Sunrise Enabler serves as a cognitive map to discover embedded and multiple factors related to the theory, tenets, and assumptions with the specific domain of inquiry under study. This visual diagram reminds the researcher to search broadly for diverse factors influencing care within any culture under study. The enablers do not neglect professional or etic medical knowledge about human beings in illness and health such as biophysical, social, and nursing or medical factors, but focus mainly on total lifeways and care or caring factors influencing health and-or wellbeing, disabilities, and death. Traditional emic medical and nursing knowledge exists but it is often lodged in social structure, ethnohistory, and environmental factors. These emic sources of knowledge (limitedly discovered in the past) are now providing very rich and new insights about people in their familiar and general cultural holistic contexts with specific cultural needs.

Researchers' openness for discovering different influencers on care and caring is imperative with this theory and method. The Culture Care Theory is neither a grand theory nor a middle range theory even though some nurses may try to place the theory in these reductionistic categories. Researchers wed to middle range theories tend to reduce data to specific variables and fail to grasp holistic and multiple, related factors about human care behavior as known and explained by informants. Middle range theory generally limits exploration to a few variables and leads to a study of narrow, restrictive, and specific variables that tend to fit the researchers' interests or problems. Holistic discoveries and their interrelationships as explained by informants are essential for discovering fully both culture and care phenomena. The ethnonursing method was designed so the researcher could discover both macro and micro phenomena depending on the researcher's stated domain of inquiry within the tenets of the Culture Care Theory. The theory with its broad holistic focus can provide both particular and general care data with relationship to social structure and other factors. Both rich descriptive subjective and objective culture care phenomena are the informants' authentic *truths* to explain care and culture phenomena within their world. In addition, the theory provides the framework to abstract phenomena discovered from the use of the <u>Observation, Participation, and Reflection Enabler</u>. Such detailed observations and shared information from key and general informants provide scientific and humanistic data as macro or micro findings when using the qualitative ethnonursing method and its paradigm enablers. Nursing students who have used the theory and method become very excited when discovering social structure factors related to specific care phenomena such as kinship and religious ideas that explain care and care practices. Care constructs such as comfort, succorance, nurturance, presence, comfort, respect, and many other specific care expressions have been discovered over the past many decades largely by using the enablers (Leininger 1991a/b, 1997b; Leininger & McFarland, 2002). Although the ethnonursing method was designed to focus on culture care phenomena, many new insights and findings have been discovered with the method and theory related to nursing, care, and health–illness practices. Credible and accurate data are sought from the informants using verbatim statements and other data, along with symbolic referents and ways to heal and care for people of specific cultures. Such findings provide both depth and breadth research knowledge about human care phenomena (Leininger 1985, 1991a/b, 1995, 1997a; Leininger & McFarland, 2002).

The <u>ethnonursing method</u> is a <u>qualitative nursing research method focused on naturalistic, open discovery, and largely inductive [emic] modes to document, describe, explain, and interpret informants' worldview, meanings, symbols, and life experiences as they bear on actual or potential nursing care phenomena</u> (Leininger, 1985, 1995; Leininger & McFarland, 2002). This method is valuable for discovering both <u>emic</u> generic and <u>etic</u> professional data. It is a natural and familiar people centered method that informants enjoy—finding the open and informal discovery process comfortable and natural. They like to talk about their views and to lead the discussion focused on their culture. Fresh informant ideas, practices, and beliefs from the culture and their care world along with a wealth of related data are discovered using the theory and the ethnonursing method. The Culture Care Theory is a highly rewarding and valuable theory and the research method fits the theory. The indepth, diverse, and rich descriptive data are valuable for discovering care and cultural findings. Informants seldom withdraw from studies as many are pleased that this is *the first time they could tell their story about their culture and lifeways.*

Criteria to Evaluate Ethnonursing Research Findings

In the mid 1950s, the theorist was confronted with a major dilemma as many nurses were already wed to the use of quantitative methods for obtaining and evaluating so called *scientific* nursing and largely medical data. Using quantitative methods they often missed rich data that comes from qualitative methods, purposes, and related philosophies. With the Culture Care Theory and the ethnonursing method, qualitative criteria were chosen to explicate largely covert, detailed, and meaningful data on care, culture, and nursing. If one relied on the quantitative criteria, many findings would be lost, omitted, or reduced to almost meaningless numbers and sometimes unreliable explanations. Quantitative criteria such as Hardy's (1974) or other similar criteria that emphasized operational definitions, logical inferences, and numerical outcomes often missed data related to cultures and care. Reducing data to measurable indicators related to the five senses and using narrow experimental quantitative numerical formulas seemed inappropriate to study care and health. Moreover, narrow hypotheses and measurement scales and specific statistical formulas did not always lead to meaningful outcomes about cultures and care. After rigorous study of many diverse qualitative research methods and evaluation criteria, the author identified and defined qualitative research criteria to fit the theory goals and the new ethnonursing method to tease out largely embedded detailed, covert, and complex explanatory findings about culture and care phenomena (Leininger 1985, 1991a/b, 1995; Leininger & McFarland, 2002).

After considerable study and use with several ethnonursing studies, the six ethnonursing method criteria were developed to systematically examine and discover indepth care and culture meanings and interpretive findings. These six criteria remain in use:

1. <u>Credibility</u> refers to the *accuracy, believability, and truths* of findings largely from the informants.
2. <u>Confirmability</u> refers to repeated direct and documented objective and subjective data confirmed with the informants.
3. <u>Meaning-in-context</u> refers to findings that are understandable to informants studied within their natural and familiar environmental context(s).
4. <u>Recurrent patterning</u> refers to the repeated instances, patterns of expression, and patterned occurrences over time.
5. <u>Saturation</u> refers to the exhaustive search from informants of data relevant to the domain of inquiry in which no new findings were forthcoming from informants.

6. Transferability refers to whether the findings from a particular qualitative study can be transferred to or appropriately used in another similar culture or cultures and within their context (Leininger, 1985, 1991a/b, 1995, 1997a; Leininger & McFarland, 2002). The last criterion of transferability is the most difficult to use and often necessitates a good mentor to prevent inappropriate uses.

Each of these criteria meets the purposes and philosophy of qualitative research analysis and the purposes of the ethnonursing method. While some numerical informant data are included, they are used primarily to confirm data or for directional findings alone. Numbers may be used for weighing interpretive statements or the extent of influences as provided by the informants. The above six criteria address internal and external dimensions of discovering care phenomena but must not be dichotomized or reduced to numbers without qualitative indicators. Leininger holds one does not have to always measure every thing or all phenomena to know or understand them. Lincoln and Guba (1985) use several of these criteria but did not use meanings-in-context and recurrent patterning criteria which Leininger has held as critical for culture care discoveries.

Domain of Inquiry

Discoveries within the theory begin by the researcher making a statement of the domain of inquiry (DOI). This domain must be carefully stated and then rigorously and fully examined with the theory tenets using the six criteria as previously described. The tenets, predictions, and the goals of the theory are foremost in the researcher's mind. The use of the word *tested* is inappropriate for qualitative paradigmatic studies; instead the phrases *indepth examination of data* or *confirming the findings* are used. Indepth, detailed, supportive data are used to report findings with qualitative methods such as ethnonursing. Data from indepth interviews and direct and indirect observations of informants are documented and used to confirm findings. Both material and non-material evidence such as informant biographies, photos, written or verbal stories, and other kinds of qualitative data are used to confirm the findings for the ethnonursing method.

Most ethnonursing studies usually cover an extended period of time, often six months to a few or several years. Much depends on the scope of the domain of the inquiry and whether the researcher desires to conduct a study over time. The six standard enablers of the theory, along with recurrent observations of covert and complex phenomena, are used to document and confirm data with informants. The ethnonursing researcher seeks to grasp the <u>world of the informants and the totality of their culture with care meanings and life experiences</u>. The Sunrise Enabler and the other enablers focus on theory tenets to provide a full and accurate picture of the domain of inquiry. Diverse and similar findings must be documented to remain within the theory tenets. Both <u>key</u> and <u>general</u> informants of the culture are purposefully selected focusing on the criteria and the domain of inquiry. For example, one might study Amish mothers and their care or caring patterns during pregnancy as a domain of inquiry. Every word from the informants is focused on within this domain of inquiry. The theory findings often provide rich practical ideas, but also data to explain the meanings and practices. Symbolic and abstract data may be discovered in a culture and studied for their care meanings. Most importantly, the criteria of *credibility, confirmability, and meaning-in-context* must be used from the beginning to the end of the study with documentation. Rich and meaningful *truths* from cultural informants are largely emic data. The cultural truths are known and held by the informants over time, which gives constancy and credibility. All data obtained are discussed, confirmed, and even analyzed with the informants for accuracy and to fulfill the confirmability criterion.

The research enablers, as part of the ethnonursing method, have been extremely valuable for teasing out hidden and complex data. The enablers, as the name implies, facilitate the informants to share their ideas in natural and casual ways. With the ethnonursing method, the researcher is expected to develop enablers that fit the domain of inquiry on culture and care. The six enablers are facilitators and not models per se. They are also not *tools* or *scales* but ways to examine the major tenets of the theory and the domain of inquiry. New data from informants obtained in naturalistic [largely informal modes] are also sought without the researcher controlling the informants' views. The informants are encouraged to be open and spontaneous in sharing their knowledge. The researcher encourages informants 'to tell <u>their</u> stories' from their life experiences. Several interviews and observations are done with key and general informants in their natural and familiar living or working contexts. The six major enablers designed to facilitate ethnonursing data are:

1. <u>The Sunrise Enabler</u>. This enabler is used as a major guide throughout the study to explore comprehensive and multiple influences on care and culture. These major dimensions can be seen in Figure 1-1. Further information on the use of the Sunrise Enabler can be studied in Leininger & McFarland (2002, pp. 79–83).

Leininger's Sunrise Enabler to Discover Culture Care

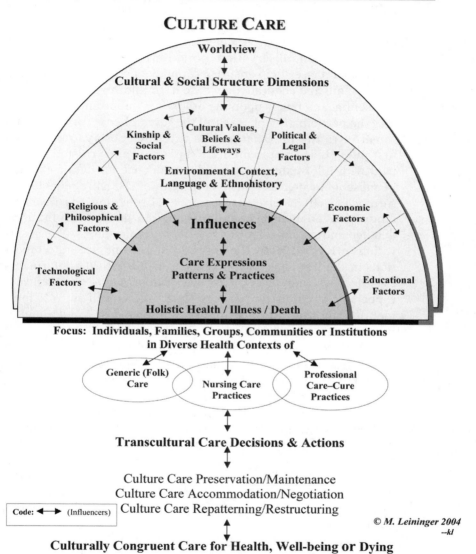

CULTURE CARE

Worldview

Cultural & Social Structure Dimensions

Kinship & Social Factors

Cultural Values, Beliefs & Lifeways

Political & Legal Factors

Environmental Context, Language & Ethnohistory

Religious & Philosophical Factors

Influences

Economic Factors

Care Expressions Patterns & Practices

Technological Factors

Educational Factors

Holistic Health / Illness / Death

Focus: Individuals, Families, Groups, Communities or Institutions in Diverse Health Contexts of

Generic (Folk) Care

Nursing Care Practices

Professional Care–Cure Practices

Transcultural Care Decisions & Actions

Culture Care Preservation/Maintenance
Culture Care Accommodation/Negotiation
Culture Care Repatterning/Restructuring

Code: ◄──► (Influencers)

© M. Leininger 2004
--kl

Culturally Congruent Care for Health, Well-being or Dying

Figure 1-1   Leininger's Sunrise Enabler to Discover Culture Care

2. <u>The Observation-Participation-Reflection Enabler.</u> (Leininger &
   McFarland, 2002, p. 90). This enabler guides the researcher to
   obtain focused observations of the informants in their familiar
   and natural living or working environments. The researcher gradually moves from the <u>observation</u> to <u>participation</u> phase and still
   later to full <u>reflection</u> and <u>confirmation</u> of data collected with
   informants. The researcher continually confirms findings during
   and after each observation period with informants. These
   sequenced phases help ensure a sound data collection process to
   obtain a full and accurate data base from informants. Each phase
   is essential and builds upon the other. It is important not to move
   into the participation phase until the researcher is trusted by and
   sensitive to the informants. The extensive observations in the
   first phase help the researcher to later become a trusted participant with informants and provide confidence for data collection
   in subsequent phases. This enabler can offer highly reliable culturalogical client care assessments. Throughout the research
   study this enabler becomes a valuable guide for obtaining
   detailed and systematic observations with informants. The observations are essential as the bases for sound and accurate reflections in the last phase. Reflections are done with the informants
   to verify the accuracy of their views or information obtained, and
   especially to confirm what was observed, as well as to help to
   identify any gaps and research biases related to the domain of
   inquiry (Leininger & McFarland, 2002, pp. 92–97).
3. <u>The Researcher's Domain of Inquiry Enabler (DOI).</u> Most importantly, researchers develop their own Domain of Inquiry (DOI).
   Each researcher's enabler is designed to cover every aspect
   (words or ideas) stated in the DOI, and is focused primarily on
   the researcher's major hunches and general interests about care
   and culture. At all times, the researcher keeps focused on the
   DOI and the general tenets of the Culture Care Theory and the
   theory goal (Leininger, 1991a/b; Leininger & McFarland, 2002).
   The reader may refer to dissertations and studies cited in the
   Appendix for further information and examples.
4. <u>Stranger to Trusted Friend Enabler.</u> This enabler was developed
   by the theorist as she worked around the globe in both Western
   and nonWestern cultures. It has been a powerful means for self-
   disclosure, self-reflection, and assessment. It guides the researcher
   while working with informants to become a trusted friend, and is
   used from the beginning of the research until the end. (Leininger,
   1991a/b; Leininger & McFarland, 2002). Data from this enabler
   can provide high reliability and confirmability with informants as

the researcher carefully moves from a stranger role to becoming a trusted research friend. Entering the world of the key and general informants to learn about care meanings and practices is obtained with this enabler. Based on the theorist's experience of working with diverse cultures and in using the enabler, meaningful and credible data can be obtained, especially when signs of trust between researcher and informant prevail. This enabler was developed to obtain authentic emic data for understanding care meanings and lifeways. It has also been a valuable means for mentoring transcultural nurse students as they perfect their transcultural nursing clinical skills. Most importantly, this enabler assists the researcher in becoming reflective of and honest about one's own behavior as one moves from a stranger to a trusted friend. For only when one is trusted by informants can one be confident about obtaining the *truths* or authentic emic data from informants. Accurate, consistent, and meaningful data can be obtained using this enabler. If one remains a stranger to informants, one will discover data having less reliability and accuracy and with limited details being shared by informants. When mistrust prevails, the informants are not comfortable sharing detailed, personal, and intimate data (Leininger & McFarland, 2002, pp. 90–92). The reader is also encouraged to read Leininger's work with the Gadsup of New Guinea where this enabler was first developed and refined with approximately 200 informants over several years (Leininger & McFarland, 2002).

5. Ethnodemographic Enabler. This enabler is used as a guide to tap general ethnographic data about key informants with respect to their environment, history, and related factors. Ethnodemographic factors include social and cultural factors, ethnic orientation, gender, and geographic locations where the informants are living or have lived. Family data, the geographic area, and general environmental factors such as water supply, buildings, and other factors may be included. Specific ethnodemographic facts of different cultures and within a historical context can help to understand the meaning of care and care practices. This enabler is generally used during the interviews with key and general informants and while talking to informants about their family origins, general history, and current or past living and working environments; the present and past history are part of the data obtained during these open ended interviews.

6. Acculturation Enabler. The purpose of this enabler has been to identify the extent to which informants are more traditionally or nontraditionally oriented to their culture (Leininger, 1991a/b,

pp. 98–103; Leininger & McFarland, 2002, pp. 92). The researcher uses all of the above enablers, by using open ended questions or open frames related to all areas identified and related to the stated domain of inquiry (DOI). A frame such as "Tell me about ____" [let informant finish the statement] must be thoughtfully used to ensure the researcher covers the DOI as stated in order to fully assess the acculturation and life style patterns of the informant(s).

Key and General Informants

Selecting key and general informants for interviewing, observation, and indepth study is very important. The selection criteria for the informants often includes that the informant: (a) is associated or identifies with or is a member of the culture being studied; (b) is willing to participate in the study and be interviewed; (c) speaks English or the researcher can understand the language spoken; (d) volunteers time to visit with the researchers and be observed; and (e) has lived in the community or country for at least 5 to 10 years. Leininger and McFarland (2002) provides excellent examples of factors in selection of informants and guidelines for the interviews.

1. The key informants are those who are generally the most knowledgeable about the culture and interested in the DOI. This information comes from the researcher's casual visits in the village, town, hospital, or community, as one talks and listens attentively to suggested informants for the study and inquires about their interest to participate in the study. For example, a DOI may be focused on child care patterns and practices of mothers who are working outside of the home. The researcher will seek to find key informants among mothers who may have had several years of employment as well as other mothers who have been employed fewer years and spend more time with their children. Selected mothers who are interested and volunteer to share their ideas with the researcher about the DOI are usually asked to participate in the study. The study must be clearly discussed with potential key and general informants about what they might expect during the research process.

2. The general informants, like the key informants, are thoughtfully and purposefully selected. General informants usually have only general knowledge about the DOI; however, they have some knowledge about the research topic and will likely be able to offer relevant reflections and cultural insights.

A mini [small scale] ethnonursing study has approximately six to eight key informants who are interviewed and observed over approximately 6 to 8 months. A maxi (large scale) ethnonursing study has approximately 12 to 15 key informants and 24 to 30 general informants. The researcher spends approximately 30 minutes with general informants in their home or other familiar settings. Key informants are visited more often than general informants and also observed more often, sometimes six or seven times over a 6-month period. The length of time with key informants may vary until indepth and accurate data has been obtained as stated in the DOI. The researcher searches for indepth knowledge about care and confirms ideas with both key and general informants. Voluntary consent to talk with the informants is obtained at the outset and reaffirmed throughout the study. Key and general informants are always free to withdraw at any time without negative consequences. If the study is conducted in a hospital, clinic, or community setting, it is necessary to obtain agency as well as individual consent to protect both informant and agency rights.

Selected Research Findings from the Culture Care Theory

The first transcultural nursing study was conducted with the Gadsup people of the Eastern Highlands of New Guinea in the early 1960s by Leininger and was an approximately two year indepth ethnonursing and ethnographic study (Leininger, 1991a/b, 1994b; Leininger & McFarland, 2002). The researcher–theorist has made a few visits to the Gadsup people in subsequent decades (1960–2001) to discover culture changes in care beliefs and practices. Culture care findings, beliefs, and values with major care meanings and action modes of the Gadsup were initially discovered in the 1960s and several informants have been assessed over time to determine changes in what they believe and practice. The findings from the Gadsup have been used in nursing practice and education today. From indepth study over time the researcher–theorist found that the dominant Gadsup core care meanings and practices were: (1) respect; (2) succorance; (3) differential gender roles; (4) nurturance [ways to help people grow and survive]; (5) watchfulness and surveillance nearby and at a distance; (6) male protective caring with women and children in nurturant modes; (7) prevention as care from illnesses and to prevent death; (8) touching as caring; and (9) presence. In addition, nearly 35 transcultural care practices were observed in the culture. The meaning of cultural pain, suffering, cultural touch, spiritual care, and many transcultural care principles and practices were discovered. The researcher discovered a very rich body of new knowledge for nursing and health care personnel while living in this nonWestern culture. These findings were within the culture's special ethnodemographic living context in the Eastern Highlands of New Guinea. Many social structure factors influenced care but especially mother and father care roles, kinship, and strong cultural values. This was the first maxi transcultural nursing study; since then Leininger has studied about 25 Western and nonWestern cultures (Leininger, 1991a/b, 1995).

The New Guinea findings were a major breakthrough in nursing and health knowledge from a nonWestern culture. The care constructs gave new hope for the discovery of the beliefs within a specific culture and for seeing cultural values preserved over many years. The care values were assets and contributed to the health and wellbeing of the Gadsup. The theory tenets were confirmed using the ethnonursing method with the Gadsup people.

Since the early 1960s, nearly 100 definitive care constructs within the meanings and practices of diverse cultures have been discovered (Leininger 1991a/b, 1995). Most importantly, the care meanings were largely embedded in kinship, politics, gender roles, cultural values, environment, politics, economic, and historical factors. These factors were major influencers of care patterns and outcomes for healing, helping others, and maintaining or preserving healthy lifeways as confirmed by the informants and researchers' repeated observations (Leininger & McFarland, 2002). There was a wealth of other findings from the use of the theory and method from the Gadsup and many other cultures (1960 to present). The theorist and others continue to study and compare culture care findings in Western and nonWestern [nontechnological cultures] looking at similarities and differences among and between cultures. Such studies and others have confirmed care phenomena with some unique cultural attributes, adding to the body of transcultural nursing knowledge and practice.

These care meanings and dominant care constructs were unknown in nursing and health services. This new knowledge for transcultural nursing and for nursing education and practices has the potential to transform nursing. Since the first New Guinea transcultural nursing study, nurses have been studying culturally based care and are excited about the field of transcultural nursing. This first study was also a major breakthrough for encouraging nurses to study cultures indepth and over time for their culture care values, beliefs, and practices in both Western and nonWestern cultures. Today, more nurses are using the theory and the ethnonursing method to study complex and embedded care findings with different cultures in order to provide culturally congruent and mandated care—the goal of the theory. Interestingly, other health personnel are becoming interested in the theory and the ethnonursing method. The enablers and the qualitative criteria for congruent care knowledge and practices are being adopted by many health researchers. Indeed, qualitative data is becoming more and more used and valued in the health services. Other disciplines are finding that the theory and method are natural ways to relate to cultures and can lead to a wealth of meaningful data to improve care to cultures that have been neglected in many health institutions. The theory and method can be used by other health disciplines if they focus on the distinct features of their specific discipline.

Wenger's ethnonursing study of the Old Order Amish was another landmark research investigation. It was the first maxi Western transcultural nursing investigation to examine indepth the care meanings and action modes using the Culture Care Theory and ethnonursing method (1988a/b/c, 1991a/b). This indepth emic study of the Amish revealed that generic care meanings and practices were important, such as care as anticipatory care used within a community context. Amish care was tightly embedded in their worldview and in several social structure factors such as religion, kinship, cultural beliefs, and values. Within the Old Order Amish's unique environment and lifeways, care was seen as essential to *community* based daily modes of healthy living. *Care* meant giving to others, sharing with others, and anticipating care needs of others in the home and community. Using technology in health care and daily living was contrary to the Amish cultural lifeways and was not viewed as a caring modality. This finding contrasted sharply with Anglo American care practices and beliefs. The dominant culture care constructs with meanings and action practice modes discovered for the Old Order Amish were:

1. Providing anticipatory care: anticipating the needs of others and their cultural care needs;
2. Practicing principled pragmatism care: doing practical acts for family and friends in their traditional and simple ways; and,
3. Being an active care participant in daily community-based life activities and in religious activities was important to promote group, family, and community wellbeing and health (Wenger, 1991).

These were major discoveries by Wenger that showed culturally based care and were new insights about the Old Order Amish care.

In addition, Wenger (1988) found care for the Old Order Amish was *high context* in meanings and practices. The community lifeways were of major importance for giving meaning to care. Grandparents were greatly respected and were the major caregivers in the Old Order Amish culture. Amish culture care acts were found to be universal in the communities studied, but there were some signs of slight intergenerational differences. There were many other new insights discovered. Providing nontechnological care was difficult for nonAmish nurses. To prevent cultural imposition practices, the Old Order Amish study findings were used to help these nurses to understand a culture often viewed as strange in the United States and helped to prevent cultural imposition practices. This study revealed how care could be discovered and how it was culturally practiced. Culture specific generic care values among the strong Old Order Amish people had been practiced for many years. The care findings of this transcultural nursing study have expanded nursing knowledge and provided better understanding of Old Order Amish cultural lifeways and care patterns.

Luna's (1989) study was another major and early investigation. She used the Culture Care Theory to conduct a 3-year indepth study of Lebanese Muslim immigrants living in a large urban Midwestern city in the United States. It was another first of its kind. Observation and study of the provision of professional health services to Lebanese Muslims while in hospitals, clinics, and their homes she found marked differences in informants' generic care values from professional nursing and medical practices (Luna, 1989). Gender role practices within the family and in religious and political activities and care practices were extremely important to understand in providing care to Lebanese Muslims. This study clearly discovered that generic care practices were preferred in the home and in the community, and were different from professional care practices in hospitals and clinics. Generic care was the dominant care which was limitedly known and understood by nurses, physicians, and other staff in hospitals and clinics. This lack of transcultural nursing knowledge and skills led to many cultural conflicts and clashes when Lebanese people were cared for in institutional contexts. Their Lebanese traditional beliefs and practices were very different and strongly held. Their care modes were used in daily life for keeping well and for healing practices. Again, the Lebanese values, beliefs, and practices were in marked contrast with Anglo American ones, most notably in regard to food, infant bonding, religion, health, and healing practices. Cultural imposition, stresses, and other noncaring practices were clear discoveries in nurses who were not knowledgeable about Lebanese care. Such imposition practices often led to nontherapeutic actions when these nurses cared for Lebanese Muslims. Luna (1998) found an urgent need for nurses to become educated about this culture and to learn some transcultural nursing principles and care constructs specific to the Lebanese culture. This study emphasized the critical need for nurses to change their practices and focus on ways to provide transcultural culturally congruent care using knowledge and practices learned through study of the Lebanese Muslim cultural values and beliefs. Luna's (1989) study offered excellent examples of ways to provide Lebanese care using the three modes of care practices and actions (Leininger, 1989). Most of all, nurses needed to incorporate Lebanese Muslim <u>generic care constructs into professional nursing care for safe and beneficial outcomes</u> and to prevent unethical and destructive outcomes (Luna, 1989).

In the early 1990s, MacNeil studied the Baganda people with Acquired Immunodeficiency Syndrome (AIDS) in Uganda, Africa (1998). This was another major and important first transcultural nursing study in Africa, which focused on the care meanings, patterns, and expressions of Baganda women as AIDS caregivers. This indepth ethnonursing study used both the Culture Care Theory and ethnonursing method. MacNeil relied on general knowledge of transcultural principles from her doctoral study to guide her investigation and actions. As a transcultural researcher, MacNeil lived in the country and near the people for approximately two years. This is another example of an <u>immersion</u> field study. Such detailed indepth observations and direct, first person experiences with the Bagandan women were essential for discovering many indepth care beliefs and practices of these people that previously had not been revealed to professional nurses and others. Several universal themes were repeatedly documented from key and general informants along with many other general transcultural care discoveries. Some of the major universal or common theme discoveries were:

1. <u>Culture care meant responsibility, love, and comfort measures as teased out from the Baganda kinship, religious, cultural beliefs, and values, and from generic folk health care beliefs;</u>
2. <u>Culture care meant cultural survival for the next generation through education and land claims;</u>
3. <u>Culture care meant preserving and continuing to care for others (especially kin members), despite great adversity and the tremendous burden of caring for many AIDS victims over time</u> and in different villages;
4. <u>Culture care meant respecting generic role differences and caring values and beliefs for others after the death of loved ones;</u> and
5. The dominant care concepts of <u>being fully involved with</u> and <u>offering care as presence and persistence in care giving for others</u> were discovered as deeply held care values (MacNeil, 1998).

Some culturally <u>diverse care</u> themes were identified among Bagandan women such as the belief of *making the most out of life for the HIV-positive women.* MacNeil's (1998) indepth transcultural AIDS study was detailed, descriptive, and an excellent first study for discovering specific cultural care [emic] knowledge with AIDS victims in Africa. This important study serves as a guide for nurses and others giving AIDS care for Bagandans and other African peoples. Learning about the complex ethno-historical and social structure factors of the African Bagandan women and their families was essential for the discovery of their generic care practices and beliefs. The use of the Culture Care Theory and ethnonursing method, especially the Sunrise Enabler, helped to identify comprehensive, covert, and meaningful data from these nonWestern people.

McFarland (1995, 1997) conducted a 2-year ethnonursing study using both the theory and method to study Anglo and African American clients living in an institutional residence home for the elderly in a large Midwestern city. The purpose of this comparative maxi research study was to explore the indepth emic and etic cultural care of two cultures living in the shared setting of a residential facility. Many significant findings were discovered, such as:

1. Anglo and African elderly expect their preadmission generic (folk) care patterns to be practiced, respected, and maintained by nurses;
2. Doing for others [rather than a self care focus] was a major care value for both cultures;
3. Protective care was more important for African American than Anglo American elders;
4. African American nurses combined their generic and professional care values and practices, whereas Anglo American nurses were less aware of generic culture care values;
5. The institutional home for elders had definitive subcultural values reflecting unique institutional care patterns and practices; and
6. The three modes of culture care actions and decisions of the theory were invaluable means to discover and find ways to provide culturally congruent health care practices for the elderly of both cultures within the institution (McFarland, 1995, 1997).

An extension of this unique study was repeated by McFarland (1997) studying *care as the essence of nursing with the two cultures.* Several institutional care policies were developed to guide professional care for the elderly in this institutional setting. This study confirmed the Culture Care Theory tenets and several care patterns that Leininger discovered in an early comparative study of Southern and Northern African Americans and Anglo Americans in two Southern United States villages (1985, 1988c, 1991a/b, 1998a).

George (2000) conducted a 2-year study focused on the domain of inquiry of the culture care meanings, expressions, and experiences of a subculture of chronically mentally ill people living in alternative community settings in a Midwestern United States city. The purpose of the study was to discover knowledge to guide nurses in providing culturally congru-ent care for the chronically mentally ill within a community context so that the clients could maintain and-or regain their mental health and wellbeing. The theory of Culture Care Diversity and Universality and the ethnonursing method were used and the findings clearly reaffirmed the importance of obtaining subtle, complex, and covert data with the use of the six enablers of the ethnonursing method. George (2000) recom-mended fresh new approaches for psychiatric and mental health nursing practices by incorporating transcultural factors into nursing care. Cultural factors have been limitedly known, valued, and used by nurses in mental health or psychiatric care practices. The care meanings and expressions related to mental health were clearly embedded in social structure factors as well as the patterns of living with the identified sub-culture of the chronically mentally ill. The findings of this study revealed that the worldview, cultural and social structure factors, and environmen-tal context of the chronically mentally ill markedly influenced their care meanings, expressions, and experiences related to regaining and main-taining mental health. Three new and recurrent care constructs discov-ered in the subculture of the chronically mentally ill were:

1. Survival care referred to the essential features of care that were needed to assist a chronically mentally ill person to live or make it through daily living, and also for a period of time outside the mental institution in the community and culture;
2. Constructive care was identified and referred to as the recognition and use of clients' strengths and assets to maximize their health and wellbeing over time and to emphasize the clients' strengths that were beneficial to chronically mentally ill individuals within the subculture in order to survive in the dominant culture; and
3. Inclusive care referred to inclusion of assistive, supportive, and enabling actions and decisions that promoted the participation by members of the subculture of the chronically mentally ill in the dominant culture.

The discovery and formulation of these three new care constructs of knowledge were viewed as essential for nurses to use along with the three modes of action and decision for therapeutic transcultural mental health care practices with the chronically mentally ill, especially when living in an urban community.

These transcultural caring research investigations are excellent examples of comprehensive ethnonursing studies to demonstrate the use of the Culture Care Theory. They are valuable for understanding and practicing nursing in new ways among the diverse cultures of the United States. They provide new knowledge for old practices and professional modes of helping clients. The findings emphasize the importance of generic care that contrasts with professional nursing care for therapeutic outcomes.

Stitzlein's (1999) study discovered the <u>nature of moral caring by nurses</u>. The domain of inquiry was to discover if moral caring knowledge existed in nursing education, practice, and administration settings in the United States. The Culture Care Theory was used toward the goal of promoting <u>morally congruent nursing care and professional satisfaction</u>. Stitzlein (1999) documented shared narratives of moral caring and nonmoral caring in nurse practice situations. Twelve master's degree-prepared nurse clinicians practicing in the United States were key informants in this study and represented African Americans and European Americans of both sexes. They participated in an open ended discovery process using the ethnonursing method through indepth interviews conducted from 1996 to 1998. Five dominant moral caring themes were discovered:

1. <u>Moral caring</u> was nursing action emanating from personal, generic, and professional characteristics of the nurse and focused on a meaningful nurse–client relationships;
2. <u>Moral caring was derived from family</u>, religious, and philosophical [generic] and professional role modeling influences on the development of the nurses' commitment to moral caring actions;
3. Professional experiences of <u>personal satisfaction, intense moral distress, and moral conflict were major attributes discovered</u> along with moral caring;
4. <u>Economic, technological, political/legal, religious, and human environmental factors</u> all greatly and repeatedly influenced the nurses' ability to provide moral caring;
5. <u>Moral caring</u> influenced the nurses' professional role satisfaction as reflected in the employment and employee retention patterns.

From Stitzlein's (1999) important study, three new transcultural nursing care themes were identified:

1. A need for a <u>unified ethic of moral nurse caring</u>;
2. Nurses' pursuit of <u>professional care satisfaction</u> was based on moral caring; and
3. Nurses' expressions of <u>many unresolved moral care distress factors</u> in providing nursing care.

The findings of this study were congruent with the tenets of virtue ethics and confirmed Leininger's theoretical assumption that care is the essence of nursing with diverse expressions and values. The findings supported the Stitzlein's (1999) hunches that <u>moral caring is a virtue</u>. The complementarity of virtue ethics, obligation based ethics, principle based ethics, and the relational ethic of care were demonstrated. Social structure factors, especially generic and professional values and experiences, were powerful influencers on the moral caring practices of participants and showed the importance of using Leininger's theory for discovering the multiple dimensions that influence moral caring, and thus confirming the theoretical tenets and predictions of the Culture Care Theory.

In conclusion, these cited examples of transcultural nursing research using the Culture Care Theory demonstrate diversities, some universalities or commonalities, and the relevancy and meaning of culture care as discovered through transcultural study using the ethnonursing research method. The theory and the method were crucial for discovering new care constructs and their meanings in an era when <u>self care</u> by professionals dominated nursing. Leininger (1991a/b) has found in her many studies that *other care* was held to be far more important than *self care*. These findings are important to advance the body of transcultural nursing knowledge and practices into broader areas of nursing thought, knowledge, and practice. The reader is encouraged to read the full text of the studies summarized herein to grasp fully the use of the theory and the wealth of data obtained through the ethnonursing method. In addition, several dissertation studies are listed in the Appendix, which were conducted using the Culture Care

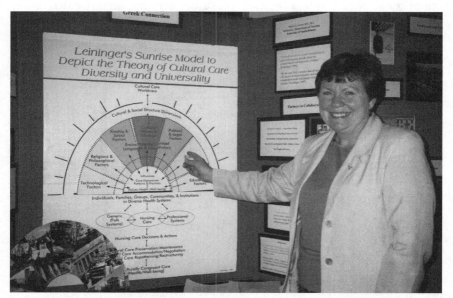

Figure 1-2 A Graduate Student Creatively Using Dr. Leininger's Sunrise Enabler

Theory and ethnonursing method under the mentorship of the theorist, Dr. Madeleine Leininger. Most of these studies are, again, first breakthroughs in care and health knowledge for nurses and other health care disciplines. The reader is also encouraged to read the dominant culture care published findings of the research conducted by Leininger over the past five decades with approximately 80 cultures (Leininger, 1998b).

Summary

In this chapter, the nature, importance, and major features of the theory of Culture Care were discussed. The ethnonursing research method and the enablers were presented to show the fit between the theory and the method. Knowledge of both the theory and the method are needed before launching an ethnonursing study. Fully understanding the theory and method leads to obtaining credible and meaningful research findings. Transcultural research becomes meaningful, exciting, rewarding, and understandable as the researcher develops confidence and competence in the use of the theory and method.

Culture Care Theory is becoming valued worldwide. With slight modifications, other disciplines have found the theory and method most helpful and valuable. Nurses who use the theory and method over time frequently communicate how valuable and important it is to discover new ways to know and practice nursing and health care.

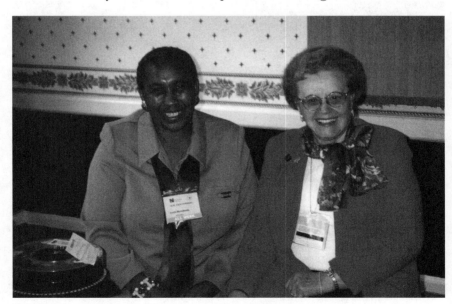

Figure 1-3   Dr. Leininger Mentoring an African Student

Practicing nurses can now use holistic, culturally based research findings to care for clients of diverse and similar cultures or subcultures in different countries. Contrary to some views, the theory is not difficult to use once the researcher understands the theory and method and has available mentorship guidance if needed. Newcomers to the theory and method can benefit from experienced and expert mentors in addition to studying published transcultural research conducted using the theory and method. Most importantly, nurses often express that the Culture Care Theory is *the only theory and method that makes sense for use in nursing*. They also hold that the Ethnonursing Method is a very natural and humanistic method to use in nursing, and helps one to gain fresh new insights about care, health, and wellbeing. The theory is the relevant theory of today and tomorrow and one that will grow in use far into the future in our increasingly multicultural world. The research and theory provide new pathways to advance the profession of nursing and the body of transcultural knowledge for application in nursing education, research, and clinical consultation practices worldwide.

References

Faucett, J. (1984). The metaparadigm in nursing: Present status and future refinements. *The Journal of Nursing Scholarship, 16*(3), 84–87.

Faucett, J. (1989). *Analysis and evaluation of conceptual model of nursing* (2nd ed.). Philadelphia: FA Davis.

Fitzpatrick, J., & Whall, A. (1989). *Conceptual models of nursing: Analysis and application.* Bowie, MD: Brady.

Gaut, D. (1984). A theoretical description of caring as action. In M. Leininger, *Caring: The essence of nursing and health* (pp. 17–24). Thorofare, NJ: Charles B. Slack.

George, T. (2000). Defining care in the culture of the chronically mentally ill living in the community. *Journal of Transcultural Nursing, 11*(2), 102–110.

Hardy, M. (1974). Theories: Components, development, evaluation. *Nursing Research, 23* (March–April), 100–107.

Leininger, M. (1963). [Transcultural nursing: A new field to be developed]. Address for Minnesota League for Nursing, Northfield, MN.

Leininger, M. (1973b). Culture Care Theory: An evaluation process. Paper presented at the group meeting of the Minnesota National League for Nursing, Northfield, MN.

Leininger, M. (1976). Transcultural nursing: A new area of study. National League for Nursing Report.

Leininger, M. (1977). Transcultural nursing: A promising subfield of study for nurse educators and practitioners. In A. Reinhardt, & M.D. Quinn (Eds.), *Current Practice in Family Centered Community Nursing.* St. Louis, MO: C.V. Mosby.

Leininger, M. (1978). *Transcultural nursing: Concepts, theories, and practices.* New York: John Wiley & Sons.

Leininger, M. (1980). Caring: A central focus of nursing and health care services. *Nursing and Health Care, 1*(3), 135–143, 176.

Leininger, M. (1984). *Reference sources for transcultural health and nursing.* Thorofare, NJ: Slack.

Leininger, M. (1985). Qualitative research methods in nursing. Orlando, FL: Grune & Stratton.

Leininger, M. (1988a). *Caring: An essential human need.* Detroit, MI: Wayne State University Press.

Leininger, M. (1988b). Leininger's theory of nursing: Culture care diversity and universality. *Nursing Science Quarterly, 2*(4), 152–160.

Leininger, M. (1988c). *Care: The essence of nursing and health.* Detroit, MI: Wayne State University Press.

Leininger, M. (1989). Transcultural nursing: Quo vadis (Where goeth the field?). *Journal of Transcultural Nursing, 1*(1), 33–45.

Leininger, M. (1991a). *Culture care diversity and universality: Theory of nursing.* New York: National League for Nursing.

Leininger, M. (1991b). The theory of culture care diversity and universality. In M. Leininger (Ed.), *Culture care diversity and universality: Theory of nursing* (pp. 5–68). New York: National League for Nursing.

Leininger, M. (1991c). Ethnonursing: A research method with enablers to study the theory of culture care. In M. Leininger (Ed.), *Culture care diversity and universality: Theory of nursing* (pp. 73–117). New York: National League for Nursing.

Leininger, M. (1993a). Quality of life from a transcultural nursing perspective. *Nursing Science Quarterly, 7*(1), 22–28.

Leininger, M. (1993b). Culture care theory: The comparative global theory to advance human care nursing knowledge and practice. In D. Gaut (Ed.), *A global agenda for caring* (pp. 3–19). New York: National League for Nursing.

Leininger, M. (1994a). *Nursing and anthropology: Two worlds to blend.* Columbus, OH: Greyden Press. (Original work published 1970; New York: John Wiley & Sons.).

Leininger, M. (1994b). *Transcultural nursing: Concepts, theories and practices.* Columbus, OH: Greyden Press.

Leininger, M. (1995). *Transcultural nursing concepts, theories, research and practices.* Columbus, OH: McGraw-Hill Custom Series.

Leininger, M. (1997a). Overview of the theory of culture care with the ethnonursing method. *Journal of Transcultural Nursing, (8)*2, 32–52.

Leininger, M. (1997b). Transcultural nursing research to transform nursing education and practice: 40 years. *Image, 29*(4), 341–347.

Leininger, M. (1997c). Founder's focus: Transcultural nursing: A scientific and humanistic care discipline. *Journal of Transcultural Nursing, 8*(2), 54–55.

Leininger, M. (1997d). *An essential human need.* Detroit, MI: Wayne State University Press.

Leininger, M. (1998a). The theory of culture care with selected research findings with method and uses in professional transcultural nursing. In *Jurgen Osterbrink*. Symposium conducted at the meeting of the First International Nursing Theory Congress, Nuremburg, Germany.

Leininger, M. (1998b). Special research report: Dominant culture care (emic) meanings and practice findings from Leininger's theory. *Journal of Transcultural Nursing, 91* (3), 45–46.

Leininger, M. (2002). The theory of culture care and the ethnonursing research method. In M. Leininger, & M. McFarland (Eds.), *Transcultural nursing: Concepts, theories, research and practices* (3rd ed., pp. 71–116). New York: McGraw-Hill.

Leininger, M., & McFarland, M. (2002). *Transcultural nursing: Concepts, theories, research and practices* (3rd ed.). New York: McGraw Hill.

Lincoln, Y., & Guba, E. (1985). *Naturalistic inquiry*. Newbury Park, CA: Sage.

Luna, L. (1989). Transcultural nursing care of Arab Muslims. *Journal of Transcultural Nursing, 1*(1), 22–26.

Luna, L. (1998). Culturally competent health care: A challenge for nurses in Saudi Arabia. *Journal of Transcultural Nursing, 19*(2), 8–14.

MacNeil, J. (1998). Use of culture care theory with Baganda women as AIDS caregivers. *Journal of Transcultural Nursing, 7*(2), 14–20.

McFarland, M. (1995). Culture Care Theory and Elderly Polish Americans. In M. Leininger (Ed.), *Transcultural nursing concepts, theories research and practices* (pp. 101–425). New York: McGraw-Hill.

McFarland, M. (1997). Use of culture care theory with Anglo and African American elders in a long-term care setting. *Nursing Care Quarterly*, Fall.

Ray, M. (1987). Technological caring: A new model in critical care. *Dimensions of Critical Care Nursing, 6*(3), 166–173.

Stitzlein, D. A. (1999). *The phenomena of moral care/caring conceptualized within Leininger's theory of culture care diversity and universality*. Unpublished doctoral dissertation, Wayne State University, Detroit, MI.

Watson, J. (1985). *Human science and human care: A theory of nursing*. Norwalk, CT: Appleton Century Crafts.

Wenger, A. F. (1988). The phenomenon of care in a high context culture: The Old Order Amish. Unpublished doctoral dissertation, Wayne State University, Detroit, MI.

Wenger, A. F. (1991) Role in context in culture specific care. In L. Chinn (Ed.), *Anthology of Caring* (pp. 95–110). New York: National League for Nursing.

CHAPTER TWO

Ethnonursing: A Research Method with Enablers to Study the Theory of Culture Care

[Revised Reprint]

Madeleine M. Leininger, PhD, LHD, DS, CTN, RN, FAAN, FRCNA

> *The ultimate goal of a professional nurse–scientist and humanist is to discover, know, and creatively use culturally based care knowledge with its fullest meanings, expressions, symbols, and functions for healing, and to promote or maintain wellbeing (or health) with people of diverse cultures in the world.*
>
> —Leininger

In the history of nursing, nurse–theorists and researchers have borrowed and depended on research methods from other disciplines to study or test nursing phenomena. Nurses developing their own nursing research methods to study nursing phenomena and specifically nursing theories has not been a dominant practice until recently. There are a few nurse–researchers who are beginning to realize that nurses may need to develop their own research methods and strategies to study particular nursing domains, problems, or questions. This awareness has occurred largely because of the inadequacy of borrowed methods to study highly complex, covert, and embedded nursing phenomena such as human care and wellbeing.

When considering past norms of nurse-researchers, it is clear that nurses rely strongly on established research methods in order to adhere to the tenets of logical positivism or the 'received view' of empirical scientists (Carter, 1985; Leininger, 1985a). To develop new research methods to study nursing phenomena was untenable because nurses felt compelled to use the established scientific method to obtain reliable and valid data and to have their research recognized by other 'hard core' logical positivists. Moreover, the culture of nursing reflected largely "other-directed" (Leininger, 1970) decisions and practices until recent years, and so most nurses would not consider that they could be

---

Readers familiar with the theory and the method will find that the Sunrise diagram is now called the *Sunrise Enabler* by the theorist.

self directed and have sufficient confidence to develop their own research methods. Indeed, nurses have been quick to use ready-made methods and standardized instruments already in use and validated by largely nonnursing methodologists. Thus, the idea to develop nursing research methods to study nursing phenomena was a radical and bold new step, which the author took in the early 1960s. It was still a more courageous step to develop a research method to study a specific nursing theory such as cultural care. These and related trends set the context for discussing the ethnonursing research method as an essential nursing method to study a nursing theory.

In this chapter, the author presents the purpose, rationale, and philosophy for the ethnonursing research method. Specific features of the method are given along with the research process and principles, research enablers, and other aspects of the method. The chapter serves as background framework for several research studies that follow to demonstrate the use of the method with the Culture Care Theory. The research philosophy, process, and enabling guides are an integral and important part of the ethnonursing research method.

Purpose and Rationale for Ethnonursing Method

The central purpose of the ethnonursing research method was to establish a naturalistic and largely *emic* open inquiry discovery method to explicate and study nursing phenomena especially related to the theory of Culture Care Diversity and Universality. This research method was designed to tease out complex, elusive, and largely unknown nursing dimensions from the people's local viewpoints such as human care, wellbeing, health, and environmental influencers. In the 1950s and 1960s, there were no appropriate nursing research methods to explicate and to know and understand the nature, essence, and characteristics of human care and of actual or perceived nursing phenomena. The use of borrowed research methods was quite inadequate to study indepth human caring and from a transcultural perspective. In those days, I had already identified human care as central to nursing, but there was a critical need to know the meanings, expressions, patterns, functions, and structure of human care and caring. Without such knowledge, nursing could not support or justify its existence as a profession or a discipline. As a nurse leader eager to make nursing a legitimate, scholarly, and well-grounded discipline, I held that nurses needed research methods to establish the scientific, humanistic, epistemic, and ontologic bases for nursing's unique discipline perspectives especially focused on human care (Leininger, 1969). How people knew and experienced human care was essential for nurses to describe, document, and explain so that this knowledge could ultimately guide nursing practices. An open discovery and naturalistic people-centered research method was needed that would permit people to share their ideas about care in a spontaneous and informative way with nurse–researchers.

From my continuing clinical nursing studies, I realized that care was an ambiguous and often elusive phenomenon that was extremely difficult to study (Leininger, 1976, 1980, 1981). From an anthropological perspective, I realized that care was also extremely difficult to identify as it was embedded in the worldview, social structure, and cultural values of a particular culture. Revealing embedded and undiscovered care phenomena required an inductive and open inquiry method that was familiar to human groups. Nursing needed a research method that would help nurses discover and fully know the many elusive, culture specific, and unknown ideas about human care and caring.

Prior to the 1960s, as a nurse leader and researcher, I was cognizant that care had not been systematically explicated in nursing and different health care and cultural settings. If human care was to become the essential and distinctly claimed feature of nursing, such systematic explication was necessary. The idea of an ethnonursing research method that was people- or client-centered rather than researcher-centered also seemed necessary to know human care and its influence on the health and well-being of people from different cultures in the world. Most assuredly, quantitative research methods (e.g., the experimental method) seemed questionable at best and inappropriate at worst to study human caring. Care meanings, perceptions, patterns, and experiences hardly could be studied at a distance, or manipulated, tightly controlled, and measured by quantitative methods. To lead people to credible and meaningful insights about humanistic care based on accurate findings, the epistemics of care knowledge required another method. Indeed, researchers that treated people as objects or nonhumans could only lead to nonhumanistic care data and questionable results. Clearly, such an approach was not congruent with the nature of nursing and human care practices, or for the discovery of knowledge essential for the profession. As caregivers, nurses are expected to get close to people and to establish and maintain intimate caring relationships. Research methods that relied on creating distance and controlling informants, as in quantitative methods, would limit the discovery of and learning about care meanings, structure, and processes. Thus, the current quantitative methods in use by the scientific community were inappropriate to study human care and nursing care practices.

To study care phenomena required an openness to examining subjective, intersubjective, spiritual, or supernatural experiences as well as the caring experiences lived by cultures. In addition, a research method was needed to discover, document, preserve, and accurately interpret care meanings and experiences of different cultural groups.

This necessitated a perspective on methodology that was quite different from that prevailing in experimental and other types of quantitative methods used by nurses. The ethnonursing inductive and naturalistic research method was needed to discover the nature, essence, and distinguishing features of human care in different life contexts and cultures.

Another major reason to establish the ethnonursing research method was interest in discovering differences between *generic* or *native* folk (*naturalistic*) care [informally learned indigenous knowledge] and *professional nursing care* [learned through formal educational systems in nursing] among different cultures. I had speculated that differences between generic and professional care existed, but a research method was needed to tease out the subtle and elusive aspects of these sources of care. As a nurse–anthropologist, I was aware that folk practices (and undoubtedly folk care) had been practiced by cultures for hundreds of years, and that 'modern' professional nursing was a recent development in human history. Discovering generic or naturalistic care was held essential to know and to use in developing professional nursing care practices (Leininger, 1976, 1981). In the early 1960s, during my field study with the Gadsup of the Eastern Highlands of New Guinea (Leininger, 1966), I had come to realize that generic care was essential to know and understand in order to provide meaningful, congruent, and acceptable care—the goal of Culture Care Theory. However, generic care was unknown and had not been considered for systematic discovery in professional nursing prior to the 1960s. Therefore, I predicted that generic care would be quite different from professional nursing (Leininger, 1970, 1978, 1981).

In the late 1950s, I learned by chance about Pike's (1954) use of the terms *emic* and *etic* in linguistic studies and thought that they would be most helpful to explicate and understand human care transculturally. At that time, although *emic* and *etic* were unknown in nursing, and had not been used in anthropological field research, I could see their usefulness as part of the ethnonursing research method to study care and other nursing phenomena. According to Pike, *emic* referred to the local informants or inside views of people whereas *etic* referred to the outsider's views of a culture. While studying the Gadsup of New Guinea, I had used these concepts (*emic* and *etic*) and found they greatly helped to reveal the meanings of ideas regarding the values, beliefs, norms, rituals, and symbols of care, health, and illness (Leininger, 1966, 1970). *Emic* ideas about Gadsup spiritual or ancestral beliefs became known to me with an *emic* focus on traditional ideas and experiences of the people. It is clear that the *emic* view also was needed to discover human care with other cultures regarding their history, social structure, environment, biological, ecological, and many other factors. *Etic* knowledge about professional nursing views also was needed to obtain a full understanding about human caring or care.

Most importantly, the ethnonursing method was conceived and developed to overcome the limitations and philosophical tenets of logical positivism, the use of the prevailing scientific method, and other conventional features and goals of the quantitative paradigm to study nursing phenomena. Nursing was different from many established disciplines and its researchers needed better ways to discover its distinctive body of care knowledge. Thus, the ethnonursing method was viewed as the answer to discover the true essence, nature, patterns, and expressions of human care among others to advance nursing care knowledge (Leininger, 1969, 1978, 1981, 1984).

Ethnonursing: Its Major Features

Since the ethnonursing research method was the first of its kind developed to study nursing phenomena, it was conceptualized and developed from a nursing perspective (Leininger, 1978, 1985b, 1987, 1990a). The prefix *ethno* was chosen to refer to people, or a particular culture, with a focus on their worldview, ideas, and cultural practices related to nursing phenomena. Ethnonursing was developed as a research method to help nurses systematically document and gain greater understanding and meaning of the people's daily life experiences related to human care, health, and wellbeing in different or similar environmental contexts (Leininger, 1980, 1985b, 1987, 1990a). My anthropological experiences with ethnography, ethnoscience, and ethnology in the early 1960s provided some rich insights of ways to study people and as a basis to develop the ethnonursing method. People centered research with an *emic* focus required a friendly naturalistic approach that permitted people to share their ideas, beliefs, and experiences with research strangers or investigators unknown to the people being studied. It also was clear that the goals, purposes, and phenomena of anthropological research were different from those of nursing. As a result, the ethnonursing method was oriented to discover nursing's central interests or phenomena within the scope of human caring.

Discovery of *actual* or *potential* people centered care, wellbeing, and health phenomena as well as noncaring practices predicted to lead to illness, disability, or death was the primary purpose for developing the ethnonursing method. New insights from diverse cultures obtained from a holistic care perspective (biophysical and psychocultural) were needed to establish professional nursing within a discipline perspective both humanistic and scientific. I defined *ethnonursing* as a qualitative research method using naturalistic, open discovery, and largely inductively derived *emic* modes and processes with diverse strategies, techniques, and enabling guides to document, describe, understand, and interpret the people's meanings, experiences, symbols, and other related aspects bearing on actual or potential nursing phenomena (Leininger, 1978, 1985a, 1990a).

Establishing the ethnonursing research method required an approach radically different from the traditional quantitative paradigm (Leininger, 1985a). In the early 1960s, while the qualitative and quantitative paradigms and their features were largely unknown to nurses, their attributes were becoming identifiable. The ethnonursing method was designed to discover how things really were and the way people knew and lived in their world. The method focused on *learning from the people through their eyes, ears, and experiences* and how they made sense out of situations and lifeways that were familiar to them. The method required direct naturalistic observations, participant experiences, reflections, and checking back with the people to understand what one observed, heard, or experienced. It required that the ethnonurse–researcher enter into a largely unknown world, remaining with the people of concern for an extended time, to learn firsthand meaningful constructions specific to the natural context or lived environment of peoples. It meant that the realities of individuals, groups, or collectives were developed over time by enculturation or socialization processes and influenced by a variety of cultural and environmental factors. The use of *a priori* judgments, scientific hypotheses, and the testing of the researcher's interests or variables was not congruent with the ethnonursing method. Instead, with the ethnonursing method, the researcher had to suspend or withhold fixed judgments and predetermined truths to let the people's ideas come forth and be documented (Leininger, 1985b, 1987). Exploring the informants' world to discover vaguely known or unknown ideas about human care and other nursing phenomena was a dominant focus. The researcher had to be sensitive and responsive to the people's ideas and to interpret ideas that gave meaning to the informants' views and cultural lifeways about human care or noncaring along with the factors influencing the phenomena discovered.

Since the mid 1950s, I had perceived care as the essence of nursing, which distinguished nursing from other health professions (Leininger, 1967, 1970, 1976, 1980, 1984). However, I realized that human care required systematic investigation with a method appropriate to discover the full subjective and objective human meanings, patterns, and values of care in different cultures. This research goal was essential to establish the epistemics or roots of nursing knowledge for the discipline and profession of nursing. Because nurses claimed to care for all people, a research method was needed to discover what was universal or diverse about human care transculturally. Generic or people-based care could only be fully known by studying care from the people in their natural contexts such as the home, workplace, or wherever people lived and functioned each day and night, and in different cultures. Thus, the ethnonursing method functioned as a means to obtain new foundational or substantive nursing knowledge to establish human care as the discipline's knowledge base. While this goal was yet to be recognized by nurse researchers and scholars, it remained for me a preeminent guide to differentiated nursing care decisions and actions in professional practices.

As a nurse and anthropologist, I pondered why human care had not been systematically studied and why it remained a largely unexplored area in the 1950s. I also wondered why human care transculturally had not been studied by nurses and anthropologists. I soon realized that care and its relationship to wellbeing was awaiting discovery by nurses. But, again, to study the ambiguous and invisible phenomenon of human care from a transcultural perspective (Leininger, 1978, 1980) required a uniquely focused research method that included transcultural human care phenomena as well as other largely unknown dimensions of nursing such as *health, wellbeing,* and *environmental contexts* in their historical, religious, kinship, language, technologic, environmental, biocultural, and other aspects. To obtain care knowledge from such broad dimensions of social structure and other factors required an inductive ethnonursing approach to grasp the totality of cultural care and to establish ultimately holistic nursing care practices over those practices derived from the fragmented, predetermined, disease, and symptom medical model then in use.

From my perspective, nursing in the 1950s was far too narrowly oriented and ethnocentric to discover holistic care in cultural and social contexts and to discover transcultural human care. Cultural care within the tenets of the theory provided the broadest and most comprehensive holistic means to discover care and related nursing knowledge. Most importantly, my anthropology field experiences had led me to realize that care, wellbeing, health, illness, and other related aspects of nursing were largely embedded in worldview and complex social structure factors related to kinship, cultural values, religion, environmental, worldview, biological, and language expressions, and so these dimensions had to be explicated and fully known in nursing.

While developing and refining the ethnonursing method in the early 1960s, I found myself quite alone in the study of human care from a transcultural nursing perspective. I also realized there were no research mentors or professional nurses available or interested in examining my new ethnonursing method. As a result, I developed and refined the method largely from my ongoing ethnonursing research experiences and with graduate students whom I encouraged to study care from a transcultural nursing viewpoint. These realities required that I spend considerable time establishing the method and educating students, which delayed the sharing of ideas with other nurses. However, the method was developed, refined, and did attract many nurse–researchers whose feedback was helpful. Unquestionably, nurse–researchers who were firmly entrenched within logical positivism and the quantitative scientific methods in the 1950s and 1960s regarded the ethnonursing qualitative method as 'too soft.' It did not have measurable and statistical outcomes as required by the received view of the logical positivists (Carter, 1985; Leininger, 1985b, 1987, 1990a; Watson, 1985). Moreover, the idea of nursing developing its own method to study nursing phenomena was not acceptable in those early days. Nursing as a profession was then trying to become 'scientific' by joining the league of other 'hard-core' quantitative scientists and emulating their ways.

It is of historical interest that before going to the Eastern Highlands of New Guinea, I conceptualized the ethnonursing method and developed some enabling guides such as the *Stranger–Friend Model* (Figure 2-1) and the *Observation-Participation-Reflection Model* (Figure 2-2). These enablers helped guide me in entering and remaining with the people to study their lifeways in relation to nursing care phenomena in a systematic and reflective way. The *Stranger–Friend Model* became an important part of the ethnonursing method and has been an essential guide for the researcher to obtain accurate and credible data. It was a fascinating and rewarding research experience to discover rich and meaningful data by entering the people's world as a coparticipant. I soon realized that the ethnonursing method was important to discover caring ways of feeding infants, dealing with pain and anxiety, supporting people in lifecycle events and crises, finding different ways to help people, and instructing people to maintain their wellbeing. Explication of such caring aspects of nursing and the full epistemics of care phenomena required the ethnonursing method. Specific techniques, strategies, and the use of several enabling guides were valuable to tease out the elusive, complex, and ambiguous aspects of *care* (as a noun) and *caring* (as an action) with individuals, families, and groups of different or similar cultural care systems.

The purpose of this enabler is to facilitate the researcher (or it can be used by a clinician) to move from mainly a distrusted stranger to a trusted friend in order to obtain authentic, credible, and dependable data (or establish favorable relationships as a clinician); The user assesses him or herself by reflecting on the indicators as he/she moves from stranger to friend.

Indicators of Stranger (Largely *etic* or outsider's views) Informant(s) or people are:	Date Noted	Indicators as a Trusted Friend (Largely *emic* or insider's views) Informant(s) or people are:	Date Noted
1. Active to protect self and others. They are "gate keepers" and guard against outside intrusions. Suspicious and questioning.		1. Less active to protect self. More trusting of researchers (their 'gate keeping is down or less'). Less suspicious and less questioning of researcher.	
2. Actively watch and are attentive to what researcher does and says. Limited signs of trusting the researcher or stranger.		2. Less watching the researcher's words and actions. More signs of trusting and accepting a new friend.	
3. Skeptical about the researcher's motives and work. May question how findings will be used by the researcher or stranger.		3. Less questioning of the researcher's motives, work, and behavior. Signs of working with and helping the researcher as a friend.	
4. Reluctant to share cultural secrets and views as private knowledge. Protective of local lifeways, values and beliefs. Dislikes probing by the researcher or stranger.		4. Willing to share cultural secrets and private world information and experiences. Offers most local views, values, and interpretations spontaneously or without probes.	
5. Uncomfortable to become a friend or to confide in stranger. May come late, be absent, and withdraw at times from researcher.		5. Signs of being comfortable and enjoying friends and a sharing relationship. Gives presence, on time, and gives evidence of being a 'genuine friend.'	
6. Tends to offer inaccurate data. Modifies 'truths' to protect self, family, community, and cultural lifeways. *Emic* values, beliefs, and practices are not shared spontaneously.		6. Wants research 'truths' to be accurate regarding beliefs, people, values, and lifeways. Explains and interprets *emic* ideas so researcher has accurate data.	

*Developed and used since 1959: Leininger.

Figure 2–1 Leininger's Stranger to Trusted Friend Enabler Guide.

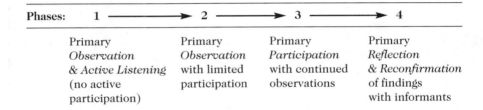

Figure 2–2   Leininger's Ethnonursing Enabler Observation-Participation-Reflection Phases

Epistemic and Philosophical Values to Support the Ethnonursing Method

Philosophically, the term *ethnonursing* was purposefully coined for this research method because *ethno* comes from the Greek word *ethos* and refers to 'the people' or culture with their lifeways. The suffix *nursing* was essential to focus the research on nursing's phenomena concerned primarily with the humanistic and scientific aspects of human care, wellbeing, and health in different environmental and cultural contexts (Leininger, 1978, 1980, 1984, 1985b, 1988). Therefore, the ethnonursing research method was designed to discover how people knew and experienced these major but insufficiently explored areas of nursing phenomena from a transcultural context and perspective in relation to the theory of Culture Care Diversity and Universality. Discovering such a potentially large base of nursing knowledge would provide the epistemic, historic, and ontological 'roots' as well as contemporary sources of nursing's discipline knowledge (Leininger, 1980, 1984, 1990a).

Philosophically and epistemologically, the sources of ethnonursing knowledge were held to be *grounded with the people* as the *knowers* about human care and other nursing knowledge. It was the ethnonurse researcher's task to learn from the people nursing phenomena and the factors influencing care and health from the local knowers' viewpoints and daily and nightly lived experiences. The knowers were teachers who could share their experiences, insights, and other knowledge of interest with the researcher. Obtaining such grounded data was essential to establish the epistemics and ontological nature and features of human care. Grounded data discoveries had long been part of ethnographic method as a way of knowing and generating theoretical data since the early, creative work of Bronislaw Malinowski (1922) with the Trobrianders in the mid-nineteenth century and with Franz Boas (1924) and his detailed work with the North American Indians. These pioneers set the idea of grounded, detailed, and epistemic sources of knowledge from 'the people' long before the work of Glaser and Strauss (1967) and other later qualitative methodologists. While I valued grounded discovery with the ethnonursing method to obtain full, rich data directly from people about human care and related nursing phenomena, I used both the *emic* (local) and *etic* (nonlocal) methods to obtain a more complete understanding of the phenomena of interest to nursing. This philosophical posture, that indigenous or local people were able to cognitively describe, know, explain, interpret, and even predict human care patterns, was an entirely new perspective to nurses in the 1960s and remains so with some nurses. Indeed, some nurses question this philosophical posture believing that professionals are the knowers of care and medical truths and that their mission is to instruct or teach clients who are nonknowers of what is best for them. Granted, nurses have professional knowledge, but it may not reflect culturally based knowledge that largely guides human decisions and actions.

The ethnonursing method, therefore, was a way of discovering, knowing, and confirming people's knowledge about care, and ways to keep well, or how they become ill or disabled. For the ethnonurse–researcher, the challenge is to be an interested friend of the people and to participate with them in discovering their past and current cultural beliefs, values, and ideas about human care, health, wellbeing, and other nursing dimensions. The ethnonurse–researcher develops skill in teasing out or explicating the people's ideas about human care meanings, expressions, forms, patterns, and general care experiences as lived. This required the use of relaxed, open ended inquiry modes approached in nonaggressive or nonconfrontive ways. It also required a genuinely interested mode of listening to and confirming informants' ideas. This approach was held as essential for informants to become the primary sharers and definers of ideas in discussion with the researcher, which could ensure accurate and meaningful interpretation of those ideas. Being a humble and open learner is as vital to this research method as it is a reversal of roles from the conventional scientific method, which assumes that the researcher holds—by logical inferences, other research studies, or from previously learned professional expertise—superior knowledge. Keeping an open mind and suspending personal beliefs, past professional experiences, and research experiences were essential attributes of the method and philosophy.

More specifically, as launched in the early 1960s, this ethnonursing research method had several general philosophical and research features to study ideas related to the theory of Culture Care Diversity and Universality (Leininger, 1966, 1970, 1978, 1985b, 1987, 1990a). First, the method required the researcher to move into familiar and naturalistic people settings to study human care and related nursing phenomena. The use of contrived, artificially controlled settings or being manipulative was not acceptable to obtain credible and accurate people-based data. Likewise, a tightly or rigidly controlled research design was not desired as the nurse researcher was expected to 'move with the local people or situation' as the informants told their past or present story, events, or lived experiences. The researcher was challenged to enter the *emic* or local world and to gradually become an active and genuinely interested learner. The Ethnonursing Method guided the researcher to *move with* the people or local informants in their lifeways and their patterns of knowing and sharing ideas bearing on human caring within their local environmental context, human ecology, or framework.

Second, by necessity, the ethnonursing method reflected detailed observations, reflections, descriptions, participant experiences, and data derived from largely unstructured open ended inquiries, or from enabler strategies. Open statements such as, "I would like to learn about your views, ideas, or experiences about caring for others or self, in this setting or culture," are used (Leininger, 1985b, 1987, 1990a). An open ended frame such as, "I would appreciate it if you would tell me more about _____ " [whatever is being shared], or on a special event also is used. In addition, *emic* local folktales, stories, or spontaneous narratives are elicited as well as *etic* ones to show any contrasts and similarities. Many additional examples of inquiry modes are given in other works (Leininger, 1984, 1985b; Wenger, 1985). Some suggestions from Spradley's (1979) ethnographic interviews are helpful, but his participant-observation research method is not the same as the ethnonursing method. In addition, learning to enter into a strange world requires some willingness to risk uncertainties and to become comfortable with strangers. It means developing skills to be an astute observer, listener, reflector, and accurate interpreter by taking a learner's role in the most naturally possible way. Being able to tolerate highly ambiguous, uncertain, subjective, or vaguely known complex sets of ideas requires patience, time, and genuine interest in others as essential features of the ethnonursing method. Some of these attributes can be found with people sensitive nurses who have developed these skills in their clinical practices and in teaching.

Third, the ethnonursing method requires that the researcher's biases, prejudices, opinions, and preprofessional interpretations be withheld, suspended, or controlled so that informants can present *their emic ideas and interpretations* rather than those of the researcher. Learning to value and respect the people's views and experiences when well, sick, disabled, oppressed, dying, or whatever human condition they are experiencing is an important skill with the method. Being cognizant of the researcher's views and any prejudices requires centering on the informant, active listening, and self reflection, often with a research mentor. The philosophical position that the individuals and cultures 'can make sense out of their world' is often difficult for any professional nurse because of past dominant emphases on 'knowing all about people being ill or having a specific diseased condition.' However, informants can share ideas that make sense to them and are important to them whether ill or well. Avoiding an interpretation of the informant's ideas to fit professional knowledge and expectations is important. As such, research mentors prepared in the method are extremely valuable for the conduct of this method. Experienced ethnonurse researchers who have lived through and used the method can deal with the novice researcher's tendencies related to ethnocentrism, biases, prejudice, and reinterpretation tendencies. The mentor can help the researcher remain sensitive to research proclivities in order to obtain accurate and credible ethnonursing knowledge. Mentors experienced in the ethnonursing method are extremely important to assess ethical and moral issues related to informant 'secrets,' confidentiality, the process of obtaining consent, and recording of detailed people data. They are especially useful in teasing out *generic* and *professional* care findings from large volumes of qualitative data and in analyzing all data collected. Having external nurse panelists who are not prepared in the method or in the culture are of limited use and may impose their ideas onto rich and new findings from an ethnonursing study.

Fourth, the ethnonursing method requires that the researcher focus on the cultural context of whatever phenomena are being studied. The cultural context refers to the totality of the situation or lifeway at hand (Leininger, 1970, 1987, 1990a). To discover and fully understand cultural context includes both contemporary and ethnohistorical underpinnings to consider. Since the 1960s, and in order to interpret cultural research findings accurately, I have held the idea of cultural context as an extremely important focus of my thinking and research. Grasping the full meaning of cultural context means examining historical, biosocial, cultural values, language expressions, technology, material, and symbolic referents in the environment of the people being studied. Any removal of cultural contextual data, or 'surgical pruning,' can markedly reduce the credibility, accuracy, and meaning of what was seen, heard, or experienced. I have used the qualitative criterion of meaning-in-context in all of my field research emphasizing the importance of describing and detailing diverse factors impinging on the meanings of human care, health, or wellbeing of cultures. Inclusion of cultural context remains an essential aspect of ethnonursing research. Contextual data also provides thick descriptions to establish the study's credibility. Thick descriptions about human care with multiple external or internal cultural factors, symbols, and beliefs will help the researcher identify embedded 'truths' about human care, wellbeing, and the lifeways of the people. However, teasing out contextual data from the social structure and worldview takes time, patience, and cultural sensitivity.

Allowing the people themselves to come forth to take control of their knowledge and experiences to share their *emic* cultural viewpoints, values, and lifeways are important. The inductive *emic* approach helps to prevent researchers from using preconceived judgments or *a priori* views of modifying informants' ideas. In general, obtaining full, thick, and detailed accounts of cultural care situations, events, or happenings through direct observations, participation, and interviews over time is critical to confirm and establish meaningful patterns of culture care. The ethnonurse–researcher remains a coparticipant with informants to discover these detailed accounts and to see how the people practice human care in their daily lives.

With ethnonursing research, it is important to obtain indepth particularistic or diverse accounts while searching for commonalities (Leininger, 1988, 1989). Ideographic or particularized patterns and situations are usually considered more important than broad sweeping generalizations with qualitative studies (Lincoln & Guba, 1985; Reason & Rowan, 1981). Arriving at generalizations to be applied to large numbers of people or population groups is not the goal of qualitative or ethnonursing research, and is, therefore, very different from quantitative research goals (Lincoln & Guba, 1985; Leininger, 1985b, 1990a). Instead, the goal of ethnonursing research is to know as fully as possible actual or potential nursing phenomena such as the meanings and expressions of human caring in different or similar contexts.

By focusing on some phenomena, the researcher often discovers new insights and ways people interpret and explain their world of knowing. For example, I discovered that there were gender differences between the adult Gadsup men and women regarding protective and surveillant care. Gadsup men had different ways to provide public protective care that contributed to the wellbeing of the extended clan members, and males felt a responsibility to provide protective care. Women also provided some protective care, but they were skilled in providing nurturant and surveillant domestic care activities, and not public care (Leininger, 1970, 1978). I also discovered that the Gadsup do not follow Erikson's (1963) stipulated stages of growth and development. Instead, the Gadsup had several phases of human development that were part of Gadsup caring and nurturance and surveillance through the lifecycle. These comparative emic and etic differences have provided refreshing new lifecycle insights that care expressions, meanings, and interpretations were different from those in our Western culture. Such ideographic or particularistic findings have provided some entirely new perspectives to transcultural nursing knowledge. I also realized that many New Guinea findings were not generalizable to other cultures, but were more culture specific or relativistic as to the

Gadsups due largely to enculturation, social structure, and ethnohistorical factors. Such findings of a particular culture provide indepth quality data, rather than generalized data about thousands of unknown people which limits understanding of them.

An important characteristic in the use of the ethnonursing method is to give attention to the sequence of events or the ethnohistory of how care lifeways and patterns developed over time. Discovering how human care was traditionally viewed and how it may have changed with individuals and groups often provides fresh insights about cultural changes and variabilities in the culture. The use of ethnohistorical data from anthropologists or social science historians can be useful as background information to show how changes have occurred over time and under different circumstances. It is the task of the nurse–researcher, however, to focus specifically on nursing phenomena in relation to ethnohistorical data. For example, human care practices often change drastically due to certain cultural events, such as major wars, feuds, coups, or major migrations to a new culture. The people's interpretations or explanation of these changes can provide meaningful explanations of the dynamic aspects of the culture. Such interpretations of historical changes contrast sharply with quantitative studies in which historical data are viewed as threats to the validity and reliability of a study and must be avoided or controlled (Polit & Hungler, 1983).

In conducting an ethnonursing study, the researcher uses a broad theoretical framework to guide the study such as the theory of Culture Care. These theoretical frameworks should be broad enough to accommodate local or particular cultural care factors while serving as a general guide to inquiry. The researcher remains active to identify whether the data supports or refutes the general or specific theoretical premises and remains alert to the theoretical assumptions or presuppositions of the study. Although ethnonurse–researchers usually have a general theoretical framework in mind with a domain of inquiry, it remains possible to conduct the study without any theory, and generate the theory in the process of conducting the study (Leininger, 1985b). Culture Care Diversity and Universality helps the researcher reflect on the theoretical tenets as well as the assumptions and major components of the theory such as worldview, social structure, cultural care values and beliefs, environment, and other dimensions held to influence human care. The theoretical framework serves as an important guide to search for holistic and particular cultural factors about human care and caring. Accordingly, a specific method of data analysis was developed as part of the ethnonursing method to provide systematic data analysis in relation to theoretical assumptions. Enablers were developed to explicate or tease out data related to the social structure and other components of the theory.

Research Enablers to Discover Human Care and Related Nursing Phenomena

In accord with any method, the methodologist develops not only the major features of the method but also techniques, strategies, and ways that can be used with the method to attain envisioned purposes. It is the methodological features with specific techniques and guides that differentiate one research method from others. In the late 1950s and before conducting my first ethnonursing and ethnographic studies, I conceived of the idea 'enablers' as ways to explicate, probe, or discover indepth phenomena that seemed as complex, elusive, and ambiguous as human care. I disliked the terms <u>tool</u> or <u>instrument</u> as they were too impersonal, mechanistic, and fit with objectification, experimentation, and other methods and logical features of the quantitative paradigm. I also disliked the idea of the researcher being 'the instrument' as it, too, harked of a cold, detached, and impersonal investigator. The idea of enablers and friendly researchers communicated a participatory and cooperative way to obtain ideas that were often difficult to know immediately without gentle probing of informants willing to share their ideas. Enablers were congruent with the qualitative paradigm and as a means to explicate cultural care. In this section, some major enablers will be discussed briefly as I developed them and as part of the ethnonursing research method. Although I have developed several unique enablers during the past three decades, I will present only those of major importance that are frequently used by ethnonurse–researchers to study comparative culture care. The ethnonursing research studies that follow this chapter have used these common enablers, and some researchers have developed their own specific enablers for a particular focus of their study.

Leininger's Stranger–Friend Enabler

I developed this model, the first enabler, before conducting my first ethnonursing and ethnography field study in the Eastern Highlands of New Guinea in the early 1960s (see Figure 2-1) (Leininger, 1985b). Although some aspects of the enabler were stimulated from reading Berreman's (1962) paper *Behind Many Masks*, it was reconceptualized with new practical indicators to help ethnonurse researchers move from a stranger to friend role when studying people to discover nursing phenomena. The enabler was designed with the philosophical belief that the researcher should always assess and gauge the relationships with the people being studied in order to enter or get close to the people or situation under study. It was anticipated that the researcher needed to move from a stranger or distrusted person to a trusted and friendly person during the ethnonursing research process to obtain accurate, sensitive, meaningful, and credible data. Based on my extensive fieldwork, I held that researchers, usually as *etic* strangers (outsiders), needed to be trusted *before* they would be able to obtain any accurate, reliable, or credible data. Initially, most cultures or informants find the researcher an outsider or a distrusted stranger until proven otherwise and someone to watch in regard to actions, motives, and behaviors. While the researcher remains a distrusted stranger, the people are generally quite reluctant to share their ideas with the researcher. On repeated occasions, and while a distrusted stranger, I have found that initial research data are often superficial, inaccurate, and incomplete (Leininger, 1970, 1978, 1985a). This is understandable—culture informants must protect themselves, their people, and their ideas until the informants know the researcher(s). This was further evident with psychological 'standardized' tests, such as Holtzman, Thematic Apperception Test (TAT), and Rorschach, which I administered to the Gadsup and from which I received nontruths while in the stranger phase.

The pattern of moving from stranger to trusted friend can be identified in all research studies that I have mentored over the past three decades with 15–20 cultures (Leininger, 1970, 1978, 1985a/b). The purpose, therefore, of the Stranger–Friend Enabler is to serve as an assessment or reflection guide for the researcher to become consciously aware of one's own behaviors, feelings, and responses as one moves with informants and works to collect data for confirmation of cultural "truths" (Leininger, 1985b). Each of the indicators or characteristics for the stranger or friend in Figure 2-1 are used and studied over time to identify patterned behaviors and expectations of people-centered studies. They have been established as credible and reliable indicators with multiple cultures over many years (Leininger, 1985a/b).

The Stranger–Friend Model also serves as a gauge for the researcher's progress, with some researchers remaining in the distrusted role longer than others. In using the model, the goal is to move from stranger to friend in order to help ensure a credible, meaningful, and accurate study. The model can be used by the researcher in hospital settings, in community contexts, and in many other places where nurses study nursing phenomena. Becoming aware of self-behavior as a researcher as well as observing those being studied is a major task for the researcher while actively participating with the people. This Stranger–Friend Enabler is especially useful as nurses study nurse–client, nurse–group, nurse–family relationships in the hospital or home. The researcher learns to appraise the progress in the study by remaining sensitive to verbal feedback or responses from the people. This enabler is essential to all people-centered investigations, and, therefore, has been used by many nonnurse researchers besides nurses involved in qualitative investigations. It is an enabler that can be used for all humanistic qualitative studies to facilitate the research process, get close to people, and to obtain accurate data in a sensitive and skilled manner within different life contexts.

Observation-Participation-Reflection Enabler (OPR)

I developed the Observation-Participation-Reflection Model in the early 1960s, and have refined and used it for five decades along with many graduate students. The enabler was partially derived from the traditional participant-observation approach used in anthropology, but was modified in several ways with the added focus on *reflections* to fit the philosophy, purposes, and goals of ethnonursing method (see Figure 2-2). The enabler also is different from the conventional anthropological participant-observation approach in that the process was *reversed*. With the OPR Enabler, the researcher is expected to devote a period of time making observations before becoming an active participant. This resequenced role serves the important function of allowing the nurse researcher to become fully cognizant of the situation or context before becoming a full participant or 'doer.' In addition, the reflection phase has been added to provide important and essential confirmatory data from the people studied. Reflection is done throughout the research process, but especially during the last phase of research. Thus, there are four phases rather than two phases found in traditional anthropological participant observation. These phases were especially conceptualized and developed to fit with the people-centered nursing ways that professional nurses are expected to work within their daily experiences.

To perfect the OPR Enabler for ethnonursing studies, I, with many graduate students, have refined it several times during the past five decades (Leininger, 1978, 1985b, 1990a). The users find that the enabler provides a most helpful and systematic way to enter into, remain with, and conclude an ethnonursing study with individuals, groups, communities, and cultures related to human caring and nursing. This enabler helps the researcher get close to the people, study the total context, and obtain accurate data from the people. The most difficult phase for most nurse researchers is the first phase of observation because most nurses find it difficult to remain in a focused observer role before becoming a participant. Nurses who are active doers and who have not learned to do sustained observing before acting find that this model helps them learn about the importance of observing for a period of time before becoming an active participant and centering on context.

Reflection is an integral part of the ethnonursing method. Reflection on the phenomena observed or ideas heard helps the nurse to focus on all contextual aspects of the research before proclaiming or interpreting an idea or experience. At the conclusion of the study, the researcher reflects back on all findings to recheck and confirm them, primarily with key informants. Reflection on small and large segments of the data is essential at every phase of the research process as it helps one to study meanings-in-context and other aspects of the data. The OPR phases are a critical and important feature of the ethnonursing research method to ensure accurate and systematic observations and interpretations of findings. This enabler has been described in other sources (Leininger, 1985b, 1987; Wenger, 1985), and by researchers who have used the ethnonursing method in this book.

Leininger's Phases of Ethnonursing Data Analysis Guide as an Enabler

A major concern of qualitative researchers has been to find ways to systematically analyze large amounts of field data. To meet this challenge, I developed and refined the Phases of Ethnonursing Data Analysis Guide (see Figure 2-3) as another enabler to facilitate the research process. This guide was refined during the past several decades as a part of the ethnonursing method to provide rigorous, indepth, and systematic analysis of qualitative ethnonursing research data, and especially research findings bearing on the theory of Cultural Care (Leininger, 1987). This enabler has been used by many nurses and by other researchers to analyze qualitative data, and remains an important systematic data analysis method for qualitative studies. Currently, this method is replacing qualitative data analysis that is vague, ambiguous, or questionable such as doing a "content analysis" in which all data are analyzed in nonsystematic ways.

The Data Analysis Guide offers four sequenced phases of analysis. The researcher begins data analysis on the first day of research and continues with regular data coding, processing, and analysis of all data until all data are collected. The researcher uses the four levels of data analysis as seen in Figure 2-3. The data are continuously processed and reflected on by the researcher at each phase (originally, in 1965, the enabler had six phases, but it has been refined to four).

As one examines the four phases in Figure 2-3, the major characteristics of each phase are presented (Leininger, 1987). In Phase I, the researcher analyzes grounded and detailed raw data before moving to Phase II. In Phase II, the researcher identifies the *descriptors, indicators,* and *categories* from the raw data in Phase I. In Phase III, the researcher identifies the *recurrent patterns* from the data as derived from Phase I and II. In Phase IV, *themes* of behavior and other *summative research findings* are presented and abstracted from the data as derived from the three previous phases. At all times, research findings from the data analysis can be traced back to each phase and to the grounded data in Phase I. This interphase check is essential to preserve emic data and to confirm findings by checking back on the findings at each phase. The systematic data analysis process is extremely detailed and is essential to understand the data and to trail back on the findings or conclusions. This process of data analysis is detailed and rigorous but essential to meet the criteria of qualitative analysis showing how the researcher met the criteria of credibility, recurrent patterning, confirmability, meaning-in-context, and other criteria of a qualitative study.

Fourth Phase (Last Phase)

Major Themes, Research Findings, Theoretical Formulations, and Recommendations

This is the highest phase of data analysis, synthesis, and interpretation. It requires synthesis of thinking, configuration analysis, interpreting findings, and creative formulation from data of the previous phases. The researcher's task is to abstract and confirm major themes, research findings, recommendations, and sometimes make new theoretical formulations.

Third Phase

Pattern and Contextual Analysis

Data are scrutinized to discover saturation of ideas and recurrent patterns of similar or different meanings, expressions, structural forms, interpretations, or explanations of data related to the domain of inquiry. Data are also examined to show patterning with respect to meanings-in-context and along with further credibility and confirmation of findings.

Second Phase

Identification and Categorization of Descriptors and Components

Data are coded and classified as related to the domain or inquiry and sometimes the questions under study. *Emic* or *etic* descriptors are studied within context and for similarities and differences. Recurrent components are studied for their meanings.

First Phase

Collecting, Describing, and Documenting Raw Data (Use of Field Journal and Computer)

The researcher collects, describes, records, and begins to analyze data related to the purposes, domain of inquiry, or questions under study. This phase includes: recording interview data from *key* and *general* informants; making observations, and having participatory experiences; identifying contextual meanings; making preliminary interpretations; identifying symbols; and recording data related to the DOI or phenomenon under study mainly from an *emic* focus. Attention to *etic* ideas is also recorded. Field data from the condensed and full field journal can be processed directly into the computer and coded, ready for analysis.

Figure 2–3   Leininger's Phases of Ethnonursing Analysis or Qualitative Data

Data from ethnonursing interviews and the enablers such as the Observation-Participant-Reflection Enabler, Stranger–Friend Enabler, Health Care Life History Enabler, and others are incorporated in the total ethnonursing mode of data collection and analyses. The culminating abstraction and identification of themes in Phase IV constitute the highest level of data analysis. This phase also is the most difficult level of analysis as it requires critical analysis of all data and keen intellectual abilities to synthesize data and abstract meanings from the four phases so that conclusions are credible and understandable. Phase IV of data analysis also requires skill to synthesize findings related to contextual factors, cultural interpretations, language analysis, social structure, and other influencers of human care and wellbeing. To conduct an accurate synthesis, the researcher must be fully immersed in the data and know the data well. The researcher must carefully preserve relevant verbal statements, meanings, and interpretations from informants in a meaningful way and not reduce data to spurious or questionable themes. Attention is given to special linguistic terms and verbatim statements, subjective and experiential data of *emic* and *etic* content. In addition, the key informants' interpretations of diverse themes and commonalities are identified. Ethnohistorical facts, artistic expressions, worldviews, material cultural items, values and beliefs, and many other aspects influencing culture care and health are presented. Each phase of analysis builds on and supports previous phases of analysis so that confident, accurate, and meaningful findings are evident. When the data analysis is completed in a systematic way, the researcher feels strongly and convincingly that the analysis is credible and fully reflects the domain of inquiry with research questions related to the theory and DOI.

A caveat should be noted with research assistants and nurses who have had no preparation with the ethnonursing method and this data analysis—they will have difficulty unless prepared by a teacher experienced with the method. Questionable findings can be identified using research assistants and analyzers who have not had experience and who have not studied the method. For those prepared in the method, it offers a highly rewarding process to make sense out of large or small volumes of ethnonursing qualitative data. Luna's (1989) study of American Lebanese Arab-Muslims and other studies in this book provide examples of detailed and rigorous analyses of data using the four phases of Leininger's data analysis. These studies have provided new knowledge and insights about culture care transculturally.

Leininger–Templin–Thompson Ethnoscript Qualitative Software (LTT)

To facilitate the above systematic mode of data collection, processing, and analysis, the Leininger–Templin–Thompson Ethnoscript Qualitative Software (LTT) was developed around 1985 (Leininger, 1990b). The LTT Software was designed as a tailor-made means to process large amounts of ethnonursing data for the Culture Care Theory (Leininger, 1987). This software was historically used with some ethnonursing data analysis in that the researcher could directly process large amounts of detailed qualitative data by use of computers. Data focusing on the worldview, social structure, cultural values, language, environmental context, historical facts, folk, and professional health care systems, specific caring modes, and other data were computer coded and processed (Leininger, 1990b). Other software has been explored and further developed to preserve all key and general informant data, and other field data collected from the enablers. Researchers can process field data directly to their laptops or desktop computers. With the development of these new and different types of data processing software, researchers are able to explore them for use in ethnonursing data analysis.

Acculturation Enabler Guide

An Acculturation Enabler Guide was created by the author to help assess the extent of acculturation of an individual or group with respect to a particular culture or subculture (see Figure 2-4). This enabler was developed as part of the ethnonursing research method to assess the extent to which individuals or groups of a particular culture are more traditionally or nontraditionally oriented, and to identify cultural variability or universality features (Leininger, 1978, 1991). The acculturation enabler was developed with thought to the components of the Culture Care Theory in order to assess cultural variabilities of individuals and groups of a particular culture along major lines of differentiating cultural experience.

During the past five decades, this enabler has been used, modified, confirmed, and perfected with many informants and in diverse contexts so that acculturation factors such as social structure, worldview, and human care factors. With this enabler, the researcher can obtain a profile of the extent and areas of acculturation with respect to traditional and nontraditional cultural orientations. Data from the enabler guide are analyzed and reported in the findings in different creative ways such as pictorial graphs, bar graphs, narratives, or informant or group profiles. There is provision for written narrative statements to support the cultural assessments in each area. The researcher may want to use percentages or simple numerical data to show the direction or degree of acculturation which is in keeping with qualitative analysis. To date the acculturation enabler has high credibility, reliability, and confirmability as it has been used with many cultures over the past five decades to identify specific characteristics or patterns of a culture bearing on cultural aspects, care, and related nursing phenomena. It is one of the few major acculturation enablers available in nursing, anthropology, and the social sciences.

Life History Health Care Enabler

As previously published and discussed in *Qualitative Research and Nursing* (Leininger, 1985c, pp. 119–133), the reader is referred to this publication for a full account of the enabler's purposes and uses in ethnonursing and related qualitative research studies. The Life History Health Care Enabler is a guide to obtaining longitudinal data from

---

Name of Assessor _____ Date: _____

Informants or Code No. _____ Sex: _____ Age: _____

Place or Context of Assessment: _____

Directions: This enabler provides a general qualitative profile or assessment of traditional or nontraditional orientation of informants of their patterned lifeways. Health care influencers are assessed with respect to worldview, language, cultural values, kinship, religion, politics, technology, education, environment, and related areas. This profile is primarily focused on *emic* (local) information to assess and guide health personnel in working with individuals and groups. The *etic* (or more universal view) also may be evident. In Part I, the user observes, records, and rates behavior on the scale below from 1 to 5 with respect to traditional or nontraditionally oriented lifeways. Numbers are plotted on the summary Part II to obtain a qualitative profile to guide decisions and actions. The user's brief notations on each criterion should be used to support ratings and reliable profile. This enabler was not designed for quantitative measurements, but rather as a qualitative enabler to explicate data from informants.

(Continues)

Figure 2–4   Leininger's Acculturation Health Care Assessment Enabler for Cultural Patterns in Traditional and Nontraditional Lifeways*

*Note: This enabler has been developed, refined, and used for five decades (since the early 1960s) by Dr. Madeleine Leininger. It has been frequently in demand by anthropologists, transcultural nurses, and others. It has been useful to obtain informant's *orientation* to traditional or nontraditional lifeways. It provides qualitative indicators to meet credibility, confirmability, recurrency and reliability for qualitative studies. This copyrighted enabler may be used if the *full title* of the enabler, recognition of *source* (M. Leininger), and *publication outlet* (*Journal of Transcultural Nursing*, 1991) is cited. The author would also appreciate a letter to know who has used it with focus and summary outcomes.

Part I: Rating of Criteria to Assess Traditional and Nontraditional Patterned Cultural Lifeways or Orientations

Rating indicators:	Mainly Traditional 1	Moderate 2	Average 3	Moderate 4	Mainly Nontraditional 5	Rater Value No.

Cultural Dimensions to Assess Traditional or Nontraditional Orientations

1. Language, Communication & Gestures (Native or Nonnative).

   Notations: _____

   _____

   _____

2. General Environmental Living Context (Symbols, material & non-material signs). Specify: _____

   _____

   _____

3. Wearing Apparel & Physical Appearance. Notations: _____

   _____

   _____

4. Technology Being Used in Living Environment. Notations: _____

   _____

   _____

5. World View (How person looks out upon the world). Notations: _____

   _____

   _____

6. Family Lifeways (Values, beliefs and norms). Notations: _____

   _____

   _____

7. General Social Interactions and Kinship Ties. Notations: _____

   _____

   _____

8. Patterned Daily Activities. Notations: _____

   _____

9. Religious (or Spiritual) Beliefs and Values. Notations: _____

   _____

Figure 2–4   Leininger's Acculturation Health Care Assessment Enabler for Cultural Patterns in Traditional and Nontraditional Lifeways *(Continued)*

Rating indicators:	Mainly Traditional 1	Moderate 2	Average 3	Moderate 4	Mainly Nontraditional 5	Rater Value No.
10. Economic Factors (Rough cost of living estimates and income). Notations: _____						
11. Educational Values or Belief Factors. Notations: _____						
12. Political or Legal Influencers. Notations: _____						
13. Food Uses and Nutritional Values, Beliefs, & Taboos. Specify: _____						
14. *Folk* (Generic or Indigenous) *Health Care* (*-Cure*) Values, Beliefs & Practices. Specify: _____						
15. *Professional Health Care* (*-Cure*) Values, Beliefs & Practices. Specify: _____						
16. Care Concepts or Patterns that.guide actions, i.e. concern for, support, presence, etc.: _____						
17. Caring Patterns or Expressions: _____						
18. Views of Ways to: a) Prevent illnesses: _____ b) Preserve or maintain wellness or health: _____ c) Care for self or others: _____						
19. Other Indicators to support more traditional or non-traditional lifeways: _____						

(Continues)

Part II: Acculturation Profile from Assessment Factors

Directions: Plot an X with the value numbers rated on this profile to discover the orientation or acculturation gradient of the informant. The clustering of numbers will give information of traditional or nontraditional patterns with respect to the criteria assessed.

Criteria	1 Mainly Traditional	2 Moderate	3 Average	4 Moderate	5 Mainly Nontraditional
1. Language & Communication Modes					
2. Physical Environment					
3. Physical Apparel & Appearance					
4. Technology					
5. World View					
6. Family Lifeways					
7. Social Interaction & Kinship					
8. Daily Lifeways					
9. Religious Orientation					
10. Economic Factors					
11. Educational Factors					
12. Political & Legal Factors					
13. Food Uses					
14. Folk (Generic) Care-Cure					
15. Professional Care-Cure Expressions					
16. Caring Patterns					
17. Curing Patterns					
18. Prevention/ Maintenance Factors					
19. Other Indicators					

Note: The assessor may total numbers to get a summary orientation profile. Use of these ratings with written notations provide a wholistic qualitative profile. More detailed notations are important to substantiate the ratings.

Figure 2–4   Leininger's Acculturation Health Care Assessment Enabler for Cultural Patterns in Traditional and Nontraditional Lifeways *(Continued)*

selected informants of their 'lived through life span experiences,' and with focus on care and caring (or related nursing aspects). Life histories have long been of value in anthropology. Ideas for this enabler were derived from several authors' experiences and from anthropological life histories. Nurses are now learning how to use full life histories to study nursing and health care practices.

It is of interest that clients and families often enjoy talking about their life history accounts, and especially with the middlescent and elderly adults. Hence, this enabler was designed to obtain a full and systematic account from informants about their caring healthy, or less healthy, lifeways and how care beliefs and practices influenced their wellbeing. Enormously rich and detailed data have been obtained from the use of this enabler especially with respect to human caring and health values, expressions, and meanings (Leininger, 1985c). Nurse–researchers using the ethnonursing method are encouraged to use this enabler to tease out historic insights about health care values and practices, especially related to generic and professional care patterns and practices throughout the life cycle. The life history guide has been useful in obtaining longitudinal narratives about the informants' special experiences in folk and professional health systems in homes and institutions.

Other Enablers: Options for the Researcher

Over time, I have developed other enablers such as those focused on: (1) Cultural Care Values and Meanings; (2) Culturalogical Care Assessment Guide; (3) Audio-Visual Guide; and (4) Generic and Professional Care Enabler Guide (Leininger, 1985a, 1988). Due to space limitations, these enablers will not be presented here. It is important to note, however, that the researcher who uses the ethnonursing method to study Cultural Care Theory can develop different kinds of enablers to study diverse cultures in different domains of inquiry related to Cultural Care Theory.

Ethnonursing Research Process

With the above philosophy, rationale, and enablers in mind, the ethnonursing research process is presented. Nurse–researchers need to envision the general research process of conducting an ethnonursing study. Figure 2-5 is presented as a visual guide to the general sequence of an ethnonursing research process. While this sequence offers general guidelines, the researcher may modify the process to fit with the research setting or context. Most importantly, the ethnonursing process

1. Identify the general intent or purpose(s) of your study with focus on the domain(s) of inquiry phenomenon under study, area of inquiry, or research questions being addressed.

2. Identify the potential significance of the study to advance nursing knowledge and practices.

3. Review available literature on the domain or phenomena being studied.

4. Conceptualize a research plan from beginning to the end with the following general phases or sequence factors in mind.

    a) Consider the research site, community, and people to study the phenomena.

    b) Deal with the informed consent expectations.

    c) Explore and gradually gain entry (with essential permissions) to the community, hospital, or country wherever the study is being done.

    d) Anticipate potential barriers and facilitators related to: gatekeepers expectations, language, political leaders, location, and other factors.

    e) Select and appropriately use the ethnonursing enablers with the research process, e.g., Leininger's *Stranger–Friend Guide* and *Observation-Participation-Reflection Guide* and others. The researcher may also develop specific enablers or guides for their study.

    f) Chose key and general informants.

    g) Maintain trusting and favorable relationships with the people conferring with ethnonurse research expert(s) to prevent unfavorable developments.

    h) Collect and confirm data with observations, interviews, participant experiences, and other data. (This is a continuous process from the beginning to the end and requires the use of qualitative research criteria to confirm findings and credibility factors.)

    i) Maintain continuous data processing on computers and with field journals reflecting active analysis and reflections, and with discussions with research mentor(s). Computer processing with Leininger–Templin–Thompson's software is a helpful means to handle large amounts of qualitative data.

    j) Frequently present and reconfirm findings with the people studied to check credibility and confirmability of findings.

    k) Make plans to leave the field site or community by informing people in advance.

5. Do final analysis and writing of the research findings soon after completing the study.

6. Prepare published findings for appropriate journals.

7. Help implement the findings with nurses and others interested in findings.

8. Plan future studies related to this domain or other new ones.

Figure 2–5   Leininger's Phases of Ethnonursing Research Process

needs to remain flexible so that the researcher can move with the people and in accordance with the naturalistic developments and human research conditions. As the researcher moves from a stranger to a friend to collect and process data, flexibility and modifications in the research plan often are needed. Nonetheless, the ethnonursing research process as depicted in Figure 2-5 helps the researcher to perceive him- or herself when entering, remaining in, or leaving informants as part of the research sequence whether in the hospital, community agency, urban street clinic, rural community, or other places. Careful use of the ethnonursing research process helps the researcher to ensure a complete and comprehensive study by being attentive to areas that need to be considered to systematically and fully study. Any credible research method contains desired ways to carry out a sound method of investigation for a complete, credible study, and this process is offered to help the researcher attain this goal.

Although the particular phases of the ethnonursing research process are not discussed here, they have been identified and discussed in other publications, and readers are encouraged to study these sources (Leininger, 1985a, 1985b, 1987, 1989, 1990a). Derived underpinnings and general philosophical premises to support the ethnonursing process also are discussed in the works of Guba (1990), Lincoln and Guba (1985), Reason and Rowan (1985), Heron (1981), and Spradley (1979).

General Ethnonursing Principles to Support the Research Method

In light of the philosophical, epistemic, and ontological bases and the purposes for the ethnonursing method, some general summative principles can be stated to guide the nurse–researcher in using the method. The first principle the ethnonursing–researcher requires is to *maintain an open discovery, active listening, and a genuine learning attitude in working with informants* in the total context in which the study is conducted. The researcher's attitude and willingness to be an active learner and to discover as much as possible from the informants and the culture is extremely important for a sound ethnonursing study. The researcher remains an active learner about the people's or client's world by becoming involved in and showing a willingness to *learn from the people.* Discovering and learning about the meanings, expressions, values, beliefs, and patterns of human care also requires active listening, suspended judgments, and reflection about informant ideas. Informants usually are willing to respond to an active listener who is genuinely interested in them, their lifeways, and viewpoints. Learning from the knowers (informants) may be difficult for some nurse–researchers who are skilled clinicians, administrators, or in other roles where subject matter expertise prevails. The nurse–researcher, therefore, needs to be aware of ethnocentric views and biases. Being a humble learner is not always easy if female nurses are eager to assert their rights and knowledge, especially to patriarchal informants. Learning from strangers and respecting what is shared without moral (right or wrong) judgments and respecting cultural secrets is essential.

The second principle the ethnonurse researcher requires is to *maintain an active and curious posture about the 'why' of whatever is seen, heard, or experienced, and with appreciation of whatever informants share with you.* Being an active participant and reflector about phenomena means becoming sensitive to the local emic viewpoints and reflecting on etic professional ideas. Searching for the why means remaining interested in the informant's views different or similar to those of the nurse. It means a willingness to explore new or different ideas about human caring from folk (generic) and professional viewpoints. Observing and pondering about the why of care expressions and action modes from both indigenous and professional caregivers often provides new insights about unknown aspects of care. Exploring caring behaviors related to care constructs such as touch, assisting others, protection, support, comfort, and other largely undiscovered culture-specific care concepts necessitates time, patience, and teasing out of vague ideas to get to the epistemics or knowledge sources.

The ethnonurse becomes an unrelenting researcher to obtain specific meanings, functions, and expressions of care with their relationships to wellbeing, health, illness, death, or to any human condition.

The third ethnonursing principle is to *record whatever is shared by informants in a careful and conscientious way with full meanings, explanations, or interpretations to preserve informant ideas.* This means that the nurse–researcher needs to value whatever is shared and try to grasp the diverse and common linkages about human caring. It also means that informants and others in the culture usually are able to interpret and make sense out of their beliefs, experiences (subjective and real), and decision modes if permitted to do so by the researcher. Sometimes it is difficult for the researcher to make sense out of cultural data of what one sees and hears, but the more one trusts local informants the more one can learn about cultural care and health patterns or experiences. Patience and a willingness to listen and reflect on informant ideas are essential to comprehend and fully understand care and related phenomena. For example, the researcher often records deviant, ambiguous, or questionable ideas with interpretations suspended or withheld until their meanings become understandable with help from informants' diverse expressions. Such diverse expressions must be preserved as well. Not only do they provide significant help in the understanding of informant ideas, often they are indicators of cultural changes, areas of conflict, or special modes of expressing cultural care practices.

The fourth ethnonursing principle is to *seek a mentor who has experience with the ethnonursing research method to act as a guide.* An experienced mentor who has conducted ethnonursing studies can be most helpful in examining the research process at hand. He or she also can help to reduce biases, prejudices, prejudgments, and questionable interpretations that do not support grounded data. An experienced research mentor provides an opportunity for the researcher to reflect on the findings and to make meaningful linkages with diverse and similar findings. Moreover, an experienced qualitative mentor can help process large amounts of qualitative data when the researcher feels overwhelmed and not able to move or 'get hold of the data.' Often, when cultural linkages may be difficult to make, the researcher mentor can reflect on the ideas in a way that facilitates the researcher's analysis. Finally, the research mentor can be very helpful in presenting and publishing ethnonursing research findings which are often issued in long, detailed reports.

A fifth ethnonursing principle is to *clarify the purposes of additional qualitative research methods if they are combined with the ethnonursing method such as combining life histories, ethnography, phenomenology, or ethnoscience.* Such combinations are possible, but the reasons and purposes for combining several methods must be made clear at the outset and with the domain of inquiry, the theory, and the research purposes. Actually, the nurse–researchers do not need to use additional research methods unless absolutely necessary, and if another method is used it should fit the paradigm and study purposes. Nurses who have not been well prepared in qualitative research methods may fail to realize that the qualitative and quantitative paradigms have very different goals and purposes (Leininger, 1985a; Lincoln & Guba, 1985). Ethnomethods and paradigms should not be mixed. As I have stated in other publications (Leininger, 1987, 1990a), *one can mix methods within a paradigm, but not mix methods of different paradigms as it violates the purposes and integrity of each paradigm.* If methods are used from different paradigms, then the researcher does not fully understand the purposes and philosophy of each paradigm. Currently, there are a host of serious problems with nurses using 'triangulation,' mixing both qualitative and quantitative methods and paradigms with limited rationale stated. As a consequence, much confusion prevails and such study results are very questionable and have limited credibility. It is possible, however, to do sequential qualitative or quantitative studies (or the reverse), but not simultaneously by merging methods and paradigms. For further guidance on the rationale and focus of the two paradigms and mixing methods, the reader is encouraged to read reliable and substantive articles on ethnomethods (Leininger, 1990a, pp. 40–51), and other writings by other qualitative experts (Guba, 1990; Lincoln & Guba, 1985; Reason & Rowan, 1981).

Informants: Key and General

Key and general informants are important in any ethnonursing research study. The ethnonurse researcher, however, does not have *samples*, *objects*, *subjects*, *cases*, and *populations* (Leininger, 1985b), but does work with key and general informants such as *individuals, families*, and *groups* of people in diverse contexts, institutions, or communities. Key and general informants become a major source for nurse researchers to learn about people and their cultural care, wellbeing, health, and general lifeways as influenced by a variety of factors.

Key informants are persons who have been thoughtfully and pur-posefully selected (often by people in the culture or subculture) to be most knowledgeable about the domain of inquiry of interest to nurse researchers. Key informants are held to reflect the norms, values, beliefs, and general lifeways of the culture, and are usually interested in and willing to participate in the study. In contrast, general informants usually are not as fully knowledgeable about the domain of inquiry, but do have general ideas about the domain, and are willing to share their ideas. After the researcher has involved key informants in several ses-sions, general informants are used to reflect on how similar or different their ideas are from key informants. Such information from key and general informants helps to identify the diversity or universality of ideas about human care and other nursing phenomenon.

During the past many decades of ethnonursing research, I have dis-covered that it requires from three to five informant sessions of approx-imately one to two hours to obtain indepth insights, full meanings, interpretations, and other data that are often embedded in diverse social structure factors and in different human care experiences (Leininger, 1989, 1990a). Since general informants provide reflective information and are not key informants less time is given to them. Ethnonursing studies in which the researcher spends limited time or only one or two sessions with key informants can result in unreliable and inaccurate data. As a result, the researcher does not get backstage or to the 'cultural secrets' of informants, and the findings may be ques-tionable. Key informants are the main source to check and recheck data collected as to its internal [*emic*] and external [*etic*] relevance, meanings, accuracy, and dependability because they [key informants] are the indepth source of information along with the researcher's direct observations and participant experiences.

When conducting a *maxi* or *macro ethnonursing* study, 12 to 15 key informants are needed or approximately twice the number of key informants to general informants. If a mini or macro ethnonursing study is being conducted (or one smaller in scope), the researcher needs 6 to 8 key and 12 to 16 general informants. A ratio of 1:2 is the general rule to follow for key to general informants with three to five sessions with the former and one session with the latter. These numbers of key and general informants have been established through many decades of research and in accord with other nurse researchers. We must remember, however, that large numbers of informants alone are not the rule; instead, the focus is on obtaining indepth knowledge to understand fully the phenomena under study (Leininger, 1985a, 1987; Lincoln & Guba, 1985). The use of large samples for qualitative studies generally leads to superficial knowledge, less credibility on interpretations and explanations, and limited insights about the why and how of particular care phenomena.

The ethnonursing method also requires that the nurse have appropriate language skills to communicate with people in the culture and to interpret ideas and written documents. The researcher must be able to cue in to what informants are talking about relative to the topic under discussion. This may require nurses to learn the language of a culture to study cultural care phenomena as language and culture are closely linked. Language becomes the means to understand meanings, patterns, and other emic or etic expressions and interpretations so critical to ethnonursing studies. Many different meanings, kinds, and patterns of care are often found in special language expressions that must be carefully written out with detailed interpretations. Ethnohistorical data about care, health, wellbeing, or illnesses also are expressed in special language statements over different time spans that the researcher must know how to explore with informants in written and spoken language. Most importantly, the nurse researcher needs to be aware of not imposing professional or personal language ideas on the data, or not interpreting the data using the researcher's linguistic expressions, professional viewpoints, or phrases. When this occurs, one can anticipate less accurate knowledge of culture care meanings from the people. In general, language skills with attention to the informants' ways of expression are essential to conduct a successful, accurate, and credible ethnonursing study.

Keeping a field journal with condensed and expanded notes with focus on the theory and the Sunrise components is essential to a comprehensive ethnonursing study (Leininger, 1985a/b, 1988, 1990a). The field (or clinical) journal offers the researcher the means to record data directly from the people in both condensed and expanded forms. The Sunrise Enabler serves as a comprehensive guide to the ethnonurse–researcher while recording grounded or raw field data and when checking on areas not fully explored. The Sunrise Enabler also serves as a cognitive map that covers the major components of the theory while collecting and analyzing the findings. The field journal covers data related to the worldview, social structure, ethnohistorical, environmental factors, folk, and professional features as areas to be explored as potential influencers of human care. The field journal remains the primary data source along with computer data processing of all field data. As discussed earlier, ethnonursing data can be collected and processed with the use of the Leininger–Templin–Thompson Ethnoscript Qualitative Software, or with other available computer software. However, the LTT was designed especially to code, classify, and process data bearing on Culture Care Theory.

Qualitative Criteria to Ethnonursing Research Studies

Since qualitative and quantitative paradigms have very different purposes, goals, and predicted outcomes, the nurse researcher must be knowledgeable about and use qualitative criteria for ethnonursing studies. Since the purpose of ethnonursing research studies is to discover the nature, essence, attributes, meanings, characteristics, and understandings of particular phenomena under study, use of qualitative criteria is imperative. The researcher is challenged to discover diversities and universalities in relation to the theory and the qualitative paradigm (Leininger, 1987, 1990a; Guba, 1990; Lincoln & Guba, 1985; Reason & Rowan, 1981). I have developed and used specific criteria for qualitative paradigmatic investigations as presented below (Leininger, 1970, 1978, 1989, 1990a).

1. *Credibility*—refers to the 'truth,' accuracy, or believability of findings that have been mutually established between the researcher and the informants as accurate, believable, and credible about their experiences and knowledge of phenomena. These truths, beliefs, and values (largely from *emic* findings) have been substantiated through the researcher's observations and with documentation of meanings-in-contexts, specific situations, or events. In addition, direct experiences of the researcher with the people over time and the people's interpretations or explanations are used to substantiate this criterion.

2. _Confirmability_—refers to the repeated direct and documented evidence largely from observed and primary informant source data, and with repeated explanations or interpretive data from informants about certain phenomena. _Confirmability_ means reaffirming what the researcher has heard, seen, or experienced with respect to the phenomena under study. It reflects evidence of the informants restating or reaffirming ideas or instances that have occurred over time in familiar and natural living contexts. Audit trails (Lincoln & Guba, 1985) or confirmed informant checks (Leininger, 1990a) with direct people feedback are ways to establish confirmability.

3. _Meaning-in-context_—refers to data that has become understandable with relevant referents or meanings to the informants or people studied in different or similar environments. Situations, instances, settings, and life events or experiences with meanings known to the people are evident. This criterion focuses on the significance of interpretations and understanding of the actions, symbols, events, communication, and other human activities within specific or total contexts in which something occurred or happened.

4. _Recurrent Patterning_—refers to repeated instances, sequences of events, experiences, or lifeways that tend to reoccur over a period of time in designated ways and contexts. Repeated experiences, expressions, events, or activities that reflect identifiable sequenced patterns of behavior over time are used to substantiate this criterion.

5. _Saturation_—refers to the 'taking in' of occurrences or meanings in a very full, comprehensive, and exhaustive way all information that could generally be known or understood about certain phenomena under study. _Saturation_ means that the researcher has conducted an exhaustive exploration of whatever is being studied, and there is no further data or insights forthcoming from informants or observed situations. There is a redundance of information in which the researcher gets the same (or similar) information, and the informants contend there is no more to offer as they have said or shared everything. Data reveals redundancies and duplication of content with similar ideas, meanings, experiences, descriptions, and other expressions from the informants or from repeated observations of some phenomena.

6. _Transferability_—refers to whether particular findings from a qualitative study can be transferred to another similar context or situation and still preserve the particularized meanings, interpretations, and inferences of the completed study. While the goal of

qualitative research is not intended to produce generalizations but to obtain indepth knowledge of a particular study, this criterion looks for any general similarities of findings under similar environmental conditions, contexts, or circumstances that one might make from the findings. It is the researcher's responsibility to establish if this criterion can be met in a new research context.

Currently, these six qualitative criteria can be studied more fully in other publications (Leininger, 1990a; Lincoln & Guba, 1985) but also in other nurse–research studies now available. It is of interest that Lincoln and Guba (pp. 290-338) used the criteria of transferability, credibility, dependability, and confirmability, but fail to identify the importance of meaning-in-context, saturation, and recurrent patterning. These later criteria are held to be extremely important to establish the soundness of most qualitative studies. It should be noted that the use of internal and external validity or reliability measurements are not appropriate, nor can they be used meaningfully with qualitative studies as the purposes and goals of the qualitative and quantitative paradigms are very different.

Summary

In this chapter, I have provided an overview of the ethnonursing research method within the qualitative paradigm to show how this method can be used to systematically study cultures using the Culture Care Theory. While it is possible that Culture Care Theory studies can be conducted using other qualitative or quantitative methods, I believe that the latter greatly limits obtaining indepth, complex, and embedded care phenomena. Instead, the ethnonursing method has been designed to achieve this goal and to explicate largely unknown and elusive aspects of human care from transcultural perspectives. Nursing phenomena such as care, wellbeing, healing, health, environmental contexts, and other undiscovered or vaguely discovered nursing phenomena remain a challenge to document fully in regard to their epistemic, ontological, and culturally relevant forms. Over the past many decades, I have made several revisions and refinements with the ethnonursing method, the Sunrise Enabler, and the theory to perfect it so as to explicate human care and related nursing phenomena. As a result, a new and different way of discovering, knowing, and interpreting humanistic and scientific care is available. Humanistic and scientific dimensions of care are being established with research findings largely with the use of the ethnonursing research method and other methods within the qualitative paradigm. Unquestionably, the ethnonursing method has become one of the most rigorous and relevant ways to discover human care and many other untapped nursing phenomena. As the only known research method linked to a nursing theory, its use is important to discover care findings to improve people care transculturally. It is the method that is helping to establish epistemic and ontologic nursing knowledge for the discipline and profession of nursing.

References

Berreman, G. (1962). *Behind many masks*. Ithaca, NY: Society for Applied Anthropology.

Boas, F. (1924). The methods of ethnology. *American Anthropologist, 22*, 311–321.

Carter, M. (1985). The philosophical dimensions of qualitative nursing science research (pp. 27–32). In M. M. Leininger (Ed.), *Qualitative research methods in nursing*. Orlando, FL: Grune & Stratton.

Erikson, E. (1963). *Childhood and society* (2nd ed.). Toronto: W.W. Norton.

Glaser, B. G., & Strauss, A. L. (1967). *The discovery of grounded theories: Strategies for qualitative research*. Chicago: Aldine.

Guba, E. (1990). *The paradigm dialog*. Newbury Park, CA: Sage.

Heron, J. (1981). Philosophical basis for a new paradigm. In P. Reason and J. Rowan, (Eds.), *Human inquiry: A sourcebook of new paradigm research*. New York: John Wiley & Sons.

Leininger, M. M. (1966). Convergence and divergence of human behavior: An ethnopsychological comparative study of two Gadsup villages in the Eastern Highlands of New Guinea. Unpublished doctoral dissertation, University of Washington, Seattle.

Leininger, M. M. (1967). The Culture concept and its relevance to nursing. *Journal of Nursing Education, 6*(2), 27–39.

Leininger, M. M. (1969). Nature of science in nursing. Conference on the nature of science in nursing. *Nursing Research, 18*(5), 388–389.

Leininger, M. M. (1970). *Nursing and anthropology: Two worlds to blend*. New York: John Wiley & Sons.

Leininger, M. M. (1976). Caring: The essence and central focus of nursing. American Nurses Foundation, *Nursing Research Report, 12*(1), 2, 14.

Leininger, M. M. (1978). *Transcultural nursing: Concepts, theories, and practices*. New York: John Wiley & Sons.

Leininger, M. M. (1980). Care: A central focus of nursing and health care services. *Nursing and Health Care*, 135–143.

Leininger, M. M. (1981). *Care: An essential human need*. Detroit: Wayne State University Press.

Leininger, M. M. (1984). *Care: The essence of nursing and health*. Detroit, MI: Wayne State University Press.

Leininger, M. M. (1985a). *Qualitative research methods in nursing*. Orlando, FL: Grune & Stratton.

Leininger, M. M. (1985b). Ethnography and ethnonursing: Models and modes of qualitative data analysis. In *Qualitative research methods in nursing* (pp. 33–72). Orlando, FL: Grune & Stratton.

Leininger, M. M. (1985c). Life health care history: Purposes, methods and techniques. In *Qualitative research methods in nursing* (pp. 119–132). Orlando, FL: Grune & Stratton.

Leininger, M. M. (1987). Importance and uses of ethnomethods: Ethnography and ethnonursing research. In M. Cahoon (Ed.), *Recent advances in nursing* (pp. 17, 23–25). London: Churchill Livingston.

Leininger, M. M. (1988). *Care: Discovery and uses in clinical and community nursing*. Detroit, MI: Wayne State University Press.

Leininger, M. M. (1989). Ethnonursing: A research method to generate nursing knowledge. Unpublished paper of the *Proceedings of Qualitative Summer Research Conferences*. Detroit, MI: Wayne State University.

Leininger, M. M. (1990a). Ethnomethods: The philosophic and epistemic basis to explicate transcultural nursing knowledge. *Journal of Transcultural Nursing, 1*(2), 40–51.

Leininger, M. M. (1990b). Leininger–Templin–Thompson ethnoscript qualitative software program: *User's Handbook*. Detroit, MI: Wayne State University.

Leininger, M. M. (1991, Winter). Leininger's acculturation health care assessment tool for cultural patterns in traditional and non-traditional lifeways. *Journal of Transcultural Nursing, 2*(2).

Lincoln, Y. & Guba, G. (1985). *Naturalistic inquiry*. Beverly Hills, CA: Sage.

Luna, L. (1989). *Care and cultural context of Lebanese Muslims in an urban community: An ethnographic and ethnonursing study conceptualited within Leininger's theory*. Unpublished dissertation. Detroit, MI: Wayne State University.

Malinowski, B. (1922). *Argonauts of the western pacific*. New York: E.P. Dutton.

Pike, K. (1954). *Language in relation to a unified theory of the structure of human behavior*. Glendale, CA: Summer Institute of Linguistics.

Polit, D., & Hungler, B. (1983). *Nursing research: Principles and methods*. Philadelphia: J.B. Lippincott.

Reason, P., & Rowan, J. (1981). *Human Inquiry: A sourcebook of new paradigm research*. New York: John Wiley & Sons.

Spradley, J, (1979). *Ethnographic interview*. New York: Holt, Rinehart and Winston.

Spradley, J. (1980). *Participant observation*. New York: Holt, Rinehart and Winston.

Watson. J, (1985). Reflections on different methodologies for the future of nursing. In M. M. Leininger (Ed.), *Qualitative research methods in nursing* (pp. 343–351). Orlando, FL: Grune & Stratton.

Wenger, A. F., (1985). Learning to do a mini ethnonursing research study: A doctoral student's experience. In M. M. Leininger (Ed.) *Qualitative research methods in nursing* (pp. 283–316). Orlando, FL: Grune & Stratton.

Some Key Updated References

Leininger, M. (1995) *Transcultural nursing: Concepts, theories, research and practices* (2nd Edition) Columbus, OH: McGraw Hill College Custom Series.

Leininger, M. (1997) Overview and reflection of the theory of culture care and the ethnonursing research method. *Journal of Transcultural Nursing, 8*(2) pp. 32–51.

Leininger, M. and M. McFarland (2002). *Transcultural nursing, Concepts, theories, research, and practices* (Third Edition). New York: McGraw Hill.

CHAPTER THREE

The Globalization of Transcultural Nursing Theory and Research

Margaret Andrews, RN, PhD, CTN, FAAN

> *The next century will be known as the Era of Globalization, in which nurses will fully realize that the profession must be viewed as one world with many diverse cultures linked together with some common professional interest, knowledge, and goals....The world will continue to be intensely multicultural and many health professionals will scurry to learn about different cultures and to function in culturally responsible and effective ways (Leininger, 1995, p. 681).*

The purpose of this chapter is to discuss applications of transcultural nursing research and theory by transcultural nursing (TCN) experts studying transnationally. Dr. Leininger conducted the first transnational study in the Eastern Highlands of New Guinea. Since then, *transcultural nursing* theory and research have gradually spread worldwide. Much of the early transcultural nursing research by Dr. Leininger and her followers used her ethnonursing research method with cultures and subcultures in the United States and elsewhere in the world. The theory of *Culture Care Diversity and Universality* spread throughout the United States, to Canada, Australia, Europe, Asia, and other parts of the world where it was embraced by many nurse scholars. Those nurses with formal academic preparation in TCN have used the theory of *Culture Care Diversity and Universality* in lectures, research, consultation, and practice. Their ideas spread transnationally. As transcultural nursing has spread to other countries, and TCN research, practice, and education have also extended, books on diverse cultures and subcultures became meaningful. Indeed, Leininger's theory of *Culture Care Diversity and Universality* has been one of the major nursing and health theories to be used in many countries worldwide.

Leininger promoted transcultural nursing as global nursing and as the arching framework for *all* areas of nursing (Leininger, 1969, 1978, 1990, 1995; Leininger & McFarland, 2002), clarifying that transcultural nursing is "...not the same as international nursing because *inter* (Latin prefix) refers to 'between some thing or place'; whereas transcultural nursing has been viewed as a much broader concept in scope and purpose because it cuts across many cultures with a comparative perspective" (1995, p. 26). Rather than using the term *international nursing*, Leininger (1970) encouraged nurses to use *transnational nursing* because the prefix *trans* means across, and she contends that when nurses engage in activities in other nations, the term *transnational nursing* more accurately describes those activities and interactions. *Transnational* nursing has become the caring discipline of many cultures as it provides a broader perspective to complex interconnections such as politics, economics, values, health, nursing, and other dimensions which together influence care outcomes.

To arrive at transnational nursing practice, education, research, and consultation, a global perspective is essential. Leininger's (1991) theory of *Culture Care Diversity and Universality* and the use of the *Sunrise Enabler* provide rich and new knowledge in nursing. For example, nursing and health care are influenced by many of the factors presented by Leininger (1970, 1991; Leininger & McFarland, 2002) such as global economics, geopolitics, world philosophies and religions, and electronic communication technologies. The click of a computer mouse can bring together people on opposite ends of the planet, enabling educational institutions worldwide to provide students and faculty with increasing opportunities for cultural study. These few examples illustrate the transnational relevance of Leininger's theory and the *Sunrise Enabler* as transnational global imperatives for the present and the future.

Transcultural nursing has become a formal area of study and practice of great importance, with emphasis on the worldwide nature of its scope as stated by Leininger, "...the field explicitly includes all cultures and subcultures in the world" (1995, p. 22). Dr. Leininger envisioned the global scope of transcultural nursing from its inception because she recognized that nurses would be expected to serve people in all parts of the world. This was a major and new development in nursing that began with Leininger's work in the 1960s. She emphasized study of cultural similarities and differences as nurses traveled, worked, and studied in various parts of the world. A theory and a method were needed to explain such differences. Advances in contemporary communication and transportation technologies had already brought nurses and other members of society into a world that increasingly had become globally interconnected and interdependent. It was no longer possible to remain isolated from the influences of other people, other cultures, or other countries. Most importantly, Leininger stated that "...The scope of transcultural nursing goes beyond local, regional, and national views to that of worldwide nursing or the global view of nursing" (1995, p. 22). This global view has been challenging and continues to be studied by transcultural nurses.

With increasing frequency, nurses and nursing students have opportunities for transnational experiences in a variety of clinical settings and specialties. Never before in human history has there been a greater need for nurses to have formal preparation in transcultural nursing and for transcultural nurse specialists to help nurses deal with complex global issues and to provide culturally congruent nursing care around the world.

Historical Perspectives on Transnational Nursing

Leininger conducted the first *transcultural nursing* study with the Gadsup of the Eastern Highlands of New Guinea using her theory and the qualitative *ethnonursing research method* (Leininger, 1970, 1978, 1985, 1995; Leininger & McFarland, 2002). Leininger chose a nonWestern culture because she wanted to learn about people who had limited contact with Western cultures. She also wanted to systematically examine her theory of *Culture Care Diversity and Universality* in a nonWestern culture to see if the major tenets of the theory could be upheld (Leininger, 1995). From its inception in the 1950s, during the subsequent theory development phase in the 1960s, and from her research, Leininger envisioned nursing as transcultural and global in nature and scope. It has now become the new paradigm focus in nursing.

Leininger (1995) has identified three historical periods or eras in the development of transcultural nursing. During the *First Era* (1955 to 1975), *the field of transcultural nursing* (TCN) was established for the advancement of nursing knowledge and practices. Leininger (1991) recognized the relationships between nursing and anthropology, but kept a focus on nursing and the benefits of her theory. In the 1960s, Dr. Leininger conceptualized transcultural nursing a formal area of study and practice that she called *transcultural nursing*. In the early part of this era, it was imperative to develop transcultural nursing knowledge with specific concepts, principles, and potential practices. From the early 1960s to the present day, Leininger and other transcultural nurse scholars have conducted *ethnocare* studies of Western and nonWestern cultures. Leininger's position on *care* as the essence of nursing in cultures and subcultures globally became a hallmark of her research and theory (Leininger, 1984), which is continued by many nurse scholars today. By 1975, through the theory of *Culture Care Diversity and Universality* (and the use of the *Sunrise Enabler*), *care* phenomena became of general interest to many nurses in the United States, Canada, and many other places in the world.

Leininger has identified 1975 to 1983 as the *Second Era: Program and Research Expansion* in Transcultural Nursing. A growing number of nurses became interested in the valuable contribution of transcultural nursing around the world. Nurses reading about transcultural nursing in the United States and elsewhere believed that such knowledge was essential and would help them to better understand cultural similarities and differences especially as they traveled, studied, taught, and consulted in other nations. Leininger (1995) reported that many nurses who were working in Saudi Arabia, India, Africa, and other parts of the world had a new and futuristic perspective for nursing, education, and practice, and found the study of transcultural nursing meaningful and necessary.

Canadian and Australian nurses became interested in transcultural nursing through workshops, conferences, and publications sponsored mainly by the Transcultural Nursing Society. Nurses from Brazil, China, Japan, Korea, Sweden, Denmark, and the Netherlands came to the United States to study transcultural nursing with leaders in the field and to learn ways to develop educational and clinical programs congruent with the cultures in their homelands; they returned to initiate transcultural nursing in their nursing curricula. During the Second Era in Transcultural Nursing, there was considerable growth and progress in establishing transcultural nursing education, research, practice, and consultation throughout the United States, but significant inroads were also being made in other nations. The global nature of transcultural nursing became meaningful to many nurses.

Leininger (1995) has identified the *Third Era: Establishing Transcultural Nursing Worldwide* (1983 to present) as the period during which the global agenda of transcultural nursing was the primary focus. During the past two decades increasing numbers of nurses have been traveling and working in different countries and interacting with people from many different cultures electronically and face to face. They were eager to use transcultural nursing concepts, principles, and appropriate research findings in their work, and many nurses studied courses in transcultural nursing.

In the late 1980s the Transcultural Nursing Society responded to the growing interest of nurses around the world in transcultural nursing by holding its first annual conference outside the United States, first in Canada in 1988 and then in the Netherlands in 1989. These conferences attracted nurses from within the host nations but also worldwide. Transcultural nurse leaders have continued to expand their linkages with nurses worldwide and have collaborated in the areas of education, clinical practice, research, and consultation in nations on six continents. They also have been involved in developing transcultural nursing policies with selected cultural groups since 1984 to facilitate transcultural exchanges, research, and practice. As a result, the number of requests for expert consultations also increased (Andrews, 1985, 1986; Bisch, 1983).

During the Third Era, Dr. Leininger established the *Journal of Transcultural Nursing* as the official publication of the Transcultural Nursing Society. The purpose of this publication was to share scholarly work among transcultural nurses and others with an interest and to disseminate transcultural nursing knowledge. In recent years the focus of the articles in this journal has increasingly reflected the transnational expansion of transcultural nursing. For example, a growing number of nurses from various countries around the world have been publishing in the *Journal of Transcultural Nursing*, the *Journal of Multicultural Nursing & Health*, the *Journal of Cultural Diversity*, and other journals. The focus of these publications was frequently of a transcultural and global nature—reporting research findings, describing contemporary issues and trends in education, research, and practice in their nation or between their nation and other countries—thus, transnational comparative analyses contributed to transcultural nursing. Similarly, the editorial board for the *Journal of Transcultural Nursing* was comprised of representatives from diverse locations around the world.

Lastly, there has been an increase in the number of transcultural nursing workshops and conferences being held worldwide. Dr. Leininger has presented at numerous workshops, conferences, and symposia in transglobal locations since 1975; other TCN experts have also lectured extensively throughout the world. In 2004 the annual Transcultural Nursing Society conference was held in Spain; previous regional and national conferences have been held in Australia, Canada, Asia and the Pacific Rim, South America, Africa, the Near and Middle East, Europe, as well as the United States. With the fast paced advances in contemporary communication technologies and the speed with which travelers can go from one end of the globe to the other, opportunities for transcultural collaboration among nurses and health care providers from other disciplines steadily increases each year. Worldwide transcultural nursing has become truly global in focus, interest, and practice.

Transnational Nursing: Regional Updates

Leininger (1991) holds that *care* is the central and unifying domain that comprises the essence of nursing globally. She also has stated that care and caring are not universal. Most importantly, nurses need to be aware of the manner in which care is conceptualized, constructed, and practiced across cultures and within different cultures of the world (Kanitsaki, 2003l; Leininger, 1978, 1995; Leininger & McFarland, 2002). With the Theory of Culture Care Diversity and Universality and other pioneering work in transcultural nursing, Leininger has created space for nurses to "...speak, engage, debate, contemplate, deliberate, develop, and grow as they raise awareness of cultural care as a legitimate area of study and authentic area of practice" (Daly, Speedy, & Jackson, 2000, p. xiv). Leininger's focus on discovering what is universal about care amid diversity has been a major breakthrough for the advancement of transcultural nursing *but also for* nursing as a discipline.

In the remainder of this chapter, the author examines transcultural nursing advances in various regions of the world, with special emphasis on theory, research, and scholarship that has advanced transcultural nursing knowledge in clinical practice, policy development, education, consultation, administration, and in promoting inter- and multidisciplinary collaboration.

Advances in Transcultural Nursing: Australia and New Zealand

Since her initial visit to Australia in 1960, Leininger has made 15 trips to this nation and has mentored many Australian nurses (Omeri, 2003a/b). During the 26th Annual Transcultural Nursing Research Conference in 2000, Dr. Leininger was awarded the Life Fellowship and Distinguished Visiting Scholar's Award by the Royal College of Nursing, Australia—the first time the award was bestowed upon anyone outside of Australia. The October 2003 issue of *Contemporary Nurses* was dedicated to Leininger in recognition of her pioneering work and consultation with Australian nurses in supporting and promoting transcultural nursing education, research, and practice (Omeri, 2003a/b). During the past 25 years, Australian nurses have learned, taught, and conducted research in transcultural nursing, which has been a noteworthy achievement.

According to the Australian Bureau of Statistics (2001), out of Australia's population of 19 million, 4 million (21.9%) were born overseas, and 417,000 (2.2%) are indigenous in origin (Australian Aborigines and Terres Strait Islanders). These statistics reflect the growing diversity that characterizes Australia. This diversity and its associated issues are the underlying reasons for the commitment of many nurses and professional nursing organizations in Australia to the study and advancement of transcultural nursing.

Leininger's work became visible in Australia in the mid 1980s and marked the beginning of unprecedented scholarship in transcultural nursing in the country. Many scholars have promoted and contributed to the expansion of transcultural nursing in Australia; among them are Kanitsaki (1988, 1989), Idrus (1988), Omeri (2003a/b), and Omeri & Cameron-Traub (1996). In addition, influential nursing organizations such as the Royal College of Nursing, Australia (RCNA), the Australian Nursing Federations (ANF), and the Australian Council of Nursing (ANC) have all recognized the importance of culturally congruent nursing care and have developed standards and guidelines aimed at enhancing cultural competence and cultural congruence. According to Kanitsaki (2003, pp. vii–viii), the development of transcultural nursing in Australia and elsewhere in the world is a "...testimony to the futuristic and moral thinking of an ever increasing number of nurse researchers, theorists, ethicists, and social scholars who have dedicated attention to questioning the cultural assumptions underpinning nursing and its care practices." The author would like to state that transcultural nursing not only had a global impact but also gave new hope to the scientific and practice *world* of nursing.

Nurses from Australia and New Zealand have contributed to the advancement of transcultural nursing in a wide variety of areas—including better understanding of the impact of globalization, migration, colonization, social inequity, and technology on health care, health management, and health behavior of indigenous people, immigrants, ethnic groups, and multicultural societies.

The entire October 2003 issue of *Contemporary Nurse* was dedicated to Leininger's work and to advances in contemporary transcultural nursing viewed from an Australian perspective and highlighted the contributions made by Australian nurse scholars in advancing transcultural nursing practice, education, and research. The issue is divided into four sections: Globalization: Nursing Education, Research and Clinical Practice; Culture and Health (including issues affecting Aboriginal Peoples); Cardiovascular Health; and Mental Health. The issue had a compelling epilogue which addressed culture, health, and social justice, and the role of nurses in advocating for social justice for the groups and communities for whom they provide care (Jackson, 2003). It carried a global message to show ways transcultural nursing has been changing the practice of nursing by providing new ideas and practices.

Advances in Transcultural Nursing: Asia

In recent years there has been a marked increase in the numbers of Asian nurses coming to the United States to study transcultural nursing. After completing their coursework, many of these individuals return to their homelands to conduct research using Leininger's *Theory of Culture Care Diversity and Universality* and to introduce transcultural nursing into clinical practice and education. Dr. Leininger and transcultural nursing colleagues have made numerous visits to Asian nations where they have been invited to speak, consult, teach, and engage in collaborative research with Asian counterparts.

Summarized in Table 3-1 are eight articles focusing on advances in transcultural nursing in South Korea, Japan, Thailand, the People's Republic of China, and Taiwan that have appeared recently in the *Journal of Transcultural Nursing*. These articles include information about people across the life span. For example, there was a transnational comparison of cultural and technical differences in perinatal care between the United States and China (Liu & Moore, 2000); reports of research on cultural influences on symptoms experienced by South Korean women during menopausal transition (Im, 2003); a study of factors affecting maternal role attainment by HIV-positive mothers in Thailand (Jirapaet, 2001); a study of Thai elders to determine the relationship of daily living practice and perceived life satisfaction (Othaganont, Sinthuvorakan, & Jensupakarn, 2002); a study of Taiwanese who have attempted suicide (Wen-Chii, 2001); and a study of the culture bound syndrome Hwa-Byung that is prevalent among Korean women (Park, Kim, Kang, & Kim, 2001). Lambert, Lambert, Daly, Davidson, Kunaviktikul, and Shin (2004) provided a transnational comparison of women's health content in the nursing curricula in educational programs in Japan, South Korea, Thailand, and Australia. Lastly, Iwata (2003) presented a concept analysis of the father's role from a Japanese perspective. Iwata's findings will assist in future instrument development and will stimulate transnational nursing theory development and research in the important area of gender roles. Horn's (1975) early work on prenatal care of children transculturally was an important study to show the potential of global transcultural nursing in addition to Leininger's research from the 1950s and 1960s in New Guinea.

Advances in Transcultural Nursing: The Near and Middle East

Never in recorded history has the need for knowledge of Near and Middle Eastern cultures been more important and urgent. There has often been a strong interconnection between culture and religion in many Near and Middle Eastern nations. Although not everyone residing

TABLE 3-1 Articles Published in the *Journal of Transcultural Nursing* (2000 to Present) with a Transnational Focus

Author(s)/Date	Country and/or Cultural Group	Type of Article	Remarks
Australia and New Zealand			
Goold (2001)	Australia Aborigines Torres Strait Islanders	Commentary	Author provides an overview of the two groups that comprise Australia's Indigenous peoples: the Aborigines and the Torres Strait Islanders and provides guidelines for working with Indigenous peoples.
Lambert, Lambert, Daly, Davidson, Kunaviktikul, & Shin (2004)	Australia, Japan, South Korea & Thailand	General article on nursing education	Transnational comparison of nursing curricula and women's health care content.
Spence (2001)	New Zealand nurses	Research	A hermeneutic study of N = 17 New Zealand nurses was conducted to explore the experience of nursing people from cultures other than one's own with emphasis on the notions of prejudice, paradox, and possibility.
Wepa (2003)	New Zealand	Research	Study of the experiences of four cultural safety educators in New Zealand using action research methods, primarily reflective diaries.
Asia			
Im (2003)	South Korea United States	Research	Study of the cultural influences on symptoms experienced during menopausal transition by women in South Korea and Korean immigrant women in the US.

(Continues)

TABLE 3-1 Articles Published in the *Journal of Transcultural Nursing* (2000 to Present) with a Transnational Focus *(Continued)*

Author(s)/Date	Country and/or Cultural Group	Type of Article	Remarks
Iwata (2003)	Japan	Concept analysis	Concept analysis of the father's role presented from a Japanese perspective
Jirapaet (2001)	Thailand	Research	Phenomenological study of N = 39 low-income, Thai, HIV-positive mothers selected for their successful adaptation to the diagnosis. Purpose: to explore factors affecting maternal role attainment during infancy among HIV-positive mothers of low-income status in Thailand.
Lambert, Lambert, Daly, Davidson, Kunaviktikul, & Shin (2004)	Australia, Japan, South Korea & Thailand	General article on nursing education	Transnational comparison of nursing curricula and women's health care content.
Liu & Moore (2000)	China United States	General article	Authors compare cultural and technical differences in perinatal care in the United States and People's Republic of China.
Othaganont, Sinthuvorakan, & Jensupakarn (2002)	Thailand	Research	Study of 73 matched pairs of Thai elders to determine the relationship of daily living practice and perceived life satisfaction or dissatisfaction.
Park, Kim, Kang, & Kim (2001)	Korea	Research	Study of 2,807 Korean women ages 41–65 years to determine the prevalence of the culture-bound syndrome, Hwa-Byung, associated symptoms, sociodemographic factors and life style factors that contribute to it.

Author(s)/Date	Country and/or Cultural Group	Type of Article	Remarks
Wen-Chii (2001)	Taiwan	Research	Phenomenological study of N = 10 Taiwanese patients ages 20–52 years after they attempted suicide. Purpose: to determine the experiences and feelings of Taiwanese patients who have attempted suicide.
Near and Middle East			
Al-Shahri (2002)	Saudi Arabia	General article on clinical practice	A Saudi health professional describes selected cultural health beliefs & practices for the purpose of educating non-Saudi health care providers recruited from around the world to work in the Saudi Arabian health system.
Fooladi (2003)	Iranian nursing students and faculty	Research	Ethnographic study of 6 nursing faculty and 5 nursing students regarding gender in nursing education and practice in Iran.
Gharaibeh & Abu-Saad (2002)	Jordanian children	Research	Study to examine the cultural validity, reliability and preference by N = 95 Jordanian children concerning three pain assessment tools. Jordanian and Dutch university affiliation held by co-investigators.
Hattar-Pollara, Meleis, & Nagib (2003)	Egyptian women	Research	Study of role stress and patterns of coping for N = 190 Egyptian women in clerical jobs
Miller & Petro-Nustas (2002)	Jordanian women	Research	Ethnonursing, observation-participation & interview data were gathered from 15 women in two cities and three villages in Jordan to document, describe, and analyze diverse and universal care patterns for Jordanian women. US-Jordanian co-investigators.

(Continues)

TABLE 3-1 Articles Published in the *Journal of Transcultural Nursing* (2000 to Present) with a Transnational Focus *(Continued)*

Author(s)/Date	Country and/or Cultural Group	Type of Article	Remarks
Petro-Nustas (2001)	Jordanian women	Research	Descriptive correlational study of N = 76 Jordanian women to assess beliefs and identifying factors that contribute to their utilization of mammography.
Petro-Nustas, Kulwicki, & Zumout (2002)	Jordanian and U.S. nursing students	Research	An exploratory, comparative study to assess and compare US and Jordanian nursing students' knowledge, attitudes, and beliefs about AIDS and HIV/AIDS prevention.
Europe			
Davies, Deeny, & Raikkonen (2003)	Ireland, Finland, United Kingdom, Sweden, Spain, Italy, & other European nations	General article on nursing education	Description of the development and implementation of the world's first and only Master of Science (MSc) in disaster relief nursing program by cooperating partners in European countries.
Friedemann, Astedt-Kurki, & Paavilainen (2003)	Finland United States	Research	Study of the challenges associated with the transfer of a family assessment instrument developed in the United States, the Assessment of Strategies in Families-Effectiveness (ASF-E), and its theoretical basis when used in Finland.
Gebru & Willman, 2003	Sweden	Research-based didactic model for education in TCN	Model using Leininger's Theory was developed to facilitate culturally congruent care by Swedish nursing students and nurses.
Higginbottom (2000)	United Kingdom	General article on clinical practice	Author examines the breast-feeding experiences of women of African descent residing in the United Kingdom.

Author(s)/Date	Country and/or Cultural Group	Type of Article	Remarks
van den Brink, Y. (2003)	The Netherlands	Research	Ethnographic study on diversity and universality in care values and meanings of Turkish lay care givers and Dutch professional nurses caring for Turkish elders in Rotterdam
Watt, Law, Ots, & Waago (2002)	14 European countries	General article on nursing education	Description of the development and implementation of a 4-week European Nursing Module involving international student exchanges by 26 colleges in 14 European nations for the purpose of developing cultural competence in European nursing students.
Africa			
Fongwa (2002)	Cameroon	General article on the health care system	Description of the health care system in Cameroon and recommendations for quality improvement through international assistance and collaboration with more developed countries.
Lothe & Heggen (2003)	Ethiopia	Research	Participant observations and in-depth interviews at an orphanage in Addis Ababa with 8 survivors of the 1984–85 Ethiopian famine. Study focused on resilience related to childhood experiences during the famine.
Mill (2003)	Ghana	Research	In-depth interviews and focus groups with 31 HIV-positive women, 5 HIV-positive men, 8 nurses, 10 professionals, and 2 traditional healers. Two-fold purpose of study: 1) examine the experience of HIV-positive Ghanaian women; and 2) identify factors that influenced their vulnerability to infection. Participatory action research by a Canadian investigator.

(Continues)

TABLE 3-1   Articles Published in the *Journal of Transcultural Nursing* (2000 to Present) with a Transnational Focus *(Continued)*

Author(s)/Date	Country and/or Cultural Group	Type of Article	Remarks
Moon, Khumalo-Sakutukwa, Mbizvo, & Padian (2002)	Zimbabwe	Research	Study of N = 48 informants to assess the acceptability of vaginal microbicides to prevent heterosexually transmitted HIV.
Savage (2002)	Tanzania	Case Study	A case study of a member of the Chagga tribe is presented to identify guidelines for the provision of culturally congruent nursing care.
Smith, Garbharran, Edwards, & O'Hara-Murdock (2004)	South Africa	Research	Study of N = 300 heads of household to identify educational needs of African Zulu and Xhosa women concerning sanitation, hygiene and health. Multistep approach using quantitative and qualitative methods. US funding used for this joint US–South African project.
Tabi & Mukherjee (2003)	Ghana United States	Description of study abroad program	Description of a 6-credit hour, 6-week summer study abroad program hosted by University of Cape Coast (Ghana) for Georgia Southern University undergraduate and graduate students in nursing and health-related disciplines.
Central and South America			
Cesarman-Maus (2003)	Mexico	General article	Description of the Mexican Communities Abroad offices located throughout the United States and operated jointly by the Mexican government and a group of Mexicans living in the US. These offices represent an ideal site for outreach for both Mexican and US-based organizations interested in the health and wellbeing of Mexican migrants working in the US.

Author(s)/Date	Country and/or Cultural Group	Type of Article	Remarks
de la Cuesta (2001)	Colombia	Research	Grounded theory study of N = 21 Colombian adolescents regarding their perceptions of romantic love and the gender rules that guide young women's behavior.
Hoga, Alcantara, & de Lima (2001)	Brazil	Research	Ethnonursing study of 15 men ages 21–64 living in a low-income community. Purpose: to explore men's involvement in reproductive health. Leininger's culture care modes were used to explain culturally meaningful nursing care actions.
Holt & Reeves (2001)	Dominican Republic	Research	Ethnonursing study with N = 45 informants. Purpose: to explore the meaning of hope and generic care practices to nurture hope among people from a rural village in the Dominican Republic.
Kraatz (2001)	Brazil	Research	Ethnographic study of N = 10 key informants conducted for the purpose of describing the understanding of health and illness by women living in a *favela* (urban slum) in southeastern Brazil.
Purnell (2001)	Guatemala	Research	Descriptive study of N = 51 Guatemalans to examine their practices of health promotion and wellness, disease and illness prevention, and the meaning of respect.
Riner & Becklenberg (2001)	Nicaragua United States	General article on nursing education	Description of the development of a service learning course at Indiana University School of Nursing based on a sister cities' partnership between Bloomington, Indiana and Posoltega, Nicaragua.

(Continues)

TABLE 3-1 Articles Published in the *Journal of Transcultural Nursing* (2000 to Present) with a Transnational Focus *(Continued)*

Author(s)/Date	Country and/or Cultural Group	Type of Article	Remarks
Canada			
Labun (2002)	Native Canadians	General article on nursing education	Description of a program successful in assisting "Native Canadians and other disenfranchised students" to succeed academically in a baccalaureate nursing program.
Majumdar, Chamters, & Roberts (2004)	Canadian Aboriginals	Research	HIV/AIDS prevention among Aboriginal youth using a train-the-trainer educational program as an intervention
Globalization and Professional Nursing Organizations			
Pacquiao (2003a)	Globalization and the Transcultural Nursing Society (TNGS)	*JTN*—Editorial	TCNS President's Message concerning the organization's responsiveness to global challenges
Pacquiao (2003b)	Globalization and the Transcultural Nursing Society (TCNS)	*JTN*—Editorial	TCNS President's Message concerning connectedness and global influence in TCN
Purnell (2000)	Global Institute for Nursing and Health	*JTN*—International Department	Summary of the Global Institute for Nursing and Health's second annual meeting in Eskilstuna, Sweden.
Zoucha (2002)	Global Society	*JTN*—Editorial	TCNS President's Message concerning the need for global understanding and the need to address issues of racism, oppression, violence, and hatred in order to promote a safer and more secure world.

in this region of the world is Muslim, followers of Sunni or Shi'a Islam comprise the majority of the population in most nations (with the exception of Israel which is a Jewish state). It should be noted that several million Christian Arabs reside in these regions of the world, including the Maronites of Lebanon, the Chaldeans of Iraq, and Orthodox Christians in Israel.

The term *Arab* refers to people who reside in the area extending from Morocco to the Arabian Gulf, speak Arabic, and self-identify with the Arabic culture and history. Caring for Arabs—and others whose heritage is Near or Middle Eastern—poses a challenge to many nurses because Western awareness about their complex cultural beliefs, values, and lifeways has just begun to develop (Leininger, 1995; Leininger & McFarland, 2002; Luna, 1989, 1994). Kendall's (1992) research of mother and infant care in an Iranian village in the 1970s was the earliest transcultural nursing research in the Middle East.

Summarized in Table 3-1 are seven recent articles from the *Journal of Transcultural Nursing* focusing on advances in transcultural nursing in Saudi Arabia, Iran, Egypt, and Jordan. An influential nation in the Arabic and Islamic worlds, Saudi Arabia has a population of 21 million and employs more than 90,000 physicians and nurses to care for its citizens. Eighty percent of physicians and nurses come from the United States, the Philippines, and other nations; thus, the Saudi Arabian health care system is staffed primarily by non-Saudis. To foster the provision of culturally congruent care for Saudis by non-Saudi health professionals, Al-Shahri (2002) presented an overview of the Saudi culture and subcultures and health related Islamic beliefs and practices such as cleanliness, modesty, and gender specific needs to be considered when caring for Saudi Arabian clients and their families. Luna's (1998) culture care studies of the Arab culture have led the way to understanding Arab gender differences related to nursing care (Luna, 1989, 1995).

Fooladi (2003) reported the findings of an ethnographic study of Iranian nursing students and faculty concerning gender in nursing education and practice in this nation. This study underscored the cultural significance of gender issues in nursing education and practice in the Islamic Republic of Iran and raised awareness of the need for transnational knowledge about gender. Three other studies focused on gender and women. Petro-Nustas (2001) conducted a descriptive correlational study of Jordanian women to assess beliefs and identifying factors that contribute to their use of mammography to screen for breast cancer. Miller & Petro-Nustas (2002) studied Jordanian women residing in urban and rural settings to document, describe, and analyze diverse and universal care patterns among women. Noting that women are increasingly becoming significant contributors to the Egyptian workforce,

Hattar-Pollara, Meleis, & Nagib (2003) studied role stress and coping of Egyptian women employed in low paying clerical jobs. The investigators found that there was an interconnectedness among all women's maternal, marital, and relational roles when describing their stress, satisfaction, and coping; that much of their perceived stress and coping patterns were imbedded in and confined to their traditionally defined gender roles; and, that women coped through learning to be self reliant and using cognitive and emotion focused coping approaches such as problem solving negotiation with spouses and shielding of emotion and-or distancing oneself from conflicts.

Gharaibeh and Abu-Saad (2002) examined the cultural validity and reliability of three pain assessment instruments on Jordanian children—the Poker Chip, the Faces, and the Word Description Scales—tools that are used to evaluate pain intensity. Although all three instruments were found to be valid and reliable measures of pain intensity among Jordanian Muslim children ages 3 to 14 years, the investigators found that there were both cultural and gender differences in relation to scale preferences by the children in the study. Girls preferred the Poker Chip Tool whereas boys preferred the Faces Scale, a finding the investigators attributed to the socialization process within the Arab culture.

Lastly, Petro-Nustas, Kulwicki, and Zumout (2002) conducted an exploratory, comparative study of US and Jordanian nursing students' knowledge, attitudes, and beliefs about AIDS and HIV/AIDS prevention. The results indicated that the US students' responses related to knowledge of HIV/AIDS were significantly greater and their attitudes toward AIDS were more positive than their Jordanian counterparts. More US students approved of the use of condoms in preventing the spread of HIV/AIDS than Jordanian students.

Advances in Transcultural Nursing: Europe

As indicated in Table 3-1, there were five recent articles from the *Journal of Transcultural Nursing* focusing on advances in transcultural nursing in European countries. Davies, Deeny, and Raikkonen (2003) discussed the development and implementation of a Master of Science (MSc) program in disaster relief nursing established by cooperating partners in European countries. The partners included European educational institutions and aid relief agencies. The program's goal was to enhance the provision of relief aid by endorsing the role of nurses as providers of health care in disaster stricken areas around the world. Student placements have included areas such as Angola, Mozambique, the Balkans, and Taliban prison camps in Northern Afghanistan. The authors stated that "As an attempt to address the implications of globalisation in health care, the programme was established as a recognition of the rapidly developing specialty of transcultural/transnational nursing" (Davies, Deeny, & Raikkonen, 2003, p. 349). Glittenberg's (1994) study of Guatemalans who experienced the devastating effects of an earthquake was the earliest transcultural nursing disaster research.

Watt et al. (2002) described the development and implementation of a 4-week international nursing student exchange program involving 26 colleges in 14 European nations. The purpose of the program was to develop cultural competence in European nursing students. Using Leininger's *Theory of Culture Care Diversity and Universality*, Gebru and Willman (2003) developed a research based didactic model for transcultural nursing education in Sweden. To facilitate the provision of culturally congruent care for elders from the largest immigrant group in the Netherlands, van den Brink (2003) conducted an ethnographic study of the diversity and universality in care values and meanings of Turkish lay caregivers and Dutch professional nurses. Higginbottom (2000) examined the breast-feeding experiences of women of African descent residing in the United Kingdom (UK). Noting that women of African descent migrated to the United Kingdom largely for economic reasons, Higginbottom asserted that breast-feeding patterns might change as the women became more acculturated and adopted the breast feeding norms of the dominant UK culture. She concluded that midwives and health care providers were challenged to harness and sustain the breast-feeding tradition in the generations of women of African descent who are not immigrants but were born in the UK and therefore exposed early to prevailing breast-feeding socialization processes of the dominant culture.

Friedemann, Astedt-Kurki, and Paavilainen (2003) reported the findings of a study on the challenges associated with the transfer of the Assessment of Strategies in Families-Effectiveness (ASF-E), a family assessment instrument developed in the United States, and its theoretical basis when used to assess Finnish families. To improve this instrument when used with Finnish families, the researchers addressed two dimensions: family operation, and the process of resolving interpersonal crises. Although loosely connected and highly individualized, Finnish families tend to be bound by strong emotional ties that rendered separation very painful, thus necessitating modification of items on the ASF-E related to the expression of positive and negative outcomes on the two dimensions identified. The investigators also addressed the challenges associated with instrument translation and discussed additional procedures such as focus groups to let respondents express their thoughts. The researchers admonished that investigators must be vigilant and astute in observing the unique cultural patterns of the people when conducting transnational research and when using an instrument developed in another country. Lamp's (2002) study of the culture care meanings and practices of Finnish childbearing women included an excellent pictorial study of their perinatal childbearing processes in which Leininger's three care modes were beautifully identified. This study provided a means for sharing care patterns in childbearing and perinatal care practices 'in action' through the use of visual media.

Advances in Transcultural Nursing: Africa

By virtue of its multiracial and tribal differences, Africa is a continent that is characterized by extensive cultural diversity. As indicated in Table 3-1, there have been seven recent articles from the *Journal of Transcultural Nursing* focusing on advances in transcultural nursing in various parts of Africa—Cameroon, Ethiopia, South Africa, Ghana, Zimbabwe, and Tanzania. Fongwa (2002) described the health care system in Cameroon and put forth recommendations for improving the quality of care in that nation. Among the suggestions for improving care was increased international assistance and collaboration with more developed countries— nations with the financial resources to enhance the overall health care provided to the people of Cameroon. In a study on the resilience of the human spirit during and after experiences of childhood famine, Lothe and Heggen (2003) conducted indepth interviews with survivors of the 1984 to 1985 Ethiopian famine. The informants were children at the time of the famine, but researchers interviewed these survivors at an orphanage in Addis Ababa nearly twenty years after the devastating famine that affected this nation. Using US funding, Smith, Garbharran, Edwards, and O'Hara-Murdock (2004) studied 300 heads of households in South Africa for the purpose of identifying the educational needs of African Zulu and Xhosa women regarding sanitation, hygiene, and health. In a nation where communicable diseases continue to be among the major health care problems, knowledge about clean water, proper disposal of wastes, and personal hygiene can mean the difference between health and disease, and between life and death. Using a multistep approach to the investigation, researchers used both quantitative and qualitative methods to understand the educational needs of these South African women. Mashaba (2002) conducted an ethnonursing study of South African culturally based health-illness patterns and humanistic practices, and indicated the manner in which Leininger's three action modes promoted culturally congruent nursing care for South Africans.

Africa has the largest number of reported AIDS cases in the world. To examine the experience of HIV-positive women in Ghana and to identify factors that influenced their vulnerability to infection, Mill (2003) conducted indepth interviews and focus groups with HIV positive men and women, nurses, other health care professionals, and traditional healers. Mill (2003) reported that the need for secrecy in "breaking the news"—informing the woman that she was HIV positive—was one manifestation of AIDS stigma in Ghana, a nation in which the diagnosis was frequently accompanied by isolation, stigmatization, and withdrawal from family members. The Ghanaian women interviewed during this study were informed about their diagnosis in an indirect manner, often through an intermediary. Following diagnosis, it was common for the women to be told by their HIV counselor that to avoid stigma, they should keep their diagnosis secret. The informants experienced or anticipated many negative outcomes in relation to HIV disclosure. For example, some women were no longer permitted to share family meals, were isolated by community members, or were forced out of their homes. These outcomes were extremely stressful to the women and motivated them to keep the diagnosis secret. The secrecy led to some women not benefiting from financial and emotional support that might have been available from families. The investigator posited that such secrecy may have actually maintained and amplified AIDS stigma in Ghana. The investigator encouraged disclosure of the diagnosis within a trusting and supportive environment as one strategy to diffuse the stigma associated with AIDS. Mill also recommended that nurses be trained to counsel and care for patients with HIV, and that nurses should play a key role in ameliorating AIDS stigma by role modeling compassionate attitudes toward persons living with HIV and AIDS.

In a study conducted in Zimbabwe, Moon, Khumalo-Sakutukwa, Heiman, Mbivzo, and Padian (2002) investigated the acceptability of vaginal microbicides in the prevention of heterosexually transmitted HIV. Most women were enthusiastic about the microbicide products but had concerns about safety and about how the use of the products might affect their relationships with their husbands. Many men were concerned that women would be able to use the products without their consent or knowledge. The investigators concluded that several microbicides might be acceptable in this culture, but must be introduced within the existing gender power structure. This US-funded study involved collaboration by investigators from the World Health Organization and from universities in Zimbabwe and the United States.

Tabi and Mukherjee (2003) described Nursing in a Global Community, a 6-semester credit hour, 6-week summer study abroad course. This course enabled undergraduate and graduate students in nursing and other health-professions disciplines from Georgia Southern University to participate in a program hosted by the University of Cape Coast in Ghana. The program had a community health focus and was developed to give students the opportunity to "learn, observe, and experience transcultural nursing and health care at the international level" (Tabi & Mukherjee, 2003, p. 135). Students participating in the program had both acute care and community based learning opportunities. The course emphasized the use of primary health care as a framework for health promotion, health education, and disease prevention

After conducting a cultural assessment of the Chagga tribe of Tanzania, Savage (2002) presented a case study of a fictional member of the Chagga tribe. The case study method was used to introduce nurses and nursing students to guidelines for the provision of culturally congruent nursing care for the Chagga people.

Advances in Transcultural Nursing: Central and South America

The so-called Latinization of North America reflects the increased northward migration of people from Mexico and other Central and South American nations to the United States and Canada, often for economic and-or political reasons. Similarly, there has been migration to other parts of the world by people from Latin America.

Summarized in Table 3-1 are six recent articles from the *Journal of Transcultural Nursing* focusing on advances in transcultural nursing in various parts of Central and South America. Cesarman-Maus (2003), a physician affiliated with the Mexican Ministry of Foreign Affairs, described the Program for Mexican Communities Abroad and identified its offices as ideal sites for organizations committed to the improved health and wellbeing of Mexicans to establish outreach programs for Mexican migrant workers. The author described several general health and local health activities that were currently being provided by the Program for Mexican Communities Abroad ranging from health fairs to radio outreach to mobile health clinics. The organization also provided educational programs on topics such as sexually transmitted diseases, addictions, domestic violence, oral hygiene, alternative medicine, and related subjects.

In a study of Colombian adolescents, de la Cuesta (2001) reported findings of an investigation on perceptions of romantic love and the gender rules that guide the behavior of women in male-female relationships. The study revealed that adolescent pregnancy occurred in the context of a 'genuine love affair' in which the ideas of romantic love and gender rules guided young people in their sexual decision making and behavior choices. Ideas of romantic love and gender rules were powerful influences on those who unintentionally became pregnant. Nurses with knowledge about these Colombian cultural beliefs and gender rules can be instrumental in counseling young women about ways to avoid unwanted pregnancies such as educating them about sexual abstinence, adoption, the use of oral and intrauterine contraceptives, and other methods for dealing with an unplanned pregnancy. There have been a number of other clinical field studies by transcultural nurses in Central America over the past two decades.

Hoga, Alcantara, and de Lima (2001) conducted a study of men ages 21 to 64 years living in a low income community in Brazil. The purpose of the study was to explore men's involvement in reproductive health. Leininger's (1991) culture care modes were used to explain culturally meaningful nursing care actions. Also concerned about the relationship between health and low socioeconomic status, Kraatz (2001) conducted an ethnographic study of women living in a *favela* [urban slum] in southeastern Brazil. The purpose of the study was to describe the women's understanding of health and illness. Data analysis yielded a taxonomic structure for the domains of health and illness. The researcher reported that six components played a part in both health and illness: cleanliness, nutrition, visits to a physician, herbal remedies, sympathetic magic, and spirituality. The investigator recommended integrating the indigenous components of health into health teaching in order to enhance the congruence between nursing care and the worldview of *favela* residents.

With a focus on rural health care, Holt and Reeves (2001) explored the meaning of hope and generic care practices for people living a rural village in the Dominican Republic. The investigators examined ways to nurture hope among these poor rural villagers. Purnell (2001) studied Guatemalans for the purpose of examining their practices of health promotion and wellness, and disease and illness prevention. Among the important findings reported by the investigator was the meaning and significance of respect in the Guatemalan culture—especially the demonstration of respect by nurses and other health care providers for the client and his or her cultural values, beliefs, and practices.

Riner and Becklinberg (2001) described a partnership between Indiana University School of Nursing in Indianapolis, Indiana (USA) and the Bloomington, Indiana-Posoltega, Nicaragua Sister City Organization to provide an international service learning course in nursing. Service learning courses engaged students in meaningful voluntary service to a community and at the same time facilitated students' achievement of course objectives. Over a period of four years the Indiana University School of Nursing faculty developed an independent study option for a single student into an elective course with N = 10 students enrolled. Student learning activities for this course included: developing relationships with Posoltega community residents; providing prenatal classes; supporting nursing scholarships; and participating as interdisciplinary, multicultural team members. The authors reported that the Sister Cities International partnership provided nursing students with opportunities to learn about and participate with Nicaraguan and international health care workers in meeting population health needs in stable communities and refugee environments in Posoltega, Nicaragua.

Advances in Transcultural Nursing: Canada

Summarized in Table 3-1 are two recent articles from the *Journal of Transcultural Nursing* focusing on advances in transcultural nursing in Canada, and one article in which a Canadian researcher reports the findings of her study of HIV-positive women in Ghana (Mill, 2003). Canadian trends and issues in transcultural nursing theory and research have been critically analyzed by Srivastava and Leininger (2002).

Recognizing that the recruitment and retention of students from culturally diverse backgrounds remains a vital and critical concern in nursing education, Labun (2002) presented an overview of the Red River College (Winnipeg, Manitoba) Model for Enhancing Success for Native Canadian and Other Nursing Students from Disenfranchised Groups. A significant proportion of nursing students of Native Canadian, refugee, and immigrant groups as well as those from poor single parent families require social, academic, financial and-or personal support to be academically successful. The author provided background information on establishing the access program and its development over a 17 year period. The author described the population served, program design, and factors that had contributed to the students' success, such as strategies for overcoming language difficulties, dealing with discrimination, harassment, and racism in both classroom and clinical settings, and keeping students focused on their original motivation for wanting to become a nurse. Since its inception, the access program had graduated 226 students at the time of the study and had significantly increased the number of Native Canadians and other minorities in the nursing profession in Canada.

Recognizing the paucity of scientific data on Canadian aboriginals and HIV prevention efforts targeting aboriginal youth, Majumdar, Chambers and Roberts (2004) delivered an educational workshop on HIV/AIDS to a group of aboriginal adolescents from a First Nations community in Ontario. Canada's aboriginals (First Nations, Inuit, and Metis) comprise 2.8% of the Canadian population, with approximately 60% of the group being less than 30 years of age. The purpose of the intervention study was to promote knowledge of HIV/AIDS among aboriginal adolescents through a cooperative venture and to encourage the sharing and perception of values among peer groups. The investigators reported that the participatory method employed in this study fostered communication and the creation of a support group among participants.

This study provided the initial basis for aboriginal adolescent–peer HIV/AIDS education and offered a group of aboriginal youth the opportunity to share, discuss, and acquire relevant HIV/AIDS information from their peer facilitators. The investigators reported that the aboriginal adolescents in the study not only gained knowledge about HIV/AIDS, but also experienced a positive change in attitude toward HIV/AIDS. The successful implementation of an HIV/AIDS intervention depended on such factors as the collaborative efforts of researchers, the cooperation of prevention service providers (health departments, community based organizations), and the target population. The aboriginal community directly involved key members of the group conducting outreach and intervention activities, and utilized local and tribally relevant forms of communication which were identified as critical factors in the prevention effort against HIV/AIDS. The researchers concluded by saying that the complex nature of HIV prevention work implied that researchers need to consider the interconnections among societal, behavioral, and emotional factors that underlie the transmission of the disease.

Concluding Remarks

Significant progress has been made to advance transcultural nursing as a discipline and a formal area of study and practice. Nursing's global agenda for transculturalism has occurred over the past twenty years, which Leininger has referred to as the *Third Era: Establishing Transcultural Nursing Worldwide* (Leininger, 1995; Leininger & McFarland, 2002). During this Third Era, transcultural nursing leaders have used strategies to establish a solid foundation in transcultural nursing on every continent—to fulfill the vision articulated by Dr. Leininger that "The needs of the world will be met by nurses prepared in transcultural nursing." These words also appear on the Transcultural Nursing Society logo. The credo has confirmed support through a considerable number of solidly conducted theory based transcultural nursing research studies that have provided sound guides for care actions and decisions.

Establishing transcultural nursing worldwide has required several key components: 1) the futuristic direction for transcultural nursing practice, education, research, and consultation transnationally, which has been articulated by the Founder of Transcultural Nursing, Dr. Madeleine Leininger, and by many of Transcultural Nursing Society Board Members; 2) nurses with formal academic preparation in transcultural nursing who exercise strong leadership and influence key health care decision- and policymakers worldwide; 3) opportunities for exchanging ideas and sharing transcultural nursing knowledge with nurses and other health care professionals from around the world—face to face through participation in workshops, seminars, and conferences and electronically; 4) a solid theoretical and research foundation in transcultural nursing and health; 5) educational and health care facilities that support transnational exchanges of nurses and other health care providers; 6) government and nongovernment organizations, international agencies, corporations, and private health care foundations that fund transnational research, education, and travel for nurses and other health care providers; and 7) transcultural nurse leaders who are creative, innovative, and visionary in planning and implementing nursing's global agenda for the 21st century.

During the past two decades, increasing numbers of nurses have been traveling and working in different countries and interacting with people from many different cultures both electronically and face to face. Each year the *Journal of Transcultural Nursing* contains important articles on transnational nursing, thus providing a venue for the exchange of ideas among transcultural scholars who contribute to knowledge in the areas of transnational clinical practice, education, research, and consultation. These full-text articles can be accessed electronically or in print format by nurses and others interested in scholarship in transcultural nursing virtually anywhere in the world. In addition, nearly 40 books and 1000 articles on transcultural nursing focus on research, theory, and practice in many global locations.

There are, however, several areas for continued growth and development despite the impressive advances in transcultural nursing around the world. First, although much transcultural nursing research has been conducted around the world, there remain many cultures and subcultures that have not yet been studied—largely due to lack of nurses with the preparation necessary to conduct these investigations. Second, educational institutions that prepare nurses around the world must integrate transcultural content and research findings into the curricula and develop graduate programs in transcultural nursing and practice, with affects on outcomes. Third, there needs to be a constructively critical ethical analysis of contemporary issues and trends in transnational nursing. Ethics provide a framework within which nurses can reflect on the moral nature of actions, i.e., their rightness or wrongness and can evaluate moral judgments, character, and proposed policies. Some examples of ethical issues include the cultural imposition of US curricula and textbooks on schools of nursing in other nations without regard for the cultural context of the host country. Another ethical issue concerns nursing consultations that advocate the use of high tech interventions that are likely to benefit a small number of the most affluent citizens of a country versus low tech solutions (e.g., immunizations for communicable diseases) that could benefit large numbers of the population at an affordable cost. Fourth, there needs to be broader assessments of people's cultural needs transnationally, including the refinement of instruments that build on the theory and research of transcultural nurse scholars. Fifth, investigations on phenomena of interest in transnational nursing need to utilize a theoretically sound transcultural nursing framework (e.g., Leininger's *Theory of Culture Care Diversity and Universality*). Too many studies fail to focus on *care* or *culture care*, the core constructs of nursing, transcultural nursing, and culture. Many studies are atheoretical or fail to clearly explicate the researcher's theoretical perspective. Using Leininger's *Theory of Culture Care Diversity and Universality* would be a way to address this and the atheoretical nature of much of the research just reviewed. Sixth, there needs to be increased emphasis on the cultural, social, and environmental aspects of global health problems rather than emphasis on the narrow biophysical aspect. Seventh, there needs to be more emphasis on what can be learned *from* people in other nations. For example, there needs to be more research on folk, indigenous, or generic healing practices studying the healers responsible, about the parsimonious use of scarce resources (e.g., water, medical equipment and supplies, energy, etc.), and about health care delivery systems that provide more efficient, cost effective, and quality nursing and health care outside of the dominant country or culture, or one's own.

Lastly, there needs to be increased transnational cooperation among professional nursing and health care organizations and consensus building about nursing's global agenda. For example, the World Health Organization, International Council of Nurses, Transcultural

Nursing Society, and many other professional organizations have identified the perils associated with the global AIDS epidemic. These professional organizations need to approach this complex, multifaceted social and health problem with a comprehensive, cohesive, multidisciplinary plan for the prevention and eradication of AIDS. The Transcultural Nursing Society continues to be positioned strategically to provide global leadership in facing the challenges associated with HIV/AIDS and other problems of global significance. The Society is a well organized, established, highly respected organization that boasts members from every continent and the majority of countries around the world. The Society can quickly and effectively communicate information through its newsletter, the *Journal of Transcultural Nursing*, and other publications; regional, national and international conferences; and its website (www.tcns.org). This information is of great value to nurses seeking to grasp the global aspects of transcultural nursing.

This chapter highlights several major and significant developments in the evolution of transcultural nursing worldwide. The reader is encouraged to read the studies in the *Journal of Transcultural Nursing* prior to 1998 when Leininger and McFarland served as editors. Approximately 85 cultures were discussed using the Culture Care Theory, some focusing on cultures outside of the United States. Space limited the inclusion of these important studies or mention of their authors.

References

Al-Shahri, M. Z. (2002). Culturally sensitive caring for Saudi patients. *Journal of Transcultural Nursing 13*(2), 133–138.

Andrews, M. M. (1985). International consultation by United States nurses. *International Nursing Review, 32*(1), 50–54.

Andrews, M. M. (1986). U.S. nurse consultants in the international marketplace. *International Nursing Review, 33*(2), 50–55.

Australian Bureau of Statistics. (2001). *Census Basic Community Profile.* Retrieved from www.abs.gov.a/ausstats/abs%40census/

Bisch, S. A. (1983). Understanding international development models. *Nursing Outlook, 31*(2), 123–128.

Cesarman-Maus, G. (2003). The consular program for Mexican communities abroad: A source of outreach for health workers. *Journal of Transcultural Nursing, 14*(3), 272–275.

Cortis, J. D. (2000). Perceptions and experiences with nursing care: A study of Pakistani (Urdu) communities in the United Kingdom. *Journal of Transcultural Nursing, 11*(2), 111–118.

Davies, K., Deeny, P., & Raikkonen, M. (2003). A transcultural ethos underpinning curriculum development: A master's programme in disaster relief nursing. *Journal of Transcultural Nursing, 14*(4), 349–357.

de la Cuesta, C. (2001). Taking love seriously: The context of adolescent pregnancy in Colombia. *Journal of Transcultural Nursing, 12*(3), 180–192.

Daly, J., Speedy, S., & Jackson, D. (2000). *Contexts of nursing: An introduction.* Sydney: Maclennan & Petty.

Douglas, M. (2000). Effect of globalization on health care: Double-edged sword. *Journal of Transcultural Nursing, 11*(3), 85.

Fongwa, M. N. (2002). International health care perspectives: The Cameroon example. *Journal of Transcultural Nursing, 13*(4), 325–330.

Fooladi, M. M. (2003). Gendered nursing education and practice in Iran. *Journal of Transcultural Nursing, 14*(1), 32–38.

Friedemann, M., Astedt-Kurki, P., & Paavilainen, E. (2003). Development of a family assessment instrument for transcultural use. *Journal of Transcultural Nursing, 14*(2), 90–99.

Gebru, K., & Willman, A. (2003). A research-based didactic model for education to promote culturally competent nursing care in Sweden. *Journal of Transcultural Nursing, 14*(1), 55–61.

Gharaibeh, M., & Abu-Saad, H. (2002). Cultural validation of pediatric pain assessment tools: Jordanian perspective. *Journal of Transcultural Nursing, 13*(1), 12–18.

Glittenberg, J. E. (1994). *To the high mountain and back: The mysteries of Guatemalan Highland family life.* Prospect Heights, IL: Waveland Press.

Goold, S. (2001). Transcultural nursing: Can we meet the challenge of caring for the Australian indigenous person? *Journal of Transcultural Nursing, 12*(2), 94–99.

Hattar-Pollara, M., Meleis, A. I., & Nagib, H. (2003). Multiple role stress and patterns of coping of Egyptian women in clerical jobs. *Journal of Transcultural Nursing 14*(2), 125–133.

Higginbottom, G. M. A. (2000). Breast-feeding experiences of women of African descent in the United Kingdom. *Journal of Transcultural Nursing, 11*(1), 55–63.

Hoga, L. A. K., Alcantara, A. C., & de Lima, V. M. (2001). Adult male involvement in reproductive health: An ethnographic study in a community of Sao Paulo City, Brazil. *Journal of Transcultural Nursing, 12*(2), 107–114.

Holt, J., & Reeves, J. S. (2001). The meaning of hope and generic caring practices to nurture hope in a rural village in the Dominican Republic. *Journal of Transcultural Nursing, 12*(2), 123–131.

Horn, B. M. (1975). *An ethnoscientific study to determine social and cultural factors affecting Native American Indian women during pregnancy.* Unpublished doctoral dissertation, University of Washington, Seattle.

Idrus, L. (1988). Transcultural nursing in Australia: Response to a changing population base. *Recent Advances in Nursing, 20*, 137–155.

Im, E. (2003). Symptoms experienced during menopausal transition: Korean women in South Korea and the United States. *Journal of Transcultural Nursing, 14*(4), 321–328.

Iwata, H. (2003). Concept analysis of the role of fatherhood: A Japanese perspective. *Journal of Transcultural Nursing, 14*(4), 297–304.

Jackson, D. (2003). Epilogue: Culture, health and social justice. *Contemporary Nurse, 15*(3), 347–348.

Jirapaet, V. (2001). Factors affecting maternal role attainment among low-income, Thai, HIV-positive mothers. *Journal of Transcultural Nursing, 12*(1), 25–33.

Kanitsaki, O. (1988). Transcultural nursing: Challenge to change. *Australian Journal of Advanced Nursing, 5*(3), 4–11.

Kanitsaki, O. (1989). Clinical nurse teaching: An investigation of student perceptions of clinical nurse teaching behaviours. *Australian Journal of Advanced Nursing, 6*(4), 18–24.

Kanitsaki, O. (2003). Transcultural nursing and challenging the status quo. *Contemporary Nurse, 15*(3), v–x.

Kendall, K. (1992). Maternal and child care in an Iranian village. *Journal of Transcultural Nursing, 4*(1), 29–36.

Kraatz, E. S. (2001). The structure of health and illness in a Brazilian favela. *Journal of Transcultural Nursing, 12*(3), 173–179.

Labun, E. (2002). Red River College model: Enhancing success for Native Canadian and other nursing students from disenfranchised groups. *Journal of Transcultural Nursing, 13*(4), 311–317.

Lambert, V. A., Lambert, C. E., Daly, J., Davidson, P. M., Kunaviktikul, W., & Shin, K. R. (2004). Nursing education on women's health care in Australia, Japan, South Korea, and Thailand. *Journal of Transcultural Nursing, 15*(1), 44–53.

Lamp, J. K. (2002). Finnish women in birth: Culture care meanings and practices. In M. M. Leininger and M. R. McFarland (3rd ed.), *Transcultural nursing: Concepts, theories, research & practice*. New York: McGraw-Hill.

Leininger, M. M. (1969). Ethnoscience: A new and promising research approach for the health sciences. *Image: The Journal of Nursing Scholarship, 3*(1), 2–8.

Leininger, M. M. (1970). *Nursing and anthropology: Two worlds to blend*. New York: John Wiley and Sons.

Leininger, M. M. (1978). *Transcultural nursing: Concepts, theories, and practices*. New York: John Wiley and Sons.

Leininger, M. (Ed.). (1984). *Care: The essence of nursing and health*. Thorofare, NJ: Slack.

Leininger, M. M. (1985). *Qualitative research methods in nursing*. Orlando, FL: Grune and Stratton.

Leininger, M. M. (1990). The significance of cultural concepts in nursing. *Journal of Transcultural Nursing, 2*(1), 52–59.

Leininger, M. M. (1991). *Culture care diversity and universality: Theory of nursing*. New York: National League for Nursing.

Leininger, M. M. (1995). *Transcultural nursing: Concepts, theories, research & practices*. New York: McGraw Hill, Inc.

Leininger, M. M. (2001). Founder's focus: Australia: The global Transcultural Nursing Society's 26th annual meeting place for 2000. *Journal of Transcultural Nursing, 12*(2), 158.

Leininger, M. M., & McFarland, M. R. (2002). *Transcultural nursing: Concepts, theories, research & practice*. New York: McGraw-Hill.

Liu, H. G., & Moore, J. F. (2000). Perinatal care: Cultural and technical differences between China and the United States. *Journal of Transcultural Nursing, 11*(1), 47–54.

Lothe, E. A., & Heggen, K. (2003). A study of resilience in young Ethiopian famine survivors. *Journal of Transcultural Nursing, 14*(4), 313–320.

Luna, L. (1989). Transcultural nursing care of Arab Muslims. *Journal of Transcultural Nursing, 1*(1), 22–26.

Luna, L. (1994). Care and cultural context of Lebanese Muslim immigrants with Leininger's theory. *Journal of Transcultural Nursing, 5*(2), 12–20.

Luna, L. (1995). Arab Muslims and culture care. In M. Leininger, *Transcultural nursing: Concepts, theories, research & practices* (pp. 317–331). New York: McGraw-Hill.

Luna, L. (1998). Culturally competent health care: A challenge for nurses in Saudi Arabia. *Journal of Transcultural Nursing, 9*(2), 8–14.

Lundbert, P. C. (2000). Cultural care of Thai immigrants in Uppsala: A study of transcultural nursing in Sweden. *Journal of Transcultural Nursing, 11*(4), 274–280.

Majumdar, B. B., Chambers, T. L., Roberts, J. (2004). Community-based culturally sensitive HIV/AIDS education for aboriginal adolescents: Implications for nursing practice. *Journal of Transcultural Nursing 15*(1), 69–73

Mashaba, G. (2002). South African culturally based health-illness patterns and humanistic practices. In M. M. Leininger and M. R. McFarland, *Transcultural nursing: Concepts, theories, research & practice.* (pp. 325–332). New York: McGraw-Hill.

Mill, J. E. (2003). Shrouded in secrecy: Breaking the news of HIV infections to Ghanaian women. *Journal of Transcultural Nursing, 14*(1), 6–16.

Miller, J. E., & Petro-Nustas, W. (2002). Context of care for Jordanian women. *Journal of Transcultural Nursing, 13*(2), 228–336.

Moon, M. W., Khumalo-Sakutukwa, G. N., Heiman, J. E., Mbivzo, M. T., & Padian, N. S. (2002). Vaginal microbicides for HIV/STI prevention in Zimbabwe: What key informants say. *Journal of Transcultural Nursing, 13*(1), 19–23.

Nwoga, I. A. (2000). Take a village (TAV): A metaphorical model for health promotion. *Journal of Transcultural Nursing, 11*(4), 246–253.

Omeri, A. (2003a). Advances in contemporary transcultural nursing. *Contemporary Nurse, 15*(3), ii.

Omeri, A. (2003b). Meeting diversity challenges: Pathway of "advanced" transcultural nursing practice in Australia. *Contemporary Nurse, 15*(3), 175–187.

Omeri, A., & Cameron-Traub, E. (Eds.). (1996). *Transcultural nursing in multicultural Australia.* Deakin, Australia: Royal College of Nursing.

Othaganont, P., Sinthuvorakan, C., & Jensupakarn, P. (2002). Daily living practice of the life-satisfied Thai elderly. *Journal of Transcultural Nursing, 13*(1), 24–29.

Pacquiao, D. F. (2003a). President's message: Annual conference, a time for renewal and global linkages. *Journal of Transcultural Nursing, 14*(4), 367.

Pacquiao, D. F. (2003b). President's message: Organizational responsiveness to global challenges. *Journal of Transcultural Nursing, 14*(3), 282.

Park, Y., Kim, H. S., Kang, H., & Kim, J. (2001). A survey of Hwa-Byung in middle-age Korean women. *Journal of Transcultural Nursing, 12*(2), 115–122.

Petro-Nustas, W. I. (2001). Factors associated with mammography utilization among Jordanian women. *Journal of Transcultural Nursing, 12*(4), 284–291.

Petro-Nustas, W., Kulwicki, A., & Zumout, A. F. (2002). Students' knowledge, attitudes, and beliefs about AIDS: A cross-cultural study. *Journal of Transcultural Nursing, 13*(2), 118–125.

Purnell, L. (2000). Global institute for nursing and health: Second annual international conference, Eskilstuna, Sweden. *Journal of Transcultural Nursing, 11*(2), 144–145.

Purnell, L. (2001). Guatemalans' practices for health promotion and the meaning of respect afforded them by health care providers. *Journal of Transcultural Nursing, 12*(1), 40–47.

Riner, M. E., & Becklenburg, A. (2001). Partnering with a sister city organization for an international service-learning experience. *Journal of Transcultural Nursing, 12*(3), 234–240.

Savage, A. R. (2002). Providing nursing care for a Chagga client of Tanzania. *Journal of Transcultural Nursing, 13*(3), 248–253.

Smith, M. A., Garbharran, H., Edwards, M. J., & O'Hara-Murdock, P. (2004). Health promotion and disease prevention through sanitation education in South African Zulu and Xhosa women. *Journal of Transcultural Nursing, 15*(1), 62–68.

Spence, D. G. (2001). Prejudice, paradox, and possibility: Nursing people from cultures other than one's own. *Journal of Transcultural Nursing, 12*(2), 100–106.

Srivastava, R. H., & Leininger, M. M. (2002). Canadian transcultural nursing: Trends and issues. In M. M. Leininger and M. R. McFarland, *Transcultural nursing: Concepts, theories, research, & practice.* (pp. 493–502). New York: McGraw-Hill.

Tabi, M. M., & Mukherjee, S. (2003). Nursing in a global community: A study abroad program. *Journal of Transcultural Nursing, 14*(2), 134–138.

van den Brink, Y. (2003). Diversity in care values and expressions among Turkish family caregivers and Dutch community nurses in the Netherlands. *Journal of Transcultural Nursing, 14*(2), 146–154.

Wepa, D. (2003). An exploration of the experiences of cultural safety educators in New Zealand: An action research approach. *Journal of Transcultural Nursing, 14*(4), 339–348.

Watt, S., Law, K., Ots, U., & Waago, K. (2002). Reflections across boundaries: The European Nursing Module. *Journal of Transcultural Nursing, 13*(4), 318–324.

Wen-Chii, T. (2001). Being trapped in a circle: Life after a suicide attempt in Taiwan. *Journal of Transcultural Nursing, 12*(4), 302–309.

Zoucha, R. (2002). President's Message. *Journal of Transcultural Nursing, 12*(4), 333.

Chapter Four

Culture Care of the Gadsup Akuna of the Eastern Highlands of New Guinea

[Revised Reprint]

Madeleine M. Leininger, PhD, LHD, DS, CTN, RN, FAAN, FRCNA

> *You are a different kind of a woman. Will you be our friend or our enemy?*
>
> —Gadsup villagers

In the early 1960s, I left the United States of America and entered a strange new world in which there were very few familiarities or commonalities with the people, language, homes, food, land, and indigenous lifeways. There were no modern modes of transportation, telephones, appliances, electricity, indoor toilets, or running water. In general, there were no modern Western amenities or comforts which many Americans enjoy. Although it was an initial culture shock, it soon turned into a new world to discover, understand, and value.

When I entered the Gadsup village in the Eastern Highlands of New Guinea, I well remember how the people stared at me wondering perhaps where this white woman came from and why she might be interested in them. I, too, wondered about these villagers and why I came to study people who had been known as "head hunters of the Highlands." Would I survive and how could I ever learn about their world? It was a uniquely different world in which the Gadsup people and their lifeways baffled me. Their concern was reflected in their conscious but unspoken reflection, "You are a different kind of a woman. Will you be our friend or our enemy?" For this Western researcher, it was this very different world that posed a tremendous challenge: how to study and understand these people who were so different from the world I left behind.

When I went to New Guinea in the early 1960s, I was a third-year doctoral student at the University of Washington and had chosen this largely unknown culture to do an ethnographic and ethnonursing study by living alone with the villagers for an extended time. There were no anthropological writings on this unknown Melanesian New Guinean culture. I was prepared with a suitable theoretical and research background from my graduate studies as well as in psychiatric mental health nursing and as an educator ready to study and learn about strange or unexpected behaviors. My decision to go to New Guinea and study this nonWestern culture also was welcomed by the Department of Anthropology—it needed to be studied soon, before the Western world changed it.

Before I left the United States, I wondered what I could learn about transcultural nursing and human caring and health from a culture that had not been touched by Western ideologies and practices. I wondered how the people lived in their naturalistic environment and what were their actual daily and nightly lifeways. I wondered how these people could function without modern technologies. With my theoretical and research nursing interests, I was eager to study the meanings and expressions of human care and how care had influenced the people's health and wellbeing. I wanted to study human caring and health within the total lifeways of nonWestern people and in a culture where there had been little to no contact with Western people. I was curious how this nonWestern culture lived and expressed their human care needs, remained well, became ill, or faced death. I had heard that the Gadsup had survived and maintained themselves quite well over an extended time. Principally, I wanted to learn about the caring ways of the people from their *emic* (or local insider's) view, and how they would contrast with our American and other Western lifeways. In addition, I was interested in the environment or ecology of the people and how these factors influenced Gadsup lifeways.

During my graduate studies, I had already conceptualized most of the major ideas, tenets, and concepts of my theory of Culture Care Diversity and Universality, and so I wanted to examine systematically the theory with my ethnonursing qualitative research method in a relatively small community. Since the idea of developing a culturally based theory and using a nursing research method was unknown in nursing in the mid 1950s and early 1960s, I thought the Gadsup culture would be an ideal initial study group. The idea of using such study findings as knowledge for the new field of transcultural nursing was exciting to me. In those days, too, although no theoretical research studies in nursing with a transcultural perspective were available, there were several non-nurse anthropologists, such as Esther Lucille Brown (1948) and Lyle Saunders (1954), who encouraged nurses to use social science ideas in nursing education. The specific linkage of cultural knowledge to nursing, however, had yet to be developed and used. With increased world travel and with nurses working in different cultures, I was convinced that they would soon need transcultural care and health knowledge to be effective in future multicultural nursing. Nursing also needed the ethnonursing research approach to learn directly from the people of the daily lifeways of culture and to discover the role of caring in relation to health and wellbeing. For these major reasons and others, I chose New Guinea as the site for my field research.

In this chapter I will highlight my research work in New Guinea with my theory of Culture Care and with the use of the ethnonursing method which was specifically designed for the theory. Since the theory and the ethnonursing method have already been presented in Chapters 1 and 2, the focus will be mainly on the Gadsup Akunans and their culture care expressions in relation to the theory, research method, ethnohistory, and other dimensions of the Sunrise Enabler with research findings.

Research Domain, Purpose, and Questions

The domain of inquiry was the study of the meanings, expressions, and lived experiences of human care to the Gadsup Akunans. This domain was chosen to discover the epistemic and ontologic nature of human care and its relationship to health with Gadsup in their particular environmental context. The central purpose of this study was to generate new nursing knowledge by identifying, describing, explaining, and interpreting human care (and caring) from the Gadsup's *emic* viewpoints focusing on influencers of human care in relation to worldview, social structure, cultural values, ethnohistory, folk care, and environment of the people. The assumptive premises and hunches stated in the Culture Care theory were of central interest to me because of the need for new knowledge for the discipline of nursing and for the field of transcultural nursing. Ultimately, such knowledge and future findings from other cultures in the world could guide nurses to provide relevant knowledge as well as culture-specific nursing care practices related to ethnocare and ethnohealth. This study—the first nursing research endeavor toward the evolving study of the meaning and nature of human care from an *emic* viewpoint—was conducted to fulfill doctoral requirements in anthropology focusing on the general lifeways of a culture and their social structure features.

The following questions, which guided this ethnocare and ethnohealth research, did not limit my discovery of other Gadsup findings related to my theory of Culture Care and the lifeways of the people.

1. What are the meanings, expressions, patterns, and lived experiences of human care to the Gadsup Akunans and the influences on their health and wellbeing?
2. In what ways does the worldview, ethnohistory, social structure, culture values, language, and the local (folk) practices influence the health and illness patterns of the people?

3. What specific cultural care values, beliefs, and practices throughout the lifecycle tend to influence the health and illness lifeways of the people?
4. In what way does the physical environment (or ecology) influence human care, health, or illness patterns of the people?
5. Given the predicted three modes of decisions and actions in the Culture Care Theory, what nursing care modalities will most likely provide culturally congruent care practices?

Theoretical Framework, Assumptive Premises, and Orientational Questions

In conceptualizing the theory of Culture Care for this investigation, I used the major tenets, assumptive premises, and orientational definitions of the theory using the Gadsup Akunans as the study focus along with the Sunrise Enabler as a conceptual guide. Since the theory and the enabler have already been presented in Chapter 1, they will not be presented again except for specific perspectives related to the Gadsups.

I held that care was the essence of nursing, but there were different values, meanings, patterned expressions, and structure forms of care that were important to discover to establish transcultural and other comparative care knowledge. I predicted that the values, meanings, patterned expressions, and experiences of human care and caring would be influenced by worldview, social structure, ethnohistory, environmental (including ecology), and folk care practices screened through the Gadsup language and lifeways. I further predicted that care beliefs and practices would influence the health, wellbeing, or illness expectations of the people. Since nurses function in different kinds of environments with people, I was interested in the environmental context and ecological factors and I predicted these aspects would influence care, health, and illness patterns. The concepts of environmental context and worldview were new in nursing at that time, yet I believed they were extremely important to nursing. Finally, the three predicted modes for action and decision were viewed with the idea that if a non-Gadsup nurse were to function in the village, culture-specific care would be essential to provide acceptable, effective, and satisfying care. The idea of culturally congruent care was predicted to be important for nursing care practices.

Essentially, I used the same assumptive premises as stated in my theory in Chapter 1 except for these additional statements:

1. In a nonWestern culture where there has been limited external contact by Western peoples, human care knowledge would probably provide different epistemic and naturalistic care meanings and patterned expressions of a culture.
2. If nontechnological care practices exist, they will provide new kinds of knowledge of insights about human caring.
3. The ecological context of a culture will influence care meanings and health expressions.

Conceptualizing this study was difficult because there was no published literature or completed general *ethnographic* studies on the Gadsup of the Highlands of New Guinea. Therefore, I had to envision as best I could what possibly might be the lifeways of the people and prepare myself for the New Guinea culture area and its people.

Review of the Literature on the Gadsup and Culture Care

In the 1960s, no research studies had been completed on the Gadsup. The more general culture area in which the Gadsup live, the Eastern Highlands, had had few contacts with Western ideas and people—the geography and many diverse cultures therein were largely awaiting investigation. In 1959, Dr. James Watson (1963), at the University of Washington in Seattle, saw this need and began a series of multidisciplinary studies in the Eastern Highlands of New Guinea where the Gadsup lived to obtain physical, geographic, linguistic, and cultural anthropological data. I was invited to participate in this microevolution multidisciplinary study of four cultures under Dr. Watson (1963), and chose to focus on the Gadsup. A few other anthropologists also were phased in to study the other cultures in the Highlands over a ten-year period. Since the late 1960s and mid 1970s, a series of publications, the Anthropological Studies in the Eastern Highlands of New Guinea, have provided important information about some Eastern Highland cultures, including the Gadsup: McKaughan's (1973) linguistic studies on the Highland languages; Pataki's (1970) study on the ecology and geography of the Highlands; and Watson and Cole's (1977) study on the prehistory of the Highlands. In 1975, du Toit's study became available on the Gadsup, but it did not focus on my proposed study dimensions and there was limited information on folk health practices. During and since this time, I have written about some different aspects of the Gadsup, but primarily from a nursing care, health, and lifecycle perspective (Leininger 1966a, 1970, 1978b, 1979, 1985).

This study was an entirely new focus in nursing and a different approach to establish knowledge about nonWestern for transcultural nursing. Again, the nursing literature in this area was nonexistent when the study was initiated. McCabe (1960) had, however, begun to use a mental health training grant to incorporate selected social science concepts into an undergraduate program, but it was not a research study nor was it focused on human care. Later, Horn (1978) and Aamodt (1978) became interested in culture care and did research on the Muckleshoots and Papago in the United States. Since then, other care studies have been done in nursing mentored by Leininger with Bohay (1989), Gates (1988), Rosenbaum (1990), Spangler (1991), Stasiak (1990), and Wenger's (1988) research focused on the theory of Culture Care and reported in this book.

Orientational Definitions

The orientational definitions for the theory are presented in Chapter 1 except for a definition of the Gadsup: Gadsup refers to a nonWestern culture living in the Eastern Highlands of the Island of New Guinea in which their language, nontechnological lifeways, material items, social structure, ecology, and lifeways set them apart from Western cultures in the world.

Potential Significance of the Study

There were a number of potential significant features of this study for nursing and for other disciplines interested in human care and health. This was the first transcultural human care study done in a non-Western culture. The people had never seen or worked with a white, single nurse researcher. This historical study opened the door for subsequent Western and nonWestern transcultural nursing studies focused on comparative care, health, wellbeing, and illness patterns. Second, the study provided the epistemic and ontologic base of emic nursing knowledge about the meanings, expressions, and experiences of human care, and their relationship to health, illness, and wellbeing studied within the Culture Care theory. It was a first study in nursing to focus on the universals and differences within a specific culture and environment using Culture Care theory to explicate care and health knowledge in nursing. Third, the study provided the first longitudinal and comparative nursing study of culture care, covering approximately one year in two villages, and by a nurse researcher prepared in anthropology and nursing to collect and analyze the data. This study also was the first diachronic research in nursing to determine how the culture(s) changed over time, an extremely important aspect in the understanding of culture changes and nursing. Fourth, this study involved the first use of the ethnonursing method with the theory of Culture Care. Even today, this approach remains a new idea and is just beginning to be studied for its importance in nursing. Again, the method was designed to study some of the most invisible and little-known aspects of human care as the essence of nursing. Fifth, the nurse researcher lived immersed one year in the same village. The ethnonursing method provided one of the longest and most continuous observational and participatory studies in nursing, a unique feature never before done by a nurse researcher. Sixth, the first transcultural nursing study was done by the first nurse anthropologist. The study provided multidisciplinary collaborative contributions to anthropology and other disciplines. Seventh, this study was an indepth, inductive, ethnonursing comparative investigation within the qualitative paradigm. The researcher compared two village groups for differences and similarities in the same language, culture, and ecological setting and at the same synchronic time period. Due to space limitations, however, only one village (Akuna) is presented here. Nonetheless, this study remains today as the only intervillage comparative nursing study and offers a different approach to study nursing phenomena.

Research Methods, Informants, and Enablers

The ethnonursing method was purposely developed and used to discover culture care meanings, expressions, patterns, and lived experiences of a nonWestern culture with a focus on diverse influencers on health or wellbeing. (See Chapter 2 for a detailed account of the method.) Although the ethnographic method (Leininger, 1985) also was used to obtain a detailed descriptive account of the total lifeways of the people, only the ethnonursing method will be discussed here. It also is important to state that while I studied two Gadsup villages in the early 1960s in the Eastern Highlands of New Guinea, only the Gadsup Akunans data will be reported here.

After arriving in Akuna, I soon found myself surrounded by 260 Gadsup Akunan villagers who lived in an open grassland (kunai) ecological environment with a small forested area on the edge of their village. The Akunans spoke an Eastern Highland language with some dialect differences within and between Gadsup villages. I lived in a bamboo and grass hut which was given to me by the villagers. My 24-hour participation in the daily and nightly lifeways of the people provided a unique opportunity to study in considerable detail their lifeways and to obtain a comprehensive picture of practically every facet of their life. During my one-year stay, I had no major or extended leaves from the village except to go on occasion to a small trade town about 25 miles from the village.

After being in the village for about one month, I chose 35 key informants of both sexes for in-depth observations, participant experiences, and interviews. Since there were no calendars, clocks, or written records in the villages, the information sources were oral narrations, observations, and material culture items. I held at least four to five special interviews (often more) with all key informants. Among these key informants were ten children and adolescents of approximately 5 to 16 years of age. All remaining Gadsup Akunans, about 200 in number, served as general informants. I visited all villagers at least once, knew their names, kinship ties, and something about each one. The key informants met these criteria: (1) they expressed an interest in having four to five visits with me; (2) they had lived practically all of their life in the village and knew the day and night lifeways of the people; (3) they understood Melanesian Pidgin English or could communicate with a native translator; and (4) they were interested in talking about "their village ways," which included their worldview, social structure, and other components depicted in the Sunrise Enabler and bearing on Culture Care theory. I did not begin indepth interviews with key informants until after the third month and only when the people were reasonably comfortable with me as a friend. This decision was extremely important in gaining the trust of a nonWestern people whose culture was markedly different from my own.

I began the study by using the Observation-Participation-Reflection enabling guide (described in Chapter 2), a helpful adjunct in learning about the people's daily lifeways with a focus on care, health, and illness patterns. In my interaction with the villagers in their environment, I gradually learned their kinship ties, special roles, and responsibilities in the village. During this time, I took detailed field journal notes on the naturalistic and patterned lifeways of the children and adults as well as what constituted typical day and night activities. I became fully immersed in the people's lifeways, learning much about them through direct observation, gradual participation, and reflection to assess the meanings of what I saw, heard, and experienced. I observed their caring rituals, symbols, and some of their most covert, secretive practices about health care. As the villagers became more comfortable with me, they became my 'teachers' and I encouraged them in this role to learn as much as I could about them. I showed interest in all villagers and their animals, trees, gardens, mountains, flowers, huts, rituals, and anything they identified as influencing their care, health, and wellbeing.

Gradually, they described their history, legends, myths, and material artifacts—bows, arrows, war shields, sorcerer's substances. Later they described their male and female ceremonial rituals and secrets that influenced their care and wellbeing. I continued as a *learner* and *researcher*, letting the people teach me the what, why, and how of their culture, and according to their readiness to share ideas with me. The Gadsup taught me about their traditional noncaring enemies and caring friends, their past and current lifeways, and how these factors influenced caring, health, and illness patterns. My total immersion and involvement in their lifeways provided rich, dense, meaningful data from key and general informants. The inductive *emic* ethnonursing method was fully and continuously used with the Observation-Participation-Reflection Guide, which kept me focused and helped me to enter and remain in their world. It also was a valuable way to learn from and move with the people in their life rhythms rather than by more conventional Western modes.

The Leininger Stranger–Friend Guide (described in Chapter 2) was an extremely valuable enabling mode to assess my role as stranger and my movement into the village. I had developed the guide before going to New Guinea as a research aid conceptualized with the theory of Culture Care. It helped me to reflect on and gauge my behavior with the people as a stranger and as I became a trusted friend. Unquestionably, the Akunans first saw me not only as a stranger, but as a potential sorceress, with all the distrust and distancing behaviors implied by that perception. Some villagers "tested me" in several ways to determine my reaction— for example, did I value their food, their children, and general lifeways? Was I a "good woman" like their women, and how was I different? By the third month, I had become *their friend* and during my stay a 'true friend.' Indicators on the aforesaid enabler, such as sharing secrets and trusting, were important guides to measuring acceptance and trust by the villagers. In addition, such indicators were important for my survival—these people had been known as "headhunters of the Highlands." In fact it was only a few years before I arrived that the Australian government had stopped open tribal fighting in the Gadsup villages. A stranger, however, was still considered as a potential sorcerer (male) or sorceress (female) and could cause illnesses, trouble in the village, and even deaths. As a single woman without a husband and children, it was natural that I would be considered as a potential sorceress. Although I disliked this role assigned to me, it was necessary to understand it both for my survival and for a successful field study. As a result the people felt they had to watch me closely when I first arrived, so that I would not cause them harm, or become an active, destructive sorceress. Likewise, I watched their behavior to protect myself and to communicate effectively and appropriately with them. Shifting from a potential sorceress to a true friend was a formidable challenge. I also was quite aware of the potential consequences should they have declared I was a malevolent sorceress or a "no good woman." Although this nursing and anthropological research involved such "high risk," I had confidence that I could gain their trust and friendship by being alert to my own actions so they were not misinterpreted as non-caring or harmful to the Akunans. My clinical skills in psychiatric mental health nursing kept me alert to unexpected nonverbal cue behavior even though some Gadsup nonverbal cues did not have the meanings similar to those found in America. It also was difficult to "read the people" due to language difficulties—only a few men could speak pidgin English. It was only when they began to call me "their friend" and trusted me with secrets and confirmed what I had seen and heard, that I knew I had shifted from actual stranger and potential sorceress to *true friend*.

During my stay, I kept detailed, continuous, and extensive field journal notes. I sent copies of my journal to my home in the United States whenever I could find ways to mail them in order to preserve the data. I also used selected tape recordings for care narratives and used photographs of the people to document detailed and complex phenomena. The photographs were used as an enabling method to capture caring episodes and the diverse, daily environmental contexts that men, women, and children experienced. The photographs, while providing rich insight, also were intriguing. The people were initially frightened by the camera, but later treasured the photos for their dead ancestors. Other features of the ethnonursing method used are described in Chapter 2.

Gadsup Land and Ethnohistory Overview: Entering and Learning from the People

The Gadsup Akunans live on the Island of New Guinea, which is about 1,500 miles long, 500 miles wide, and only 6 degrees from the equator. New Guinea is shaped like a big bird with its tail straddling Australia and its head flying towards Asia (see Figure 4-1). It is one of the most densely populated islands in the world with nearly 600 distinct cultures and many different languages (with dialect differences) and cultures. The Gadsup territory was an Australian Trust Territory and under Australian government until it became independent as Papua New Guinea in 1964 (Leininger, 1966a, 1966b).

The Akunans live in the Eastern part of the Eastern Highlands near the Markham Valley. The country is beautiful with green grasslands, large areas of new forest, and some distant high mountain ranges. The

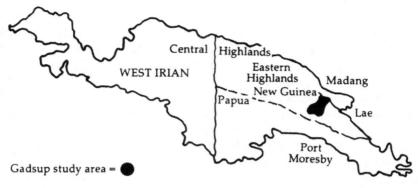

Figure 4-1 The Island of New Guinea

air was always fresh and clean with no industrial plants to pollute the
environment. The mild temperature ranged between 58 degrees
Fahrenheit at night and 85 degrees Fahrenheit in the daytime. Slight
fluctuations occurred during the dry and rainy seasons. The average
rainfall reported by patrol officers (while I was living there) was about
85 inches per year. The ecology revealed two major types of vegetation:
grassland (kunai) that the Akuna village largely represented, and the
more dense forest (bush) areas that the second village represented. The
Akuna environment was covered largely with tall kangaroo grass
(kunai) and had a few small streams about one mile from the village.
There also were dense patches of pit-pit (a reed-like grass), and a small
forested area on the edge of the village.

The Akunans had many vegetable gardens. Taro and sweet potatoes
were their main source of food. From these gardens came sweet potatoes, taro, greens, comsquash, beans, and other native vegetables.
There were many varieties of sweet potatoes along with the very old
taro plants. New gardens first were cleared by the men (slash-and-burn
method) and turned over to the women who were the managers, pro-
ducers, distributors, and controllers of the gardens. The women took
much pride in working their gardens and involved young girls (from
about seven years of age) to elderly women. When the elderly had "less
muscle" to do garden work, they would stop such work and remain in
the village plaza to care for children and provide surveillance of the
plaza for all villagers.

The small forested area on the edge of the Akuna village was largely
used and explored by men for hunting and to inspire young males to see
the forest as "their male area of intrigue." In the forest area were betel
nut, pandanus nut, fruit-bearing pandanus palms, breadfruit, banana

palms (of great variety), and bamboo in addition to birds and animals. Fruit from several of these trees was used for food. Bamboo tree products were used for house building, cooking, and as containers for carrying water from the streams to the village each day. The Akuna children often found big edible mushrooms and seasonal nuts in the bush or forest area. The young boys and men would spend many hours in the forest hunting marsupials and birds, gathering nuts and mushrooms, and searching for other food sources. They also would collect tree materials to make their bows and arrows and musical instruments. The forest area symbolized the man's world away from the women; the garden represented a woman's world and being away from men.

According to pre-historians, it is believed that the Gadsup area had been inhabited for thousands of years by their ancestors, also hunters and gatherers. There is continued speculation by anthropologists that the New Guinea people, especially the Gadsup, are a pre-Neolithic culture. The many different languages and dialects spoken by the people across the Southern, Central, and Eastern Highlands of the island of New Guinea are of interest as well as the variation in physical features and cultural lifeways of the Gadsup, and of the many other cultures who have lived in the Highlands for at least 800 years or more (Littlewood, 1972; Watson & Cole, 1977).

As the Cessna plane that first brought me to the Gadsup flew over the Eastern Highlands of New Guinea, I was struck by the dense forested area, the absence of highrise buildings, no paved roads or freeways, no billboards, and virtually no cars on the rough winding and narrow dirt roads. The ecology of the Highlands revealed much green vegetation, dense forest areas, and grasslands with high mountain ranges (some recorded at levels reaching nearly 12,000 feet) and the villages built on top of the mountain ridges. There were many active volcanoes that brought forth rich molten ash to nurture the green foliage, but there also were low intensity earthquakes (almost weekly) that the Gadsup feared.

When I first walked into the village of Akuna after a final 25-mile drive in an Australian Land Rover, I climbed over a wooden fence to the staring eyes of almost 15 dark bare-skinned people sitting around an earth oven in the village. Twenty or so bamboo and grass huts circled the village plaza. Most of the villagers were sitting around the earth oven talking and chewing on betel nut, and others (young children and adolescents) were walking about the village plaza. The wooden fence that surrounded the village divided a 'lower' and 'upper' village area which had several enclosed gardens nearby. At one end of the Akuna village was a church building, which I later found was built by Lutheran missionaries. According to du Toit (1975), the church had its history in the village some years ago. Prior to World War I the northern part of New Guinea was occupied by Germans and their missionaries, who came into the Gadsup area. With the outbreak of the war against Germany, this part of the Eastern Highlands of New Guinea was occupied by Australian forces. The Lutheran missionaries still had claims to the church, however, and occasionally a minister from the New Guinea coast came to Akuna. The religion was limitedly valued by the Akunans as it was not congruent with their beliefs.

Returning to my entry in the Akuna village, I observed that it was the Akunan men who stood up in a protective stance as the gatekeepers of the village when I entered. Three of the men spoke Melanesian pidgin as a shorthand mode of communication. After I attempted to clarify in pidgin who I was and my interest in coming to the village, I observed that they listened but did not seem eager for me to stay. I then sat with the villagers around the earth oven and let them look me over as I did likewise. The people were short in stature with dark brown skin and dark brown eyes. Their hair was short and tightly curled. The women were about 5'5" tall, while the men were about 5'8" in height.

The women weighed about 125 pounds and the men about 150–160 pounds. I saw no Akunans who were overweight or extremely malnourished. The adult women wore traditional grass skirts made out of reed grass with nothing covering the upper part of their bodies. Several women wore what later became known to me as a *mission blouse* (a blouse the missionaries felt the women should wear to cover their breasts). The men wore shorts while some older men wore traditional bark skirts. The adult and young girls always wore grass skirts from birth through old age, which changed in size and style throughout the lifecycle. In contrast, the young boys were naked until seven or eight years, after which they wore a *lap* (cloth wrap around the waist) or shorts that they had obtained at the trade store. The shorts were recent attire introduced by the Australians. If the boys had funds or could trade local homegrown foods or material village artifacts, they usually obtained a pair of shorts, which they valued. During my stay in the village, the majority of Akuna women wore their traditional grass skirts while the men wore shorts or laps. The mission blouses worn by several women were usually very dirty because the women had no means to clean them. With the women's traditional grass skirts they could be disposed of when dirty and new skirts could be made almost overnight.

After the people agreed to let me stay, they gave me an old, unoccupied hut and nothing else. Since they were skeptical of who I was and did not fully understand why I would want to live in the village with them, they offered me little else until I became their friend. They thought "my husband or kin would soon join me," and remained as curious of me as I

of them. Although I was concerned about living alone with only one suit-
case of clothes and virtually no American foods or necessities, I was
committed to learn from and stay with the villagers. My Nebraska farm
life, my own experience of hard times during the depression of the 1930s
and 1940s with the drought, plus my Irish wit and spiritual values and
German tenacity helped to sustain me while in New Guinea.

Typical Days and Nights of the Akunans

The Akunans' typical days and nights helped me to identify caring and
health patterns in their environments. I observed that the Akunans'
huts were built closely together in the village—the people had grown
quite dependent on each other over the years for protection, surveillance, and general wellbeing. Relying on their garden and forest foods
and other aspects of their ecology for their daily livelihood and for sociocultural ceremonial activities required the Akunans to know their
ecology intimately within the boundaries of the Gadsup territory.

The typical day began without the aid of any clock or watch. The
Akunans judged their time for awakening and for daily and nightly tasks
by the sun, dry and wet seasons, lifecycle events, vegetation growth patterns, earthquakes, births, marriages and death ceremonies, and by special events or happenings in the community—natural-cultural rhythms
which reduced stress and obviated time watching. After they awakened
around 5:30 A.M. (my time), the men walked about in the village plaza to
see if all was as it should be and then returned to munch on morning
foods. The women, however, were usually the first to awaken to crying
babies or children wanting food. Depending on the dry or rainy season,
the women usually started the fire within or outside their hut to cut the
coolness of the morning and to heat water. The earth oven (a shallow pit
in the ground with small rocks on the bottom) was used to cook food.
The area around the earth oven was used to observe children and pigs,
and as a social center for talking, gossiping, and planning day or night
activities. The women used small branches of trees and dry leaves for
the open oven in which they cooked yams, taro, bananas, or sweet potatoes for their two meals—a light meal in the morning and a heavier meal
at night. Most morning foods had been cooked the previous night, and
villagers munched on the cold sweet potato, taro, sugar cane, or a
slightly warmed-over sweet potato.

After 10:00 A.M. every morning, the women went to their gardens carrying young infants in their string bags and on their heads along with a big
handmade string bag filled with wooden garden tools, cold yams, sugar
cane, and wood. A few girls (ages 9–12) remained in the plaza to care for
their younger siblings or related kin's children. They were assisted in

their caregiving role by a few elderly adult men and women who watch over and protect the children and village. About 10:30 A.M., young boys and adult males strolled to the nearby forest area with their bows and arrows to hunt birds and small animals, collect mushrooms, and bamboo shoots, or to experience the mystical and powerful symbolism of the forest environment. Some men walked to nearby friendly villages to talk to their "fictive brothers or kinsmen" and then, after offering betel nut, foods or other village gifts, would return around 4:00 P.M. From about 10:00 A.M. until nearly 5:00 P.M., the village was empty except for very few people as the women were in their gardens, the men were "walking about" or making "big talk," and the small children were playing under the surveillance of older girls and the elderly. Teenage boys were free to go most anywhere and had virtually no role responsibilities. In contrast, teenage girls were either working with their mothers in the garden, collecting wood, or caring for their siblings.

Around 5:00 P.M., all the Akunans gathered around their earth ovens for the evening meal and to sing and talk about the day's happenings, a perfect time as well to care for children and to share general social experiences with other villagers. The women always prepared the evening meal in the big long oven and usually outside their hut and near those of their kinsmen or lineage. A typical evening meal consisted of baked yams, sweet potatoes, taro, breadfruit, native beans, greens, seasonal corn, squash, bananas, and sugar cane. If the men and young boys had been successful in the forest world, they may have brought back flying foxes, bird meat, and seasonal nuts. On very special occasions, wild and domestic pigs were cooked in the earth oven and especially for ceremonial lifecycle events, annual garden feasts, or for food sharing with friendly nearby villagers. The Akunans did not drink milk, soda pop, tea, or coffee, only water from a stream.

It is important to note that pigs were highly valued by all Gadsups. Pigs have long had symbolic meanings related to achieving social status, prestige, and economic gains. Pigs were owned, exchanged, and inherited individually and with lineages. It was interesting to observe the amount of care that small pigs received; the women often defined their role as caring for their children and their pigs. Small house pigs were raised in the huts by women who fed and stroked them until the pigs were able to forage for food outside the village. Attention was given to the foods pigs ate and ways to protect them. In general, pork was the only substantive animal protein eaten—infrequently—and usually prepared only for special ceremonial occasions. Pigs, it must be noted, were generally few in number and highly valued for political and ceremonial exchanges, so their consumption required a special event. The more pigs a Gadsup had, the higher that Gadsup's social status, and pigs lost or stolen were often heated legal topics in village political sessions.

There were cassowary (Wuye) and emo (turkeylike) birds that also were trapped and used for ceremonial purposes. Emo eggs were large and green (about four times the size of a chicken egg). After gaining the villager's trust, these eggs were sometimes presented to me as a special gift, along with cassowary meat. It was of interest that I was given large delicious pineapples, huge white oranges, lemons, passion fruit, and many different kinds of bananas after they trusted me as a "true Gadsup friend." The Akuna men had obtained these fruits by walking great distances (about 25 miles to the Markham Valley). During my initial period in the village, however, when the Akunans watched and distrusted me, I received many dry old sweet potatoes, wilted greens, and virtually no fruit or edible Akunan foods. Thus, one could assess my stranger–friend relationships by the quality and quantity of food given to me.

The eel, symbolic of male strength and viewed as a great delicacy, was another special village food eaten only by males. A male belief persisted that if females ate eel, they would become ill and especially if pregnant. Mushrooms and nuts were highly desired foods, but only available during certain seasons. These foods were often eaten as a midday snack with a cold yam or sweet potato. The big red seed of the pandanus tree was roasted in open fire and enjoyed while the villagers sat around the open earth pit visiting and gossiping about village affairs. All of these foods reflected the Gadsup's long history of food hunting, gathering, and having a small garden-forest subsistence economy. With no means to refrigerate or preserve such foods, they had to be collected and eaten each day. I found no evidence of cancer, heart attacks, or strokes, which I believe was related, in part, to their fresh foods, limited red meat, lots of vigorous garden work for women, and 'walk abouts' for men.

At night, the Akunans would typically sit around the open fire hearth, casually talking or telling stories, laughing, singing, and gossiping about village affairs. Males often talked about their visits to nearby villages and the women talked about their gardens, children, small pigs, and other women matters. Male and female secrets, however, were never shared between sexes. They also talked about sorcery accusations, or threats of enemy villagers, and if someone was ill or dying. Ways to revenge sorcerers and prevent further illnesses and death were discussed in hushed, low-pitched voices. Sometimes men would get their bows and arrows and demonstrate how they fought in the 'old days.' With the recent suppression of fighting, they were unable to engage in open warfare. Sorcery replaced the fighting and was more prevalent. Young male and female children and adolescents were always present at evening meals and for evening talks around the earth oven. Frequently, men and women would smoke or chew tobacco or betel nut. In the rainy season, the villagers stayed inside their family huts and talked about their dead kinsmen and about creation, myths, and about the general Gadsup lifeways that usually had caring and non-caring themes of protective care, wellbeing, and health promotion.

Around 10:00 P.M., the small children villagers went inside their huts and slept on raised bamboo platforms or mats. In keeping with past traditions and segregation of the sexes, the young boys and men went to their male huts. Earlier in the evening, however, the teenage girls and boys would walk about the village with young men trying to woo a girl for marriage. The girls and boys were lodged separately in groups of about five or six. The boys sang love songs to the girls in their family huts or as the girls sat in the village plaza. It was fascinating to hear teenage boys sing these love songs to the young girls without touching them. Sexual relations were reserved for marriage. The teenagers were always discrete, cautious, and used proper etiquette to be attracted to one another. Interestingly, the young girls remained in control of their decision of whom they would marry, and the boy was always thrilled and excited if 'chosen' by the girl. While the parents made suggestions of whom they wanted their offspring to marry, they did not make the final decision. Rather, the girl makes the final decision after talking with her female kinswomen. In addition, if the bride price was arranged satisfactorily between the two families, the wedding ceremony would occur. All Gadsup marriages occurred around the ages of 16, 18, and even older, with the mean age of 19 years. Because of a shortage of Akuna females, Akuna males had to seek marriage partners outside of Akuna. Accordingly, they would make 'afternoon and night walks' to friendly villages to woo girls. Most Akuna marriages were exogamous (marrying women outside of their lineage or clan, but some married within the village if from another clan). Other details of the lifecycle are reported in other publications (Leininger, 1970, 1978b).

To complete the typical night, about midnight or later if there were no special ceremonies requiring dancing, drum beating, and feasting, the adult married men and women went to their huts to sleep. The village elders usually went to bed earlier after the young children went to sleep. Most nights in the Akuna village were active with villagers talking and singing in their huts, or with drum beating in the plaza. There were only three or four hours of silence from about 2:30 A.M. to 5:00 A.M.

Care (Caring) with the Theory Sunrise Enabler Dimensions

Worldview and Care

The Gadsup conceive themselves as having come from 'one vine or root.' They would often say, "We are one . . . We came from the same root and we are *all brothers* . . . We all speak the same language and believe the same things." These worldview statements guided how the Gadsup related and communicated to each other, involving a community caring ethos that supported the belief that they were of one origin. Gadsups spoke of a feeling of *interconnectedness* and *belonging* to each other as a tribe or clan over a long time span despite periodic intervillage feuds and fights. Most older Akunans were aware of their tribal identity (the largest sociocultural group), clan identity, subclan identity, lineages, and of course their extended families. These clan and subclan social ties were especially loose and fragile due to potential feuds and sorcery accusations. The lineage, which could be identified by most older men and women, included those closest in social ties and interdependency along with extended families that grew out of the lineage.

Another related worldview was that there were Gadsup villages that cared about each other and would provide protection in times of threat or losses. Enemy villages, which several called 'noncaring' and which could bring harm to them by sorcery, also existed. There were periods of relation and tension with these changing views of the Gadsup world. Most importantly, they found it difficult to comprehend any world beyond that of nearby New Guineans and the fierce New Guinean fighters in the Highlands. None of the villagers had ever seen a map of the world, and none had attended a school or received a formal education. Only a few men had been to the New Guinea coast; hence, their worldview was quite small in scope. Most Akunans perceived Gadsup land as very big and their whole world. Such an ethnocentric worldview made it very difficult for Akunans to understand people who looked and acted so differently from them. As such, strangers were generally feared, and the question of where and how to place them, whether in their world or outside it, remained of concern to them.

Several key Akunan informants said, "We can have a peaceful and caring social world if we maintain good kinship ties, share foods, and perform our work . . . We must also follow the ways of our good ancestors." They also believed that they would have good health and stay well if they did not break any cultural taboos, values, and practices. When sharing their ideas about caring and health, it was clear that these went beyond individualism or self-care. Instead, they viewed caring as a way of doing good work and acts toward others and especially to other Gadsups in the Highlands. Most Akunans believed that a caring person should always watch out for others and try to protect them, especially those of close lineage and extended family members—mother's brother, father's sister, etc.—and other true Gadsup 'brothers.' They believed that caring relationships defined the particular value known as community. Feuds and sorcery accusations were noncaring and always threatening to the community. A noncaring Gadsup community did not act as 'one vine and as true brothers.' Instead, they acted in noncaring ways. Thus, caring and noncaring worldviews were closely linked together and were a source of concern that could greatly influence wellbeing and health.

Care Embedded in Religious or Spiritual Dimensions

The Gadsup Akunans held that 'true care' could be found in the way their ancestors lived in the past. They believed that when a person died their *'life essence lived on,'* which became a moral, ethical, and spiritual guide to living villagers and especially to those closest to the deceased kin. Practically all key informants said, "My good ancestor continues to care for me and others here even though they are not here." When an Akunan was in trouble, they would petition to their ancestors to guide them to do good and help them get out of trouble. They were always cognizant that if one betrayed or acted counter to the cultural lifeways or norms of the ancestors that revenge and harm could come to them. They especially feared revenge or harm from a recently deceased ancestor whose spirit was very powerful, and so they were always deferent, cautious, and careful how they behaved immediately after a recent kin death, especially a 'Big Man's' death in the village.

Although the Gadsup had no formal doctrine or organized religious beliefs, they did rely on their spiritual beliefs, which were rooted in their life essence and their worship of great ancestors in their daily lives, as guides. The spiritual caring components they spoke about were *surveillance* (to watch over them), *nurturance* (to help them grow as "good Gadsups"), and to provide protective care. These were embedded in their spiritual beliefs and served as a moral guide to prevent illnesses, harm from others, and sudden death.

Although the Lutherans and Seventh Day Adventists had tried to "teach the Akunans some Christian beliefs," they had a very difficult time. These church leaders tried to teach them about God, heaven, hell, and the devil, but these concepts were not in the Gadsup worldview nor in their spiritual ancestral views. The Gadsup found the ideas incongruous with their spiritual life and worldview perspectives. In fact, the Akunans felt at times they were coerced to attend services, learn

Christian beliefs, and had a very difficult time accepting such imported ideas. They experienced cultural imposition conflicts that some felt were non-caring ways of the ministers. The Akunans ancestral spiritual guidance was far more important than trying to learn a foreign religion. Akunans said they always had to be attentive to the spiritual power of their deceased kin as this was a community responsibility so that people's health would not be adversely affected. Akunans would appease the ancestors by offering food, making petitions, and preparing special gifts to them in order to prevent revenge, illnesses, or unfavorable life conditions in the total Gadsup community. Grief expressions for a deceased 'Big Man' of the village who had powerful life essences were observed. An elderly person who lived a full life was not grieved as much as a young child or 'Big Man.' The elderly and children had less powerful life spirits than an active middle-aged man or woman. I often observed situations in which a quick burial of these powerful dead took place within a few hours to reduce unfavorable spiritual harm or threats to their wellbeing and health status. Most importantly, Akunans firmly believed that one must always be attentive to and thus care for the dead as well as the living. To not do so exemplified a noncaring, bad person.

Kinship, Social Relatedness, and Caring Modalities

The kinship and social organizational structure of the Akunans proved to be very complex and difficult to study. From my interviews with the key informants and a number of other villagers along with many genealogies taken, I found most Akunans belonged to extended families, patrilineages, some loose subclans, and a few patricians. Practically all informants saw their identify with the Gadsup tribe as the largest social organization. Most of the older Akunans felt strong ties to the tribe that made them 'one people.' The patrician was recognized in the past as an important leader who was involved in war activities. The few subclans identified were loose in their organizational features, but did constitute groups good at feuds and some past warfare. Members of patrilineages were able to trace their kinship ties with social alignments to specific descent members some recalled, and who usually remained near the extended family in their Akuna village. Members of *extended families* were able to trace their social descent lines through the lineages and usually lived in the same village. According to most key informants, these 'nesting' social structure groupings, especially the extended families and lineages, were quite important in the daily lives of the Gadsup. However, all social structure groupings were said to be stronger in the past before warfare was suppressed. Nonetheless, they were identifiable by several older informants.

Discovering how important the extended families and lineages were in marriages, feuding, political actions, lifecycle ceremonies (birth to death), economic exchanges of food and pigs, and other material exchanges in the daily life of the people proved of great interest. I also discovered strong ethnopsychological feelings and activities between kinsmen that influenced caring and noncaring patterns related to protection, keeping people well, and preventing sorcery. Kinship ties influenced group cooperation, helping others with their work, caring for others when in need, and food exchanges. These positive caring activities maintained village wellbeing, solidarity, and protection.

While I found every Akunan had considerable freedom to make choices and decisions, still these individuals were especially influenced by the cultural values, beliefs, and practices of the extended family and the lineages. The culture identity of the Gadsup Akunan as members of the Gadsup tribe—viewed largely today as the large Gadsup community—was proudly talked about by adult male key informants and some females. While individual decisions were made, they were influenced by kinship ties and the past Gadsup image with its deep historical roots. Although a full discussion of the kinship structure of the Akunans is not possible here, the reader needs to realize that kinship ties and the total social organization present were powerful means to help Akunans feel not only united in some ways, but also 'cared for' and 'cared about' in the village. It was fascinating to hear the villagers talk about the ways kinship ties provided *protective care, surveillance care*, and *nurturant activities* to support their growth, wellbeing, and community relatedness. The informants and my observations showed evident signs of Akunan surveillance patterns and of looking after one's "brothers" (including females) as supported by extended family members still today. Caring activities and attitudes were largely embedded in kinship ties and concomitant tacit behavioral expectations. Teasing out kinship and social structure features took considerable time along with confirmation of the credibility of such kinship ties. The Akunans were not ready to share spontaneously their social or kinship ties, and always wanted me to discover them first before adding any confirmation commitments. This was an interesting challenge, but through documentation of their genealogies and action patterns each day, it was possible not only to inductively confirm these patterns, but also to obtain a picture of how the villagers functioned in terms of social relatedness. Once I had identified the major kinship features, several key informants said to me: "Now you know us and have it right. You speak true and know our ways. We have no more to tell you as you discovered our ways and we are happy." This search revealed how much they valued and kept kinship ties.

Noncaring behaviors were evident when kinship and social expectations were violated, cultural taboos overlooked, and role responsibilities neglected. Noncaring manifestations were usually altered by physical punishments to children, strong negative verbal responses to adults by the villagers, and open talks to those who violated cultural practices. When noncaring villagers caused trouble in the village, they were often denied a role in ceremonies, admonished by elders, and subject to being gossiped about by other Akunans.

Political Dimensions and Care

The Akunan 'Big Men' (as they were called) were the active and respected political orators, decisions makers, and leaders for most internal and external village affairs. Political activities such as pig and food exchanges and dealing with sorcery accusations were in the hands of the 'Big Men.' These village concerns greatly influenced Akunan caring modes and their wellbeing. Gadsup political activity largely focused on how one effectively and successfully dealt with crisis situations, maintained control, and handled local and intervillage affairs. The 'Big Men' had achieved their title and the prestige associated with it by being successful in 'watching out' (surveillance) and 'looking after' the political caring needs of the villagers. Exceptionally skilled in assessing group concerns, handling sorcery accusations, dealing with strangers, holding pig and food ceremonies, and in protecting the villagers, the 'Big Men' had earned their title by repeatedly demonstrating good decision making, proper communication skills, as well as exhibiting bravery in fights and general leadership in the village. They were skilled in handling village problems by listening, seeking different viewpoints, and maintaining a caring attitude for all villagers with equal interest and good will. These political 'Big Men,' usually aged 45–65 years, had considerable village experience dealing with outside and inside village matters in diplomatic and successful ways. They were respected by most Akunans because they used and maintained the cultural values of egalitarianism, social control, protection, moral justice, and respect for all Gadsup people, land, and their past history. At no time did they manifest showy or ostentatious behavior. When conducting political sessions in the village plaza, they exhibited an equal interest in all attending but always kept the interests of the total Gadsup villagers in mind. They were exceptionally skilled in handling matters related to stealing pigs, women, food, property, and discussing sorcery accusations. The political hearings that these political leaders conducted were always open to all Akunans and oftentimes the entire village attended these sessions. The 'Big Men' showed great acumen to handle tense matters in a protective caring way and with fairness and equal consideration to all.

Practically all key informants told me they valued the leadership of the 'Big Men,' but that they had often influenced their thinking prior to the village meetings while in the home hut. This also was an especially important women's secret—how to influence the male leaders without letting other males know. These women leaders gave accounts of how they discussed serious village matters and what they thought ought to be done while talking to their kinsmen or lineage leaders who were 'Big Men.' The women's viewpoints were taken into consideration in village political discussions and were used in some final decisions. Some of their ideas were confirmed with my observations. When the 'Big Men' gave orations about village matters in the plaza, they expressed some women's ideas discussed prior to the meeting. At political meetings, the women usually sat in the outer circle with all the males sitting or standing in the inner circle and near the leader. The women seldom spoke out in public about the issue unless it was an older woman who knew the 'Big Man' well. When asked about this behavior, the Akuna women said it was inappropriate to 'talk out' at these meetings as it was the men who would be ultimately responsible for such big decisions and actions, and besides, they contended that they had already given their ideas to the political leader and 'he usually used them.'

Political actions and good decision making were extremely valued and important to the Akunans as it provided care, protection, and security. Political activities with good leadership prevented serious intervillage feuding, fighting encounters, and curtailed ongoing discontent in the village. Key informants and all other villagers viewed this as 'protective caring.' Caring was embedded in the ways the people acted and made decisions in the village. Political caring was reinforced by the kinship system with social rules for protection and to prevent major intervillage problems from emerging. There were two men in the village, however, with different views on this matter. Both were silently jealous and wanted to be a 'Big Man' leader. A threat to village solidarity and protection, these deviant men became known as 'no goods.' When the Akuna villagers became ill during the first Australian New Guinea election (Leininger, 1966b), these deviant men were viewed as responsible, in part, for the illness problems. In general, the 'Big Men' were most effective in handling village and intervillage problems and to protect the people against threats of illnesses. Unquestionably, political caring increased group solidarity and helped the village to remain in control and maintain a positive image with other Akunans.

Economic Dimensions and Caring

Since the Akunans maintained their daily lives on a very lean subsistence economy, they were constantly attentive to the women who provided garden foods, their most reliable survival resource. Shortly before my arrival, the Akunans had begun to raise coffee trees on a few acres of land via a promotional campaign for cash income by the Australian government. Although the income from selling coffee beans was very small, it helped them to buy shorts, enamel pans, rice, canned fish, salt, tobacco, and several other items Akunans longed for at the nearest trade store. In addition, there was an exchange of money for pigs with nearby villagers—usually for ceremonial food gathering or for marriage and birth ceremonies. Pigs also were used as bride wealth. The major economic sources for wealth or subsistence were the exchange of a small margin of extra garden foods, raising coffee beans, selling or exchanging pigs, and the men and women doing periodic roadwork for the Australian government. (With the latter activity, they were seldom paid. From my experience, women were never paid by the Australian government for their roadwork, even during the rainy season when roads were completely washed out and women did most of the work.)

Reflecting on the Akunan economy and caring, I discovered that health and wellbeing were related to caring and noncaring patterns and that economics influenced care behaviors to maintain the villagers' health. There also were signs of caring patterns with women caring for small children and pigs. Intervillage exchanges of food symbolized Akunan ways of caring for their own people and other Gadsups. The women who controlled the gardens and distributed the foods demonstrated caring and noncaring expressions. Food reflected nurturance as care and provided for the health and wellbeing of their extended families each day. Garden foods, the major substance source, was collected and shared with extended family members daily, but also with lineages on special village affairs. From such sharing came nurturant and protective caring. The women also showed noncaring behaviors when they would withhold food from their husbands, children, or other kinspersons for various reasons, such as wife beating, breaking of cultural taboos, punishing children inappropriately, or neglecting social roles.

Technological Influences and Care

Since the Gadsup Akunans had no modern Western technologies, there was no use of such technologies for physical care. Instead, care was more sociocultural. The villagers had their own material or native garden and hunting technologies that included handmade tools such as wooden digging sticks, stone adzes and hoes, wooden bows, and stone arrows for hunting. In the past, there were war shields and special fighting equipment for intervillage warfare and head hunting for male honor and prestige. Women made their infant and garden string bags, their grass skirts, and pandanus mats for infants. Gadsup men made wooden vessels in which to place their cooked earth oven foods. They also made musical ceremonial instruments such as the small mouth harp, ceremonial drums, bamboo smoking pipes, big head pieces for singsings (dance festivals), and arm and leg amulets. Great care was demonstrated in making these cultural items in good artistic style and usually for practical and functional purposes. Cooperative caring and supportive village behaviors were important among the elders in making sex-linked artifacts as well. Such village artifacts were made as secret sex symbols. Through these activities, then, Gadsup villagers enjoyed their ceremonies, consumed healthy foods, and felt at home in their villages.

Educational, Language, and Caring Influences

The Akunans had only informal or local educational experiences. There was no formal educational system established for the children until the end of my field research. Informal education was largely an enculturation process of helping the child or adult to learn the Gadsup and particularly Akunan culture in order to live properly and survive. Many village kinspeople were involved in helping small children and young boys and girls become enculturated about Gadsup cultural values, taboos, and appropriate living and caring ways in order to avoid intra- and intervillage conflicts or problems. Children and adolescents had positive role models to observe and work with throughout the lifecycle. Experiential learning-in-context was the major teaching and learning mode for all villagers at different periods in the lifecycle. Informal education was achieved by using real, concrete, and practical life situations, and by talking about Gadsup village events, incidents, and ceremonies. Children and adolescents were always free to be active participants in daily and most nightly community affairs. Very few facts of life were hidden from them. A rich oral history replete with legend and information necessary to be a true Akunan was available. In the early 1960s, however, their language had not been completely analyzed by linguistic experts—a major communication handicap for me. I spoke Melanesian pidgin English and also learned some common language expressions. During the first few months, I focused on nonverbal communication and on intense observations and cue behavior to confirm with the people what I had seen and experienced. The Gadsups taught me that my nonverbal American gestures did not accurately communicate meanings to Gadsups. Learning Gadsup gestures with meanings-in-context was extremely important to grasp and understand Gadsup lifeways. It also was important to learn some Gadsup expressions of phrases for my survival, especially when I was feared as a potential sorceress who could cause village harm. Informal verbal and nonverbal learning between researcher and Gadsups occurred daily.

The Gadsups depended greatly on oral narratives to learn about their culture, their nearby world, and most everything of importance to them. As mentioned above, many oral Gadsup creation myths, historical legends, life histories, narrative events, and daily life experiences constituted some of the informal teaching and learning modes used. The Gadsup like these informal teaching and learning ways and often spoke of them as "our good ways." Caring expressions by being patient, helping others to learn, and being protective by being sure you understood the language was important. They also cared for others by sharing daily life experiences and special life events, especially ceremonies.

Caring expressions through informal educational experiences were manifested with caring behaviors related to knowing how to help others, anticipation of other's needs, learning to be a protective sharing Gadsup, groups, and by knowing how to help. others to prevent unhealthy or illness conditions. Learning to avoid violating cultural taboos and discovering ways to be a "good ethical and moral Gadsup" were frequently emphasized by all key and general village informants.

Folk (Generic) Care and Health (Wellbeing) System

For years, the Akunans have relied upon their folk indigenous care system which they claim has helped them to keep well and healthy. The concept of care was used and known in their language and actions.

While *care* and *caring* were used in different ways and with slightly different referent meanings, they generally referred "to *protective* and *nurturant* ways to enable Gadsups to grow, function, and survive" (Leininger, 1966a, 1970). Caring was primarily associated with the idea of nurturing acts to help children and adults to grow holistically; caring was not associated with an intellectual dichotomization of humans into mind and body or biopsychosocial beings. Instead, caring was documented by key and general informants as nurturant lifecycle activities related to growth and development experiences as part of living and being in the Gadsup Akunan world. In discussions with females, caring ideas came easier than in discussions with males, for caring was essential for infant survival and for raising healthy or well children. I observed caring acts of the mother and her female kinswomen in the village as they watched, protected, and held vulnerable newborns both by day and night. Women protected infants and children from external harm such as sorcery, cold air, and occasionally physical harm. Sorcery was always a threat to vulnerable newborn infants and children, especially by outside strangers who used substances such as feces, blood, or "not good foods." Maternal caring was expressed in infant breast-feeding, the mother intuitively knowing the needs of her infant and small children. Stroking, rubbing, talking, and feeding infants were nurturant caring acts. The mother and her kinsmen watched and helped the children grow properly. Such nurturant acts continued throughout the early years of childhood, but changed in form and expression for males and females at about age ten. Nonetheless, caring activities from birth to old age were held as essential for the health or wellbeing of the individual, family, and community despite slightly different processes and activities among the caregivers. Unquestionably, the women carried the heaviest responsibility for nurturant caring activities and attitudes.

While the Gadsup cared for individuals, they also always focused on the village group and what was happening to them. Caring activities for kinsmen and kinswomen were valued and expected in the village. If kin resided in another village, such as a daughter who was married and living in her husband's village (patrilocal), caring concerns prevailed for her. Caring was especially directed to families, lineages, groups, and to sociocultural institutions such as birth, marriage, and death ceremonies. The Gadsup emphases on "*other-care,*" as I referred to this in 1960, was a discovery important for its sharp contrast with present-day American nursing "self-care" ideologies and practices (Orem, 1980).

Several key informants stated, "We care for all Gadsups (referring to the "oneness and unity" concept as the broadest cultural identity of the Gadsup) just like we care for our children, small pigs, and others in our big families." Several key informants added, "It is important that we care for all kinsmen and all in our related groups (referring to the lineage) and to all in our big Gadsup community." Thus, caring was more group and other-care oriented than self-care oriented for individuals. When I asked, "How does caring help your people?", informants usually replied, "It keeps us together, well, and growing healthy . . . It helps to work in our gardens, hunt, and do our village work." While the Gadsup did not neglect individuals and their care concerns or needs, the idea of a community and village care ethos prevailed.

In attempting to discover if there were any differences between care and health, the informants replied, "Health is being able to do our work each day . . . *Health is being able to go to our gardens each day* (females)." Others said, "When we can no longer do our daily work, we have to stay in this village like our elderly men and women, then we are not as healthy." They added, "We die when our muscles are no longer able to function or if a sorcerer or sorceress kills us." Many informants said, "If we care for our people with food, watching out for them (surveillance and protection), then we can protect them from sorcery and enemies . . . But we must also watch that they do not break village taboos, so they will remain well and be healthy." The concept of health, therefore, was differentiated from the concept of care as delineated above. Care and caring remained the powerful explanatory means to keep people well, healthy, and prevent illness in the village.

Folk care practices using local material substances that included ritual caring acts were more fully known to Akunan females than males. The women were able to identify the caring acts and ways they cared for villagers to prevent potential harm and the threat of illnesses or death. In contrast, males were far more oriented to curing acts and knew how to call on curers as specialists outside the village to deal with selected illnesses, major body injuries (fractures), or to cure powerful illnesses due to male sorcery. These findings were repeatedly confirmed and established as patterns of care and cure with ethnonursing and ethnoscience linguistic analysis of village data (Leininger, 1970). Findings from this fieldwork provided the first evidence that care and cure are gender linked and that there are different ways of caring and curing with females and males. Caring was viewed as largely a female role whereas curing was viewed as a male role in Gadsup land and throughout their long prehistory. (Parenthetically, this may be a precursor to early professional Western practices in nursing and medicine.)

While special medicines were used in Gadsup caring and curing practices, emphasis was given to caring ways as a means to prevent illness and maintain wellbeing. This finding was confirmed repeatedly. It helped me realize the great importance of care and caring, and the role of nurses as care providers in illness prevention and health maintenance—an idea in direct contrast to the Western view of the nurse as a medicine dispenser, a handmaiden to physicians, or as some other "medical" technician. The Gadsup helped me to become keenly conscious of the significant role of women as caring experts.

Folk caring was symbolically expressed by selecting special foods for the pregnant spouse before, during, and occasionally after pregnancy. These food preferences surrounding pregnancy were known in the village, and it was the husband who often walked great distances to get such foods. In addition, mothers, brothers, mothers' sisters, and close kinsmen showed anticipatory and nurturant caring for pregnant women by buying or requesting special food from strangers or friends. Caring by mothers in breast-feeding their newborns and their young children (ages 2–5) were examples of caring as nurturance to help Akunans grow, be healthy, avoid illnesses, and become strong, healthy, and active men and women. These attributes also had economic benefits in the prevention of costly illnesses or death.

Folk caring modalities to prevent sickness and death and to protect the villagers from sorcery accusations and actions were documented and confirmed on repeated occasions. Many folk preventive carative measures were identified when villagers would alert other careless villagers about the disposal of their hair clippings, nails, and human excreta. They also watched for signs of the villagers violating cultural taboos or breaking village rules. Such actions were identified as noncaring behaviors and given negative sanctions by family or friends. Acts of surveillance, protection, and prevention measures were often documented within and outside the village to prevent illnesses (largely related to sorcery) or careless behaviors. Folk caring behaviors also were manifested at village ceremonies related to newborns, at marriage ceremonies, at village feasts, and at death ceremonies. For example, men's legs were pricked with leaves to reduce edema after hours of ceremonial dancing. Many other folk practices were used as caring to promote healing and wellbeing.

Unquestionably, the Gadsup were deeply interested in and concerned about *prevention* as an important caring modality. Modes of prevention were based on maintaining cultural norms and practices rather than focusing primarily on physical activities or psychological factors as emphasized in most Western health systems. Preventing children or adults from becoming physically ill or experiencing threats to health or to their lives could be prevented by maintaining cultural rules or norms. Adult key female informants often made these statements: "We must teach our children how to protect themselves so they won't get sick and die . . . We teach them our ways—the good ways to act . . ." ". . . We love our children and we do not want them to die . . ." "We must watch (surveillance) that our infants and children do not have sorcerers making them ill and die . . ." "We also must help our adolescents not get into big intervillage trouble in our own village feuds as some adults get too angry and kill each other like they did in the past. . . ." "We teach them to obey our ways." These verbatim statements and others supported evidence that watchfulness, protection, and prevention were all important caring modes in Akunan life.

Primary caregivers were adult women and young girls (7–14 years). Acutely ill males with distended abdomens, sorcery pains, and back pain would occasionally go to experienced female caregivers even though they feared possible contamination by menstrual blood. The majority of males went to male curers in other friendly Gadsup villages for curing treatments related to breaking culture taboos, broken bones, arrow tip injuries, cuts, and other unknown conditions.

Every two to three months the Australian government provided the services of a public health nurse and a "doctor boi" (a native helper who spoke pidgin English and English) at a health station nearly two miles away from the village. The Australian Patrol officers told the Akunan villagers "to bring their small children to these stations for medicines." Gadsup women were most reluctant to do this, however. They believed that the danger of their small child being exposed to sorcery and other cultural illnesses by the nurses outweighed any possible benefits of the visit. Consequently, only five or six women would go, and then reluctantly, to the nurse station. While with the nurse, the child was weighed and given immunizations. During these procedures, mothers and their infants and small children grew very frightened and they put a white powdered substance on the child's fontanel to protect the child from harm. The health nurse, usually not aware of the great fear of the mothers, was not too effective in her efforts. This nurse focused mainly on the physical condition of the child, weighing, checking his or her skin, and trying to immunize the child. The nurse had no knowledge of her client's culture and how culture influenced health and illness states.

There was a small hospital about 25 miles from the Gadsup village, but this service was seldom used by the villagers; they feared it was a "house of sorcery." Periodically, when I visited this hospital, I could see the fear of many natives who came there. Infrequently, Akunans came there for an illness that did not respond to folk practices. While in the two Akunan villages I studied, I found no evidence of cancer, mental psychoses, or heart attacks. There were, however, sorcery conditions, pneumonia (during rainy season), and gastrointestinal disturbances (i.e., villagers with diarrhea). Skin lacerations, broken bones, and head injuries were other common health conditions of the Akunans. The latter were often due to fights within or at another village and were more common in men than women. Occasionally, however, I found women with head and body injuries due to women fighting over men in adulterous relationships. The women, however, seldom went to the hospital. Children and elderly died most frequently due to pneumonia during the rainy season. During my return visit in 1978, the Akunans suffered new kinds of illnesses: drug dependency, broken bones due to car accidents (not fights), and severe malnutrition. The impact of Western contacts and a poor cash economy, plus other factors too numerous to discuss here, had markedly changed the Akunan caring and health status. Clearly, the health status of Akunans was more favorable in the early 1960s than in late 1978.

Cultural Value Influences

Thus far I have identified and discussed some of the major Gadsup Akunan cultural values as derived from grounded *emic* ethnonursing and ethnographic data. These values, extremely important to understand culture care fully, were embedded in the social structure and values of the Gadsup and can be summarized as follows:

1. *Patriarchialism* was a protective care value evident in males with decision making authority in diverse aspects of the social structure as reflected in the daily lifeways of the people.
2. *Extended family ties and social relatedness* were important culture care values which influenced Gadsup patterns of relationships to different groups, and in marriage, birth, festive, and death ceremonies. Kinship care patterns and relationships influenced what was acceptable and nonacceptable behavior in the village and with nonGadsups.
3. *Egalitarianism* was identified as a cultural value reflecting ways the villagers attempted to maintain and value equal peer relationships and to avoid 'showy man or woman behaviors.' 'Big Men' in the village had to watch their behavior in political and economic affairs and not be too different from other village men.
4. *Acknowledging gender differences* was a cultural care value held to be extremely important among the Gadsups. Males and females had different care roles related to their capabilities and responsibilities. Female and male secrets were important in all ceremonies and rituals, and were viewed as complementary attributes of the sexes. Separate material objects and symbols were valued, owned, and used by males and females for caring.
5. *Maintaining communal caring relationships* was a value upheld by the Akunans who saw themselves as part of the largest social and cultural Gadsup community. They believed they came from 'one vine' (symbol of continuity, growth, and unity) and should remain aligned. Care as hospitality and communal respect was expected among all Gadsups. Communal care values within and outside the villages were held to prevent unfavorable relationships, hostilities, open aggression, feuds, and sorcery accusations. However, open feuds did occur in the larger Gadsup communities despite efforts to suppress them. The care values of surveillance, protection, and communal assistance among 'Gadsup brothers' were expected to prevent noncaring acts.

6. *Experiential learning* was greatly valued because it was essential to help Akunans discover and know their ecology (immediate physical environments) including: trees and plants, animals, material culture, legends, and all aspects of current and past Gadsup life. Gadsups were expected to care by sharing whatever they learned with other villagers and to use their spiritual lessons from Gadsup ancestors. Concrete, practical, and mundane caring life experiences were important to know and to transmit to current and future generations. These cultural values and others (along with many beliefs) were confirmed and had meaning-in-context and shared recurrent patterning in the Akunan daily lifeways.

Thematic Data Analysis and Culture Care Theory

During the 18-month period I spent in two villages conducting this ethnonursing and ethnographic study, I gathered much new knowledge and experiences. Detailed observations and participatory experiences along with tape recordings of stories and photos brought forth meaningful data of Akuna care, health, and lifeways. The full account will be published in a forthcoming book, but here only major findings related to the theory of Culture Care Diversity and Universality will be presented.

Data analysis specific to the ethnonursing method was done in accord with Leininger's Ethnonursing Phases of Analysis for Qualitative Data Analysis already explained in Chapter 2. Data bearing on the theory were systematically examined using the five qualitative criteria discussed in Chapter 2. I systematically collected, recorded, and analyzed all raw or grounded field data beginning from the first day in the village. I also made nightly observations to obtain a full account of caring for a 24-hour period. The local people were a very rich source of data to discover themes and other findings related to the domain of inquiry. I analyzed all ethnonursing *emic* data from Phase 1 (raw data) to Phase 2 which focused on specific descriptors and components as revealed in the Sunrise Enabler. In Phase 3, data were studied for recurrent patterns, specific contextual meanings, and credibility. Finally, in Phase 4, themes were abstacted reflecting diverse or similar research findings from both *emic* and *etic* data.

In this next section, I will demonstrate how I arrived at themes from Phases 1, 2, 3, and 4 using one major theme. Space does not permit such an explication for the remaining themes. Before presenting one example of one theme and findings, however, I should discuss some culture care constructs to bring forth fuller meanings from the findings.

These *culture care emic* constructs were largely embedded in data related to the worldview, social structure, language environment, and folk care system. They would be essential to help the transcultural nurse to focus on each care construct to provide congruent care to Gadsup Akunans. Below are presented *culture care meanings and action modes* in order of greatest importance to the villagers (established largely with the criteria of credibility, confirmability, recurrent patterning, and saturation) (Leininger 1987, 1990).

1. *Surveillance* (looking out for or watching out for is surveillance care). Two kinds of surveillance were identified, namely *surveillance nearby* and *surveillance-at-a-distance*. These modes of surveillance were held important for wellbeing and health of all Akunan key and general informants. The commitment to be surveillant was seen repeatedly in practice in the village by all villagers but especially in the gardens by the women and in the forest by the men. Women were more surveillant than men; men were more watchful with protective care outside of the village.

2. *Protection* (protective care and caring). This construct was extremely important to the Akunans. It had two major features, namely (1) *protecting Akunans inside and outside the village*; and (2) *protective care of infants throughout the lifecycle*. Protective village care was manifested by daily observations and participatory activities and *obeying cultural taboos and sanctions*. Such protective care was critical to protect the villagers from sorcery, illnesses, death, and unfavorable cultural situations. Lifecycle protective care for children was well maintained by women. The men were more effective in providing protective village care with outsiders and strangers.

3. *Nurturance* (nurturant care and caring). Nurturance was manifest in women primarily with ways they helped infants and adults grow and survive in Gadsup land. The women were resourceful in providing nurturance which was an integral part of child and adolescent care. Women informants said, "We believe in nurturance for our survival . . . it helps children grow and be good strong Gadsup." Males learned how to nurture boys and young married men by teaching them hunting and forest survival skills. This concept of nurturance was the first concept identified in transcultural nursing research and it supports the epistemic roots of nursing being derived from nurturance with special meanings to the Gadsup. This was an important discovery in the 1960s, and is still little studied in nursing.

4. *Prevention* (preventive care and caring ways). This care construct was an integral part of Gadsup daily and nightly living to avoid negative sanctions, harm to people, illnesses, disabilities, and sudden death. Preventive care also was manifested by caring actions such as avoiding intervillage conflicts, problems, and stresses which could lead to feuds, potential killing, or harming of the villagers. Prevention as caring was demonstrated through cultural stories, legends, and narratives. All villagers were active supporters for preventive caring modes, and if not, one was suspected to be a sorcerer or a 'deviant person.'

5. *Respecting sex differences.* Care meant respect for and observance of differences between males and females from birth to death. Role responsibilities and other activities by each sex were features of being a caring Gadsup. Caring as respecting sex taboos reduced village stresses and illness. All villagers upheld their longstanding beliefs in sex differences in work roles, play, and other facets of Akunan life in a caring community.

6. *Touching* (touching as care and caring). Touching was expressed by bare body hugs mainly between men, and by women stroking, rubbing, and kissing infants. Women touched infants for growth, stimulation, and consolation. Intimate touching between sexes was only for married persons. If sexual intercourse occurred outside of marriage and was discovered, this led to fights and other serious repercussions. The firm shaking of a child for not obeying cultural taboos was used, but seldom were any severe punishments inflicted. Intensive touching in domestic quarrels, or in male or female feuds, was also identified. Wife and spousal abuse did occur but was viewed as noncaring behavior.

Major Theme Findings

As one examines a major theme of the Akunans in light of the theory and Leininger's mode of data analysis, one will note special features and findings.

Major Theme One

Culture care means surveillance and protective action to ensure the health or wellbeing of Gadsup Akunans.

This major theme was confirmed repeatedly as credible and important by all key informants and over 90 percent of all the village informants in Akuna village. Several said to me, "Now you speak true of us and know

our lifeways . . . This is our lifeways and what we believe is important."
Some verbatim statements with action patterns were examples establishing confirmability, credibility, and meanings-in-context of theme one at each phase of Leininger's (1987, 1990) data analysis. [Code: FAKI = Female Adult Key Informant; MAKI = Male Adult Key Informant]

Phase 1: Documentation with Raw *Emic* (Local) Care Data

FAKI: "We watch over our infants, small boys and girls and others in the village so that no harm comes to them; We keep healthy and well because we protect our children from sorcery, illnesses, and outside threats to us."

MAKI: "Akuna men know how to watch at a distance . . . We watch over the grassland, our enemies and friends, and down the road to protect our villagers from strangers and sorcerers. . ." "It is a man's protective job to do this and not a woman's."

Phase 2: Care Descriptors and Components *(only key phrases are identified from the raw data)*

FAKI: *Watching over* is important for health and wellbeing; *Watching* and *being there* and *over the person*; *Protecting* is done by *watching out for others* (demonstrated by many actions of *watching over* and *watching for* others).

MAKI: "Must *protect* our children and adults . . . *Watch out for the sorcerers* is essential . . . Our families, lineages, and villages need to be protected day and night . . . In the past we had surprise attacks and some did not watch well, we lost villagers."

Phase 3: Care Patterns and Meanings-in-Context Features *(stated as patterns from above descriptors and components)*

FAKI: *Female patterns*: (1) The researcher found that every morning for nine months the women and young girls went to the garden (universal); (2) Mothers placed their infants in net bags on a post that held the child in a pandanus mat to protect them (universal); (3) Mothers relied on young girls (7–12 years) to protect and watch over siblings to keep well; (4) Women watched over adolescent girls when delivering betel nut to strangers for their wellbeing. (The meanings-in-context can be trailed to the raw data.)

MAKI: *Male patterns*: (1) Accompanied young boys with their bows and arrows into forest area to hunt animals, to eat, to be spiritually inspired, and to be healthy; (2) Men watched over villagers and protected the males and females from sorcery in order to keep them well; (3) Males conduct male initiation rights to "protect males who still have female blood in them."

Phase 4: Stating the Major Dominant Care Theme *(it was an abstracted theme grounded in Phase 1 and could be trailed with detailed data in Phases 2 and 3):* **"Culture care means surveillance and protective actions to ensure health and wellbeing."** *This theme is grounded in Phase 1 and can be trailed in Phases 2 and 3.*

There were, of course, other interesting findings related to this theme, such as the following: (1) Young children (5–19 years) could only walk down the road to a certain place and then turn around and come back to the village (this was a strong protective culture practice still used); (2) Watching meant Akunans to be *attentive to* and *listen for sounds* across the lands; (3) Gadsup women were solely responsible for bearing healthy children to see that their children became healthy adults, got married, and had their own children. Male and female roles were very different, and yet complementary, for watching and protecting as care role activities.

Major Theme Two

Culture care means nurturance that helps people grow, perform roles, keep healthy, and survive throughout the lifecycle, and is influenced by social structure factors and folk care practices.

This theme was firmly confirmed by 95 percent of key and village informants. The credibility and confirmability of this theme was trailed from *emic* verbal statements, to daily observations, and to participatory actions by the villagers at different phases of the lifecycle, i.e., from birth, young child, older child, young man, and finally adult married men and women. It was essential to grasp the significance of the theme and to understand patterns, norms, symbols and ways that nurturance took on meaning to the Akunans as meaning-in-context. Mothers were central figures to nurture female infants (often on demand) and at birth ceremonies. Male kinsmen, especially the mother's brother, were involved in nurturance to help children grow strong and healthy. Natural garden foods were the 'best' nurturant foods, and the people valued them as safe to eat. Men provided bird meat from the forest.

This theme had evidence of saturation and recurrent patterning criteria throughout the lifecycle accounts and in social structure factors (especially political, education, and economic factors). It was extremely important that I observed their many *folk* and *generic* care practices on different occasions, in different contexts, and over an extended period of time.

Major Theme Three

Culture care (caring) means keeping 'good' culture values and life-ways based on Gadsup ethnohistory, social structure, and worldview in order to prevent illnesses, keep well, healthy, and to avoid unnecessary intervillage conflicts and stresses.

Key and village Akunan informants established as credible confirmed this theme. Saturation with recurrent patterning became evident in practically every aspect of Gadsup living. There were only slight variations or diversities. The culture history, political, kinship, and religious beliefs and practices greatly influenced direct and indirect caring patterns to remain well. Women kinfolk who married into the village (newcomers) expressed the greatest differences in their ways of viewing care and health. Folk tales, village stories, and caring narratives reinforced recurrent patterns of wellbeing, health, or illness. Noncaring ways of strangers led to or 'caused' sorcery and illnesses. Sorcery also led to feuds and intervillage accusations and caused the greatest areas of village conflict.

Major Theme Four

Care means respecting male and female sex differences in order to confirm role complimentarity, to maintain health, and to fulfill prescribed village role responsibilities.

Over 93 percent of key and village informants established as credible and confirmed this theme. I documented this theme using field journal notes after observing recurrent patterns of behavior regarding sex role attributes and action modes. Male and female role differences prevailed in every aspect of the villager's lives. The social structure, worldview, past history, folk care, and many different life span data supported sex differences at birth, marriage, and death ceremonies. Sex role performance differences were revealed in folk legends and language expressions. Such sex differences were held as essential for a division of labor and served as role modeling for children and young adults. Such gender differences had a definite impact on the quality of health and wellbeing of individuals, families, and lineage members. When sex roles were culturally violated or daily sex roles were not performed properly, cultural conflicts, potential harm, and 'deviant' individual behavior became evident. In addition, village gossip and direct actions by the 'Big Men' or other involved kinsmen occurred. Ethical sanctions related to proper sex behavior were often buttressed by the moral life principles and ethical beliefs. All criteria used for qualitative research (Leininger, 1990) supported this theme, especially *meaning-in-context* and *recurrent repatterning* in political, kinship, education, and human care expressions.

Although other qualitative findings from this study arose, the above
themes from the ethnonursing data were the most dominant and prevailing. These findings substantiated the assumptions and tenets of
Culture Care Theory.

Nursing Care Actions and Decisions for Gadsup Akunan

In light of findings from this study, the nurse is challenged to use worldview, social structure, language expressions, environment, and folk
practices to study ways to provide culture-specific and culturally congruent care. Although many nursing care actions and decisions are evident from the thick and rich inductively derived ethnonursing study
findings, only a few will be presented here. The reader will note that I
prefer not to use the term *intervention*. All too frequently this term
implies curtailing or changing the status of something or imposing a different mode of acting in a culture. As the nurse functions in different
cultures, it may be quite inappropriate to change or curtail something.
Indeed, the nurse may need to preserve or maintain that which exists as
beneficial to clients.

From this study, *generic folk care* knowledge would be essential for
professional nursing care knowledge and practices. *Emic generic care*
and caring that was largely embedded in the worldview, social structure,
and other areas depicted in the Sunrise Enabler influenced Akunans'
health and wellbeing. Interestingly, health was frequently used interchangeably with wellbeing, reflecting a comprehensive view of total
functioning within a given holistic environmental context. In addition,
health was a state of being that enabled a person to perform role functions within cultural expectations.

Turning to the three modes of decision and action, professional
nurses need to use culture-specific care knowledge that *preserves* and
maintains health. Among these expectations would be to preserve most
male and female role responsibilities that support their wellbeing. It
would be quite difficult to change male and female roles without serious
cultural conflicts and major disruptions of social structure and lifeways
of the people. Gender differences were strongly held and embedded in
the social structure. While a Western feminist nurse might be inclined
to alter gender roles "to improve Akunan women lifeways," this could
lead to major difficulties. Likewise, Akunan males generally value their
role entailments as complementary to the women. While males
expressed protective care roles, they also envied female fertility and
procreative abilities. Females believed they were a key factor in bearing

and nurturing healthy infants and children. (Future care repatterning of belief systems might be considered in gender roles if desired by the villagers.) The nurse also might be tempted to encourage Gadsup women toward overt activity in political affairs. However, Akunan women, for one, believed they were quite effective in domestic political affairs. The data gave full support for some of their beliefs as effective action modes. Women did influence men's public decisions and actions. (This finding dispels a Western belief that some women in the developing world have virtually no power.)

Given the discovery of the knowledge and importance and use of the care constructs of *surveillance, protection, nurturance, prevention*, and *appropriate touching*, such care constructs with meanings and action modes would require preservation. These care constructs have been quite effective in maintaining health and wellbeing for many years and through many generations. Knowledge of each care construct and how it could be used to preserve the ongoing health of the Gadsup for congruent care would be important.

The value of *egalitarianism* among extended family members was another major knowledge area discovered in this study. To preserve and maintain Gadsup relationships as *"true brothers"* and *equals in social and cultural relationships* would be essential to reduce sorcery accusations, conflicts, and maintain health.

Care knowledge discovered with regard to *nurturance* as a means to preserve the idea of helping Akunans to grow, survive, and stay healthy by many nurturant activities would be extremely important. Some rituals, such as feeding infants and nurturant care might be considered for *culture care negotiation* and-or repatterning by engaging young boys' involvement in these caring activities. Elders who no longer worked in the gardens cared for children in the village and were protective of the children's health; hence, care preservation would be appropriate. In a culture where sex differences predominate, the effect on health of women as *caregivers* and men as *curers* was important. When women caregivers were in control, they maintained good health; when men curers were in control, they maintained poor health. Further study of how care and cure differ with women and men in generic care is needed.

Knowledge generated from this study regarding illness and prevention modalities needs to be preserved for congruent Akunan care practices. Preventing conflicts and illness by preserving culture care values needs to be maintained. Western medications could be viewed as potential sorcery materials by the Gadsup unless the nurse develops trust with the Akunans. The nurse would also need to keep in mind that Western women may be viewed as potential sorceresses, whereas a male nurse might find their Western modalities more accepted by the Akunans. In this regard, use of the Leininger Stranger–Friend Guide in assessing his or her relationship with strangers would prove useful.

The professional nurses need to consider repatterning and restructuring with the Akunans regarding their beliefs about menstrual blood as harmful and destructive to others. Educating women would be letting them reflect on other ideas. In changing this belief, as trusting friend relationship would be necessary.

Knowledge of the many positive generic folk health practices with the use of cultural care constructs of *surveillance, protection, nurturance, prevention*, and *touching* in caring relationships with others would need to be preserved and used with professional generic care practices. Western professional values such as self-care, assertiveness, treating sexes alike, competition, and use of high technologies would be culturally incongruent with the Akunans.

The healthy foods in the Akunan culture, such as the fresh garden greens, fruits, seasonal nuts, sweet potatoes, bananas, and other fresh foods, should be preserved. Introduction of milk is inappropriate as Akunans had a lactose ingestion problem. Introducing some meat and fish was much desired and this could be done as culture care accommodation. Preventing mental illness, infectious diseases, and obesity as known in our Western world should be fully considered. We have much to learn from this culture. A number of other nursing care decisions could be considered related to the three modes predicted in the theory of culture care. The nurse would need to complete this phase of examining the theory by systematically studying what transpired with the use of each of the three modes of care and its impact to provide culture congruent care.

Conclusion

In this chapter, I have examined the theory of Culture Care with the Gadsup (Akunans) of the Eastern Highlands of New Guinea with the ethnonursing research method. The method was extremely important in teasing out and obtaining indepth data to confirm the theory.

The worldview, social structure, ethnohistory, language, and folk beliefs and practices were major factors in discovering care and caring influences on Gadsup health and wellbeing. The Gadsup universals predominated over diversities related to human care. The embedded care forms, expressions, and values were extremely important to discover culturally congruent care that would be meaningful, appropriate, and beneficial to the culture. This study reveals the importance of generic care that must be explicated to develop humanistic and scientific care

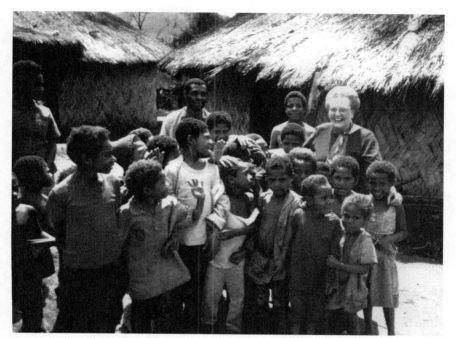

Figure 4-2   Gadsup Children with Dr. Leininger in Their New Guinea Village During Her Return Visit in 1990.

for the discipline of nursing. Such knowledge will help us shift from the traditional medical model to a true nursing model with care as the essence of nursing. This first transcultural care study should encourage nurses to realize the significance of care and why care has been difficult to explicate because of its invisible features embedded in social structure and other factors as depicted in the Sunrise Enabler. Finally, this research had a profound influence on my professional life, for it gave me new confidence about discovering care knowledge and the diverse care expressions, meanings, and forms of care. This body of knowledge provides inspiration for future nurse–researchers to become full participants and to be immersed in a culture to discover the epistemic source of generic care and its potential to advance professional nursing knowledge. Although I took a certain personal risk in doing this nursing and anthropological research in a culture that views women as potential sorceresses, I learned much from the people who became my 'true friends' and teachers by sharing their cultural secrets with me.

Notes

It should be noted that a girl is not called a woman until she has married and had a child; likewise, a boy is not called a man until he has married and had a child. Hence, the terms *girl* and *boy* were used until marriage (Leininger, 1966b, 1978).

References

Aamodt, A. (1978). Sociocultural dimensions of caring in the world of the Papago child and adolescent. In M. M. Leininger (Ed.), *Transcultural Nursing Theory and Practices*. New York: John Wiley & Sons.

Bohay, I. (1989). *Ethnonursing study: Lithuanian parent beliefs and experiences.* Unpublished master's dissertation, Wayne State University Press, Detroit, MI.

Brown, E. L. (1948). *Nursing for the future.* New York: Russell Sage Foundation.du Toit, B. M. (1975). *Akuna: A New Guinea village community.* Rotterdam: A. A. Balkema.

Dougherty, M., & Tripp-Reimer, T. (1985). The interface of nursing and anthropology. *Annual Review of Anthropology 14*, 219.

Gates, M. (1989). *Care and care meanings, experiences and orientations of persons dying in hospital and hospital settings.* Unpublished doctoral dissertation, Wayne State University Press, Detroit, MI.

Horn, B. (1978). Transcultural nursing and child-rearing of Muckleshoot people. In M. M. Leininger (Ed.), *Transcultural nursing: Concepts, theories, and practices* (pp. 223–234). New York: John Wiley & Sons.

Leininger, M. M. (1964). A Gadsup village experiences its first election. New Guinea's first national election: A symposium. *Journal of the Polynesian Society 73*(2).

Leininger, M. M. (1966a). *Convergence and divergence of human behavior: An ethnopsychological comparative study of two Gadsup villages in the Eastern Highlands of New Guinea.* Doctoral dissertation, University of Washington, Seattle.

Leininger, M. M. (1966b). *New Guinea micro-evolution studies* (memo No. 18, pp. 32–37). Department of Anthropology, University of Washington, Seattle.

Leininger, M. M. (1970). *Nursing and anthropology: Two worlds to blend.* New York: John Wiley & Sons.

Leininger, M. M. (Ed.). (1978a). *Transcultural nursing: Concept, theories, and practices.* New York: John Wiley & Sons.

Leininger, M. M. (1978b). The Gadsup of New Guinea and early child-caring behaviors with nursing care implications. In M. Leininger (Ed.), *Transcultural nursing: Concepts, theories, and practices* (pp. 375–397). New York: John Wiley & Sons.

Leininger, M. M. (1979). *Transcultural nursing*. New York: Masson Publishing.

Leininger, M. M. (1985). *Qualitative research methods in nursing*. Orlando, FL: Grune and Stratton.

Leininger, M. M. (1987). *Care: Discovery and uses in clinical and community nursing* (pp. 1–30). Detroit, MI: Wayne State University Press.

Leininger, M. M. (1988). *Care: An essential human need*. Detroit, MI: Wayne State University Press.

Leininger, M. M. (1990). The philosophic and epistemic bases to explicate transcultural nursing knowledge. *Journal of Transcultural Nursing, 1*(2), 40–51.

Littlewood, R. A. (1972). *Physical anthropology of the eastern highlands of New Guinea: Anthropological studies in the eastern highlands of New Guinea*. Seattle, WA: University of Washington Press.

McCabe, G. (1960). Cultural influences on patient behavior. *American Journal of Nursing, 60*(8), 1101.

McKaughan, H. (1973). *The languages of the eastern family of the East New Guinea Highland stock: Anthropological studies in the eastern highlands of New Guinea*. Seattle, WA: University of Washington Press.

Mead, M. (1956). Understanding cultural patterns. *Nursing Outlook, 4*(3), 260.

Orem, D. (1980). *Nursing: Concepts of practice*. NY: McGraw-Hill.

Pataki, K. J. (1970). *An environment through time: A comparison of precontact and post-contact habitats in the Eastern Highlands of New Guinea*. Boulder, CO: Institute of Behavioral Science, University of Colorado.

Rosenbaum, J. (1990). *Cultural care, culture health and grief phenomena related to older Greek-Canadian widows with Leininger's theory of culture care*. Unpublished doctoral dissertation, Wayne State University, Detroit, MI.

Saunders, L. (1954). *Cultural differences and medical care*. New York: Russell Sage Foundation.

Spangler, Z. (1990). *Nursing care values and practices of Philippine-American and Anglo-American nurses*. Unpublished doctoral dissertation, Wayne State University, Detroit, MI.

Staziak, D. (1990). *An ethnonursing study of folk care and health beliefs and practices with Mexican-Americans using Leininger's theory of cultural care*. Unpublished master's thesis, Wayne State University, Detroit, MI.

Watson, James B. (1963). A micro-evolution study in New Guinea. *Journal of the Polynesian Society, 72*(3), 188–192.

Watson, V. & Cole, J. D. (1977). *Prehistory of the Eastern Highlands of New Guinea: Anthropological studies in the Eastern Highlands of New Guinea*. Seattle, WA: University of Washington Press.

Wenger, A. F., (1988). *The phenomenon of care of the Old Order Amish: A high context culture*. Unpublished doctoral dissertation, Wayne State University, Detroit, MI.

CHAPTER FIVE

Culture Care Needs in the Clinical Setting

Debra A. Curren, RN, MS, CTN

In this chapter, client clinical care examples are provided to show how culturally competent care can occur in healthcare institutions by caregivers and staff who are prepared in transcultural nursing using the theory of Culture Care Diversity and Universality. This approach to health care will meet the growing need for transcultural care with clients now and in the future. Providing culturally congruent care with diverse cultures can be challenging, yet extremely rewarding for healthcare providers.

The need for transcultural nursing theory and practice in all areas of health care has become more evident with the changing demographics of the United States and other countries worldwide. Transcultural nursing was developed in the 1950s and has evolved into a major nursing specialty. The development of the Culture Care Theory by Leininger has led to a growing body of research-based knowledge which nurses can use to care for the culturally different (Leininger, 1991). Transcultural care has emerged as a major revolution in nursing despite the slow recognition of its value and important contributions to health care by transcultural nurses and other heath care providers. Certified transcultural nurses often work in many clinical and community settings with administration and staff not prepared in transcultural theory and research who fail to grasp the importance or acknowledge the wealth of information that could benefit clients and staff.

The word *diversity* is frequently used without recognizing that it covers many areas of a person's cultural *world*. Diversity usually includes gender, age, disability, political views, dietary habits, ethnicity, sexual orientation, education, preferred language, work status, socioeconomic factors, religious beliefs and practices, and other areas. All too often the study of these aspects of diversity occurs without a theory to guide knowledge discoveries. The theory of Culture Care Diversity and Universality has been extremely helpful in discovering similarities and differences among clients of diverse cultures. This theory is essential for nurses in order to accommodate, maintain, or repattern the client's cultural views and practices for high quality, culturally congruent health care (Leininger, 1995). Negating or ignoring important cultural differences, values, and beliefs of health care clients often leads to misdiagnoses, harmful care, and nonadherence to treatment as well as staff frustrations and anger. Nurses need theory with research findings to support their care actions and decisions.

The Sunrise Enabler (see Chapter 1) developed by Leininger, is a pictorial view of the theory and a guide for nurses to use in performing cultural assessments with clients (Leininger, 1995, 2003). This enabler assists nurses to explore various cultural areas of the client's world such as technology, religious beliefs, care expressions and meanings, economic factors, cultural history, environment, and other lifeway influencers and patterns. Such information is vital in order to provide high quality nursing care, medical treatments, and other means of holistic caring for clients of diverse or similar cultures.

The theory can also be used to assess diverse employment issues in the clinical setting. For example, some healthcare employees may feel disenfranchised and discriminated against in their employment settings given that the medical and nursing professions are predominantly Caucasian (Barton, 1999). In the United States, only 12.3% of registered nurses are from minority cultures, which can lead to feelings of exclusion from majority groups (United States Department of Health and Human Services, 2001). Physicians from minority cultures in the United States account for only 9% of all physicians (Stolber, 2002). Other healthcare professions also reflect a lack of diversity within their disciplines.

The Equal Employment Opportunity Commission (EEOC) investigates numerous claims by healthcare workers who report discriminatory incidents such as blatant racial slurs, lack of promotion opportunities, and-or working in hostile environments due to their cultural orientation (Barton, 1999). Racism is a major phenomenon that can be identified overtly or covertly in clinical settings (Vaughn, 1997). Overt forms of racism may be offensive verbal or written statements directly made to another, or may involve physical acts (even violent acts) against a particular person or group. Covert forms of racism are often subtle and difficult to identify such as the lack of advancement or promotion of a culturally diverse employee. There may be differences in sexual orientation, cultural values, age, and areas that relate to racism. Jamieson and O'Mara (1991) refer to this as *institutionalized racism*. For example, an African American orderly working in a hospital setting was denied training that others in his department received because the employer believed that it would be difficult for him to learn the content. Management assumed he was unable to learn the material because of his culture. This orderly, employed for 3 years in his department, had the most clinical experience yet twice was excluded from promotions. Moreover, other employees with less experience were promoted to comparably advanced positions. Additional incidents of discrimination occurred as this orderly was reprimanded for his cultural expressions while other employees were not reprimanded for similar expressions.

Examples of racism involving consumers of health care have also been noted. In Washington State, a family took their loved one to a local hospital. While assessing this unconscious client (behind a pulled curtain), the medical team (a physician, a physician's assistant, and a nurse) were overheard by family members making racial comments about the client and denied the client treatment due to cultural biases. As a consequence, the family sued for discrimination and won their case (American Healthcare Consultants, 2001). Another example occurred when an African American nurse brought her ill child to the pediatrician's office for treatment. After the appointment, as the nurse approached to pay her bill the receptionist asked for her MediCal (welfare) information. This clerk made the assumption that the child's mother was poor because she was African American (Tullman, 1992). Such false assumptions can be culturally offensive, damaging, and painful to the client (cultural pain). Leininger (1997) described *cultural pain* as a hurtful, offensive experience often identified in the workplace due to a lack of awareness about specific cultures. These experiences can be identified through cultural assessment and observation.

The Theory of Culture Care Diversity and Universality with the Sunrise Enabler has been invaluable in assisting the author and other employees to learn to understand one another and work in cooperative relationships with culturally diverse coworkers and clients. Transcultural education could lead to improved employee productivity and retention, less staff turnover, and reduced legal costs related to discrimination and legal suits (Cater & Spence, 1996) saving thousands of dollars for healthcare institutions. In clinical settings, the use of certified transcultural nurses knowledgeable in transcultural theory, research, and direct client care can be invaluable in building positive staff relationships, promoting positive therapeutic outcomes, and preventing unfavorable ones for clients of diverse and similar cultures.

It is of great interest that businesses such as Kodak, Hewlett-Packard, Nestle, Proctor and Gamble, and other corporations are acknowledging the value and benefit of cultural diversity programs to understand and meet diverse customer needs (Jamieson & O'Mara, 1991). One must ask why the healthcare industry lags in the area of understanding, awareness, and sensitivity in a business filled with diversity in which *people* need to be understood and respected? Human beings are different from cameras, computers, chocolate, and soap and cannot be packaged together in one homogenous group. What can be done to change this current problem in clinical healthcare settings? Given that the majority of healthcare institutions are led by predominantly Caucasian administrators, one can predict that cultural blindness, ethnocentric views, and cultural biases need to be addressed by management, human resources departments, and employees.

Understanding the culturally diverse demographics of a community is essential for staff education and therapeutic care. If the demographics reveal even a small number of a particular culture (e.g., Arab Americans or Native Americans) the clinical staff can benefit from education about these cultures within the community. There is, however, a common misconception that if minimal diversity within a community exists, then knowledge of transcultural nursing (theory and practice) is not needed. Such misconceptions can thwart progress and lead to an even greater need to learn about people from different cultures. Cultural ignorance, ethnocentrism, and narrow views can lead to many clinical problems in client care. How might these attitudes and myths be changed?

The Joint Commission on Accreditation of Healthcare Organizations (JCAHO) is a leading force behind major changes in healthcare organizations' policies and practices directing client care. Healthcare institutions often make quick and lasting changes when JCAHO mandates compliance. Unfortunately, JCAHO has yet to address transcultural healthcare diversity issues in a way that holds institutions accountable for culturally competent care. Instead, obscure standards with limited monitoring for quality care are evident. Presently, JCAHO requires healthcare institutions to assess the cultural needs of clients, but has not provided for enforced implementation of programs to meet these cultural needs. Nursing assessment forms usually have general yes–no cultural questions such as, "Do you have any cultural beliefs that you would like to tell us?" Such queries are culturally inappropriate ways to assess the client's cultural needs. Generally, nurses and healthcare providers are uncomfortable with cultural assessments as they are not adequately prepared to perform them. Moreover, staff members tend to rush through the assessment and often check *no* to avoid cultural conflicts with clients, families, and staff. Some clients from diverse cultures may also be reluctant to give cultural or personal information because they view staff as distrusted strangers. Initial encounters such as this are critical to clients who are unfamiliar with the healthcare setting and staff. If the nurse gathers specific cultural assessment information, what happens to this information? How is it interpreted and used by the clinical staff? How are cultural factors implemented and monitored in client care? In most clinical settings, the author finds the cultural assessment data are often placed in the back of the client chart behind prioritized lab reports, physician orders, and progress notes. Thus, the use and monitoring of cultural assessment data for meeting cultural needs are overlooked by staff. JCAHO needs to require ongoing education in transculturalism with clinical staff and administrators to ensure appropriate use of cultural data so culturally congruent care occurs. Policies, procedures, and evaluation of outcomes are needed in healthcare organizations to assure that meaningful and skilled cultural care is provided by transculturally prepared staff.

Some characteristics of an organization that does not tend to value diversity or provide culturally appropriate care can be identified. They include: (a) lack of administrator's understanding, involvement, and support for cultural care initiatives and practices; (b) overall absence of a culturally diverse workforce; (c) lack of a culturally diverse professional staff with minorities mainly present in menial or service oriented jobs such as laundry, food service, and housekeeping; (d) evidence of limited promotions and lack of advancement opportunities and mentorship programs for the staff of different cultural orientations; (e) lack of diverse leadership in management teams; and (f) an absence of policies, procedures, activities, and environmental ways to support culturally diverse actions and outcomes. These factors and others limit the implementation of culturally competent practices in clinical settings and healthcare organizations. Far more attention needs to be given to establishing and implementing programs supporting use of transcultural nursing theory, concepts, principles, practices, and methods. The staff needs to learn about the Theory of Culture Care Diversity and Universality and use the research findings to care for clients.

Cultural Competency Guide

Developing steps that lead to the provision of respectful, meaningful, and culturally competent care are fully discussed by Ehrmin (2002). Additionally, the author developed the Curren Cultural Competency Guide as shown in Figure 5-1 (Curren, 2003). This guide is a visualization of the transcultural education and experiential activities that the author has developed and implemented at a community hospital with positive outcomes (Curren, personal knowledge, June 2003). Each portion of the guide represents the theme of an eight step culture care program. The program includes didactic and experiential modules to demonstrate how culturally competent care can occur for clients in clinical settings and also assist employees to effectively manage cultural conflicts with clients and coworkers.

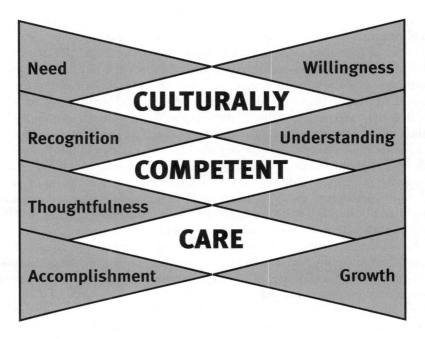

Figure 5-1   Curren Cultural Competency Guide: Phases of Development to Achieve Cultural Competency. Reprinted with permission from author of figure.

In the first session, the *need* to acquire cultural knowledge and competence is identified, which may be internally or externally driven. For example, a Christian nurse working in a community with Arab Muslims may internally recognize her need to be more culturally knowledgeable about these individuals in her care. Similarly, an externally driven need to obtain cultural knowledge could come from a manager of an employee who may be having difficulty relating to culturally different coworkers. The next session involves a *willingness* to be open to identifying one's biases and to address them. Having some ground rules agreed upon by everyone involved in these educational offerings helps to encourage open and honest communication among participants.

In the *recognition* session, self awareness is imperative. This allows staff to become aware of how one's biases and attitudes affect client care and teamwork in the clinical setting. An *understanding* session provides knowledge of different cultures and appreciation of the challenges that diverse individuals face within a dominant culture. This session may involve interviewing culturally diverse persons to gain insight and cultural exposure. The *thoughtfulness* session is one that evaluates how Leininger's nursing modalities of culture care accommodation, culture care maintenance, and culture care repatterning can improve client care and team relationships (Leininger, 1995). Analyzing client scenarios like those described in this chapter is a valuable way to increase holding knowledge of cultures and promote transcultural nursing decisions and actions that the participants can then use in *opportunity* sessions.

In the *opportunity* session, healthcare workers are given *cultural assignments* that allow participants to use Leininger's modes directly with diverse clients or staff in actual clinical situations. The *accomplishment* session evaluates the cultural assignments as experienced. These experiences are discussed in supportive ways that facilitate continued learning. The *growth* session focuses on the continued implementation and evaluation of transcultural principles toward becoming increasingly culturally competent through ongoing educational and experiential applications of skills in everyday clinical situations.

The Role of the Certified Transcultural Nurse Specialist

Certified Transcultural Nurse Specialists (CTNS) are becoming employed in many clinical settings to assist staff in providing culturally competent care and to work effectively as team members. Certification in transcultural nursing attests to the public that the nurse is an expert and qualified to guide others in providing culturally competent care. This specialist is prepared through graduate transcultural nursing education and mentoring experiences. Certified nurses are invaluable in the development of an organizational climate that values and provides culturally based care through policies and procedures that assist staff in providing culturally competent care. The transcultural nurse specialist is able to demonstrate ways to conduct cultural care assessments using the Sunrise Enabler. The specialist assists staff in developing and implementing care plans that reflect culturally specific values and practices for the client and family. Demonstrating how to use transcultural knowledge is an important role for the transcultural nurse specialist and is most rewarding. Other role responsibilities often include arranging translation services and collaborating with dietary staff to develop culturally appropriate meal plans for culturally diverse clients. Sometimes the transcultural specialist directly assists clients and families with religious services, rituals, or special ceremonies to promote culturally based care and promote healing in the clinical setting.

The certified transcultural nurse specialist is also prepared to offer educational sessions for healthcare workers in clinical areas. This involves examining cultural diversity issues in the clinical setting and then determining ways to support a climate of *acceptance* rather than *resistance* to avoid problems related to cultural differences. The transcultural nurse specialist can also implement mentorship programs in the clinical settings and the community using expert staff members to demonstrate culturally based care for diverse clients.

Another major and important role of the transcultural nurse specialist is conducting community outreach care in existing or developing minority health programs. In this role, the nurse specialist assesses, develops, and strengthens community ties, and often serves as a *cultural broker* using *emic* knowledge of clients to alter or accommodate care practices and communication processes in healthcare settings to benefit clients and staff (Leininger, 1995). Conducting research within diverse cultures in clinical and community settings is another important role of the certified transcultural specialist. Using the theory of Culture Care Diversity and Universality and the ethnonursing method for conducting transcultural research, the transcultural nurse specialist can demonstrate the effectiveness of clinical education programs and provide the organization with sound data for making clinical and organizational decisions to improve cultural congruence in client care. As a certified clinical transcultural nurse, the author has been actively supportive of the development of the transcultural nurse *generalist* role. Transcultural generalists are prepared to work primarily with culturally diverse clients and families encountered during clinical visits (Leininger, 1995). The transcultural nurse generalist assists staff in ways to communicate and establish client care practices that decrease barriers and tensions, which improves client care and staff satisfaction. Reciprocal cultural understanding often occurs and may lead to the development of additional transcultural nurse generalists or encourage culturally diverse persons to consider careers in health care. This supports the creation of a more diverse national healthcare workforce.

In 1998 the U.S. Department of Health and Human Services (DHHS) Office of Minority Health (OMH) acknowledged the need for healthcare institutions to be aware of and responsive to the cultural needs of clients by releasing the Culturally and Linguistic Appropriate Standards (CLAS; DHHS-OMH, 2001). These 14 standards address how healthcare institutions should address, monitor, and evaluate care for culturally diverse clients. Unfortunately, these government agencies did not incorporate the available and published standards of Transcultural Nursing established in 1999 by the Transcultural Nursing Society, which would have been invaluable (Leininger & McFarland, 2002; Leuning, Swiggum, Wiegert & Zander, 2002). It is hoped that regulatory agencies will apply the transcultural nursing standards to future regulations holding healthcare institutions accountable for providing culturally competent care. It is also important to note that most of the CLAS standards are recommendations (not mandates) that may be very difficult to implement in healthcare facilities with managers and staff unprepared in transcultural nursing. Interestingly, only DHHS-OMH Office standards four, five, six, and seven, which existed previously as part of the Civil Rights Act of 1964, are mandated. These four standards ensure language translation for persons for whom English is not their first language (DHHS-OMH, 2001).

In the clinical setting, there are many ways to provide translation services to meet client needs. Failure to provide adequate translation to clients and families whose primary language is other than English presents a potential liability for healthcare institutions. Some healthcare institutions have implemented telephone language translation services and contend it meets the need. However, others may hold different views. While this method may be helpful, it is far from an ideal way to provide translation services in a healthcare setting. Transcultural nurses and anthropologists recommend face to face translations with interpreters who are knowledgable about the cultures they serve. Some facilities may rely upon ancillary or nursing staff members, which may or may not be satisfactory, or they may employ certified medical interpreters, an often cost prohibitive alternative. The following scenario is offered to exemplify that telephone translation may not be useful and may be harmful.

A Spanish speaking Mexican American woman was ready for hospital discharge after the birth of her son. The nurse caring for her used the telephone language translation service provided by the hospital to complete the discharge teaching. This included information on infant care, breast care and feeding, and using a breast pump. It also included monitoring of the client's vaginal flow, care of the episiotomy, and when to safely resume sexual intercourse. The nurse gathered all the necessary papers and information for the discharge and entered the woman's room with the special language use telephone. She dialed the number and accessed a Spanish interpreter. After explaining the nature of the conversation to the interpreter, they began the process of the nurse talking to the interpreter and the interpreter then translating the information to the female client. Suddenly, the client became very upset during the conversation and loudly told the nurse, "No, no!" The nurse was unaware of the problem and terminated the discharge teaching. She then tried to calm the woman but was unsuccessful. Frustrated, the nurse discussed this baffling situation with the charge nurse. Alice, a Hispanic housekeeper who was cleaning in the client's room during the incident, overheard the conversation. Alice analyzed the situation and stated, "She [the client] cannot talk to the interpreter about such things; it is not culturally right." The nurse asked, "What do you mean Alice, who *can* she talk to?" The housekeeper stated, "It's not respectful for the client to speak with a man about such things." The nurse said, "Oh, my goodness, I never even thought about that. I thought since she had a male doctor that it would not be a problem." Alice stated, "The doctor is someone she knows and trusts, but the man on the phone is a complete stranger to her." The discharge nurse then asked Alice to join her in the client's room to prepare the client for discharge. Alice interpreted while the nurse apologized to the client for being unaware of this important cultural norm (Galanti, 2003).

Using staff members to interpret without any formal cultural or medical education (even though they may be fluent in the language) is also inappropriate. In addition, one needs to recognize that the additional workload demand placed upon staff acting as interpreters away from their regular duties may require additional compensation. Without addressing these concerns, bilingual staff may feel taken advantage of or discriminated against. If current staff are used as translators, they should be (a) educated in health terminology and transcultural communication; (b) educated about the culture they are interpreting for, and able to recognize clues that relate to cultural norms such as gender and role differences; (c) be partially relieved of other job responsibilities while translating to avoid interferences and prevent reprisal from their supervisor or peers; and (d) be rewarded for their valuable skills. These translators should be competent to interpret what transpires and accountable for accurately informing the nurse and others of client care needs. Organizations and staff need to realize and appreciate the importance of competent interpreter services.

Minor children should not be interpreters for family members as this practice may be viewed as abusive, inappropriate, or exploitive (DHHS-OMH, 2001). Interpreting for the family is usually stressful for the child and may lead to parent–child conflicts or repercussions later. The transcultural nurse specialist can collaborate with community volunteer programs and enlist the assistance of cultural brokers to provide interpreter services. Foreign language departments of local colleges and universities may be sought for their expertise and knowledge. There are also creative ways to provide linguistic interpreter services with use of grant monies. It is essential that healthcare organizations value the importance of these services and be willing to assess, support, and measure the effectiveness of qualified interpreters and other translation services.

Clinical Scenarios and Transcultural Nursing

In thinking about specific clinical situations, the following scenarios may be helpful for the reader to reflect upon and envision ways the transcultural nurse specialist can modify cultural biases to ensure culturally congruent care. These scenarios reveal common cultural biases and errors with clients. They are realistic and may occur in other clinical settings.

The Gay Client and His Partner

A young homosexual male was admitted to the hospital for supportive therapy in the last stages of Acquired Immunodeficiency Syndrome (AIDS). He had no family in the immediate area but his male partner of five years was at his bedside day and night. In the morning report, remarks were made by the night nurse finishing her shift about the partner being continuously present in the room. The day nurse assigned to the young man knew some transcultural nursing principles and identified frustration and uneasiness with her peer when the partner's presence was discussed. She asked her nursing peer, "What is it about the partner's presence that bothers you?" The night shift nurse quickly stated, "Well, for one thing, he gets very defensive when I ask him to leave the room to do my assessment and take vitals. He also doesn't need to be so *touchy-feely* with the client—I don't want to see that." The transculturally prepared nurse asked, "What do you mean?" The night nurse replied, "Well, he sits there and holds his hand, strokes his hair, and kisses him on the forehead . . . it's so disgusting." Realizing that the night nurse had very strong negative feelings toward homosexuals, the transcultural nurse respected the nurse's viewpoint, but also asked the nurse to reconsider her position if she were in the client's situation. Perhaps she would want someone . . . anyone . . . to provide care such as *touching* to convey concern which this male partner was providing. The night nurse agreed to keep this in mind and not let her biases get in the way of providing care. Later, the day shift nurse entered the client's room after gently knocking on the door. The partner was sitting at the bedside stroking the client's hair and forehead. The partner immediately began to rise from his chair as the nurse approached the bedside. The transcultural nurse said, "Oh, no, please stay where you are; I'm sure he (the client) appreciates you being there for him." The partner looked shocked as the nurse continued, "I am quite comfortable with you being present as I care for him (the client). In fact, if you would like, perhaps you can assist me in his care today." The partner arose from his chair with tears in his eyes and said, "All I want to do is to take care of the person I love more than anything in this world . . . until I'm not able to . . . any longer. . . ." The nurse, fighting back tears of her own replied, "Then today we will care for him together." The partner hugged the nurse and said, "Thank you so much."

In reflecting on this situation, respecting the *culture* of the client was an important nursing care action. In this transcultural care situation, healthcare providers need to know their prejudices and curtail them and act in the best interests of the client and family. They need to have self awareness and prevent their ethnocentric biases from unduly influencing quality care (Spinks, Andrews, & Boyle, 2000).

The Lesbian Couple

A lesbian couple was celebrating the birth of their daughter. The client had been artificially inseminated and had given birth to a healthy baby girl. The couple sat on the bed together cradling their daughter and celebrating the miracle of birth. Outside the client's room, the transcultural nurse reviewed the client's chart. One of the other nurses said, "Well, I guess that kid will become a *les-bo* too." The transcultural nurse responded, "You probably know with alcoholic families, if a parent is alcoholic this doesn't mean that the children will also be alcoholic . . . so, why do you say that?" "Well," the other nurse replied, "If that's all the kid sees, she'll probably think it's normal." The transcultural nurse said, "One should not assume that the child will only be exposed to lesbian relationships in its entire lifetime. I'm sure this couple has heterosexual friends and family members that may also be a part of the baby's life." The other nurse replied, "Well, I sure hope so, for that kid's sake!" Later, the transcultural nurse greeted the couple warmly and expressed her congratulations and happiness for the couple. The couple seemed cold at first, but realized the nurse was truly interested in expressing her caring ways. They quickly warmed to her and expressed their thanks to the nurse for "not making them feel like they had committed some kind of crime." The birth mother continued, "I heard the other nurse's comment in the hall, and I may need to have a little chat with the head nurse around here." The birth mother happened to be a lawyer in the community and her partner a landscape designer. This incident could have resulted in charges of discrimination against the nurse and the hospital. However, the transcultural nurse's cultural awareness and competence were communicated through her demonstration of respect and understanding which helped to soothe anger and avert legal actions by the couple. Respect for different cultures with their diverse lifeways is a universal transcultural nursing construct for nurses to use to prevent cultural pain.

The Native American Couple

A Native American couple was admitted to the hospital for the birth of their first baby. The mother was employed as a clerk at a department store. The father was an elementary schoolteacher. They saw themselves as a typical American family. They attended a local nondenominational Christian church. The baby's paternal grandmother maintained a strong presence in their lives and was proud to have been present for the early morning birth of her grandchild. Shortly after the baby was born, the grandmother requested to take the placenta home.

The hospital staff were alarmed and showed disbelief in their facial expressions. The delivery nurse quickly told the grandmother, "This is something we usually do not do." Later, in shift report a nurse stated, "That was such a strange expectation, what would they want to do with the placenta?" The other nurses were silent. The transcultural nurse showed respect for the family's beliefs and practices, and explained that the placenta may be used in a birth ceremony and burial ritual to pray for a healthy baby and provide proper burial of the placenta, which is an important cultural practice. The transcultural nurse also reminded the staff members that cultural differences needed to be respected. The charge nurse phoned the physician to discuss this situation. Other nurses on the unit continued to make comments about the grandmother's request and avoided the client's room whenever the grandmother was present. After several phone calls, the physician finally released the placenta to be taken home by the Native American parents. The family showed relief when they were told they would be taking the placenta home with them.

In this scenario with a Native American family, the transcultural nurse offered important cultural knowledge to help the staff nurses learn about birth expectations and practices of this culture. Later, the nurse used the Sunrise Enabler to explain to the staff nurses how one performs a cultural assessment during the admission process in order to become aware of such practices *before* the birth occurs. To obtain such culturally relevant information from this couple, one might say, "I noticed that your cultural heritage is Native American, so I am wondering if there are some special traditions you would like us to know about in your birth practices." The father might say, "We don't really have any past Indian ways. We attend a Christian church . . . however, my mom is traditional, and she will request that we take the placenta home with us." The transculturally oriented nurse would respond positively and say, "I understand and we will strive to accommodate your request." This statement represents an example of the second care mode of the Culture Care Theory, as the nursing action would demonstrate respect and accommodation for the family's cultural request through the provision of this culturally meaningful care.

After this cultural education approach was shared with the staff, they seemed more relaxed and comfortable with the family. Gradually the client's cultural wishes were accommodated by most of the clinical staff, although some staff members remained skeptical about the cultural benefits. In this situation, the staff gained new knowledge of traditional Native American birth practices and expectations through direct cultural education by the transcultural nurse.

The Asian American Client

An Asian woman had just delivered her second child and a transcultural nurse specialist was assigned to care for her. The transcultural nurse heard the following in the report by the nurse from the previous shift. The verbatim statements heard were as follows:

> Room 807 has an Asian woman who can hardly speak English, so good luck figuring out what she needs! Her oral intake is really bad. She refused her juice and milk this morning and made us stop her intravenous fluids. She even ripped the thing [intravenous catheter] out of her arm! She's not doing very well breastfeeding; she won't drink the ice water put in her room even though I keep telling her she needs the water to improve her milk supply. She also refused to get out of bed and take a shower.

The client's husband was a doctoral student at the local university. The client had no other family members in the country. The transcultural nurse began her nursing assessment with the woman by using a telephone interpreter service because there was no face to face translation available. Through the telephone service, the nurse asked, "Are you thirsty? The client responded, "Yes." The nurse asked, "What would you drink if you were in your home?" The nurse learned that the client would accept hot or warm liquids which were congruent with the cultural belief in her native hot–cold theory. With the nurse's holding knowledge, she knew that many Asian cultures deemed illnesses or conditions *hot* or *cold* and that one had to maintain a balance between *hot* and *cold* food and fluids for recovery. This Asian woman believed that pregnancy and childbirth were *cold* conditions; therefore, to restore balance in her body she needed to consume *warm* or *hot* nourishments. The transcultural nurse realized that these hot–cold ideas may have had no connection with the actual taste or temperature of the food, but referred to a cultural classification system that was a part of her Asian cultural beliefs. This belief was respected by the transcultural nurse who obtained hot drinks and foods for her client's *cold* condition. The nurse was also aware that taking showers and baths were usually not acceptable to a traditional Asian woman during postpartum because it would lead to chills and further imbalance her condition (Leininger, 2002b). Thus taking a shower would not be healthy and would not be congruent with her beliefs for the birth recovery process.

The transcultural nurse learned that the husband was home taking care of the couple's other child. Being curious, the transcultural nurse called and asked the husband about other caring measures the staff might take while his wife was in the hospital that would fit her cultural beliefs. The husband suggested offering warm blankets, a warm sponge bath, and keeping the client's door closed to prevent drafts. He said he would bring foods his wife liked and that were acceptable *hot* or *warm* foods. The husband seemed very pleased to participate in planning the care for his wife and thanked the nurse for asking about his wife's needs. According to Leininger, this *partnership care* involves the client (family) and the nurse working together and is essential in meeting culture care needs of clients (Leininger, 2002b). The transcultural nurse's cultural assessment and actions were essential for determining Asian cultural care birth practices. The cultural assessment data were used to direct client care and to teach the nursing staff ways to provide culturally congruent care that were acceptable and safe in meeting the client's cultural needs. In this scenario, it was the transcultural nurse specialist's holding knowledge gained through transcultural study that guided her nursing actions and decisions (Leininger, 1995). Cultural accommodation was clearly needed to plan and provide care for this Asian client; it was viewed as essential to her recovery and was appreciated by the client and family.

The clinical staff needed to be educated about Asian cultural beliefs and practices in order to provide culturally congruent and beneficial care. Reducing stereotyping was also needed as well as learning to accept specific cultural Asian beliefs such as the hot–cold practices. Most importantly, staff should not assume that all persons have the same beliefs and practices. Instead, individual variations exist among cultures depending on their traditional or nontraditional lifeways. Transcultural nurses learn how to discover these variations in cultural beliefs and lifeways of clients through transcultural education which includes learning how to assess client needs and respond appropriately to meet their culturally specific needs.

The Arab Client

A 50-year-old Arab woman was admitted for gallstones and subsequent cholesystectomy. In keeping with traditional Muslim practices, she was always attended by a male family member in her room. She wore the *hejab* (hair cover) whenever people entered the room. This provided her privacy and limited her body exposure; *covering* (the body) is a religious expression of her Muslim faith. To prevent a major cultural taboo, it was also important that a nurse be present when the male physician examined her abdominal incisions because the bodies of traditionally oriented Arab women are not to be exposed to men other than the husband (Lawrence & Rozmus, 2001; Leininger & McFarland, 2002).

The transcultural nurse discovered that the staff nurses were reluctant to have the Arab woman assigned to them because of the extra time it would take to accompany the physician and because of their general apprehension of the male Arab family members. There was also general fear of Muslim people since the September 11, 2001 attacks on the World Trade Center buildings.

This fear became clear in staff comments such as, "I couldn't live in an (Arab) country! Why, maybe these men were connected with those who did the bombings in our country. We really do not have time to stand around while the doctor is in the room." It was evident that the nursing staff was afraid, frustrated, and unfamiliar with providing care to Muslims and that Islamic cultural practices were difficult for the nursing staff to accept. Fortunately, the nurse caring for this woman was prepared in transcultural nursing and had holding knowledge of the culture, their Islamic beliefs, and other lifeways enabling her to provide culturally congruent care. A few examples of culturally congruent care offered by the transcultural nurse follow.

When the nurse entered the Muslim woman's room she respected that the client was intermittently wearing her *hejab* as she knew the client viewed it as a sacred practice. The nurse always waited a few seconds at the door before entering (while the woman put on her *hejab*) and would always ask if she could enter. The nurse greeted the woman in a friendly tone. The nurse was also careful not to touch the water glass or eating utensils with her left hand for she knew that the left hand is considered unclean in many Arab Muslim cultures (Lawrence & Rozmus, 2001). The nurse also accommodated the gender-appropriate behavior of avoiding prolonged eye contact with the male family members in order to prevent a cultural clash. In the room, the nurse observed a gelatin dessert on the woman's meal tray. Gelatin is generally forbidden in the diet of many Muslims due to the swine collagen used in the processing. The nurse needed to verify the woman's practices, realizing that some Arabs may not follow all Islamic beliefs. The nurse was careful not to impose her beliefs onto the client, which would be *cultural imposition*, a nontherapeutic cultural practice. The nurse said, "I notice you have a gelatin dessert on your tray; is this something that you normally eat?" The woman quickly said, "No, I eat no pork and I cannot eat the dessert." This informed the nurse that the woman and her family were following Muslim dietary restrictions (Nydell, 1996). The nurse sent for another tray without gelatin and alerted the dietary staff about other food choices congruent with Muslim diet practices as this was important for healthy outcomes with this client.

The transcultural nurse's holding knowledge was that Muslims dedicate five times per day for prayer which was very important to respect, although some Muslims may not follow traditional prayer times. The nurse said, "I learned that prayer times are important for a person in the Muslim culture . . . is this important to you?" The woman told the nurse that prayer times were very important to her. The nurse then asked, "How can I help you have these special prayer times?" The woman then told her the times of the day she usually prays and approximately how long for each prayer time she needed. The nurse told the client and the family that she would make a sign for the door that read *Do Not Disturb* and they could use it for her prayer times. The client and her son were pleased to hear this. The nurse knew it was important to also convince the staff to comply with the sign. The transcultural nurse communicated her goal to provide cultural care accommodation regarding prayer times on the care plan. The written plan was helpful for staff and demonstrated to them one way to accommodate *the client's needs for adhering to the practices of her Muslim faith*. It was of interest that a housekeeper, a dietary staff member, and a nursing assistant came to the Arab woman's door when the sign was posted but respected the sign and returned to the room later when the sign was removed. It was only the physician who insisted on entering the room despite the sign. During the course of the day, the sign went up and down at the designated prayer times. When the client and her son walked in the hallway and passed the nurses' station, they gave the transcultural nurse a friendly wave and smiled. The other nurses exclaimed, "How did you get so friendly with them? They usually don't talk to anyone!" The transcultural nurse was skilled in using Leininger's Stranger to Trusted Friend Enabler as a valuable guide to gain trust and to develop a caring relationship with the Arab client and family (Leininger, 1991, 1995). She also had Muslim-Arab holding knowledge which was essential to guide the decisions and actions of her caring ways which led to a trusting therapeutic relationship.

In this scenario, the transcultural nurse had an opportunity to educate the clinical staff about the Muslim-Arab culture and ways to use Culture Care Theory concepts and transcultural nursing principles in client care. Education of the staff about religious cultural beliefs and practices along with transcultural nursing concepts and principles was crucial.

Transcultural nurses recognize that all religions have symbols that represent beliefs and that these symbols can be very different depending on the religious group. For example, Roman Catholics are familiar with a rosary while Mormons have special undergarments worn close to their body to signify their closeness with God (Lipson, Dibble, & Minarik, 1996). Although both groups are described as 'Christian,' they have different symbols, signs, and expressions.

The Mormon Client

A Mormon woman admitted for surgery was asked to remove all her undergarments as part of her preoperative care. The woman was reluctant to comply with this inflexible hospital policy because she believed one must always wear the Mormon undergarments, especially when ill and needing God's protection. She complied and put her undergarments on a high shelf in her room where she thought no one would find them. While the woman was in surgery, a decision was made to move the client to a different room. The nurse who had been caring for this woman instructed a nursing assistant to gather all the woman's belongings and take them to the new room. The nursing assistant followed the directions and thought she had moved everything from the client's room. Later, the housekeeper who cleaned the room found the undergarments and discarded them.

When the Mormon woman returned from surgery, she immediately asked the nurse to help put her undergarments on, and found that they were gone. The Mormon woman was very upset, tearful, and deeply concerned. The woman called her husband to tell him of the incident and her concerns. This entire incident could have been prevented had the staff been educated in transcultural nursing theory with focus on the Mormon culture. A skilled cultural assessment would have disclosed the meaning of the undergarments and the woman's need to wear them especially when ill. Most importantly, Leininger's culture care accommodation and negotiation modes were needed to provide culturally appropriate care. Moreover, the nurse needed to negotiate care strategies so the Mormon woman could wear her garment during surgery. This could be accommodated by placing it on her back or other nonsurgical area. Culturally congruent care actions would have helped the client to feel safe and protected during the surgical procedure and prevented a negative client experience.

The Native American Client

On the morning John, a Native American elder, was to receive in-patient dialysis, he prayed to the Great Father to be with him and not allow any ill spirits to enter his bed during his absence. John believed that the placement of his medicine bag (a small leather bag containing sacred items) under the bed would deter bad spirits from invading his bed while he was receiving dialysis. About one half hour after he had left, the housekeeper entered his room. She did her usual tasks and removed John's beadwork from the bedside table when wiping it. In the process, several beads fell to the floor. The housekeeper swept up the beads and continued to clean the rest of the room. While sweeping under the bed she found the medicine bag. Being curious, she opened it and found a rock, a feather, a coin, a lock of hair, and some tobacco. "Strange, she thought, why would anybody keep these?" She placed the bag on the pile of beads that she had moved to the window counter and left the room.

Four hours later when John returned to his room, he saw his lunch tray on the bedside table where he had left his beadwork. John immediately asked about his beadwork and where it was. The nurse reassured him that no harm was done and encouraged him to eat his lunch. Angrily, he pushed away the tray and got up out of bed. He looked under the bed and saw that the medicine bag was gone. Frantically, he looked around the room and found the beadwork on the window counter. Though relieved to find the medicine bag there, he was very angry, sad, and fearful and wondered why it was removed from under the bed. These culturally sacred items should not have been moved without the Native person's permission (Lipson, Dibble, & Minarik, 1996). John felt he could no longer sleep in the bed because the medicine bag had been moved and therefore his bed was not protected while he was at dialysis. Hence, he called for the nurse and requested to be moved to another room. There were no empty beds on the floor. His nurse felt he was being *too superstitious*. When his family arrived (after a four hour drive from the reservation), John insisted that they take him home for he felt certain that he would die by morning. Although they knew he needed the medical treatment, they respected his wishes as he was an elder. The physician was contacted, and the client was discharged with follow-up dialysis at a clinic two hours from his home. This incident reveals the danger of cultural ignorance and cultural pain, and the importance of being sensitive to cultural knowledge about sacred cultural objects and their purposes.

The nurse learned that within three weeks of John's discharge his arterial-venous graft for dialysis had clotted and he was readmitted for fistula repair. He was very hesitant to return fearing a similar situation would again occur and that he could lose his sacred objects. So, he left his beadwork and medicine bag at home. He was very sad and depressed during his stay in the hospital, which led to a slow recovery and required extra hospital days. It was a culturally painful experience for John and led to culturally *incongruent* care (Leininger, 1997). This scenario could have been prevented had the staff been educated in transcultural nursing. All staff members providing care for persons of diverse cultures in healthcare settings need education about these cultures. Had the housekeeper been educated in Native American beliefs and practices this incident could have been prevented. The theory of

Culture Care could have guided staff to discover that culture care accommodation and negotiation were needed in this situation. Moreover, if clinical staff were knowledgeable in transcultural nursing, they would have arranged and negotiated (with John's permission) a traditional healer to perform a ceremony or ritual on the linens and cleansing of the bed to make John feel safe again. Maintaining John's Native American beliefs was essential to prevent a premature discharge leading to serious health consequences. Financial and emotional stress to the client and family was clearly evident. Transcultural nursing would have greatly reduced hospital costs, client discomfort, complications, and cultural pain.

Summary

These seven scenarios demonstrate the need for and effectiveness of transcultural nursing principles and actions in clinical settings. Transcultural nursing care knowledge is imperative to provide culturally appropriate care for people of diverse cultures. A transcultural nurse specialist and other healthcare personnel educated in transcultural nursing are needed to improve care to people of diverse cultures and to prevent disastrous situations leading to cultural harm and potential liabilities in healthcare facilities. Certified transcultural nurses are leaders in promoting culturally competent care to improve communication and understanding between clients and staff. Transcultural nurses can help to improve client adherence to care regimens and treatments, reduce recidivism, and decrease overall costs for health care (Cater & Spence, 1996; Leininger & McFarland, 2002).

The author contends that government and local agencies should hold healthcare administrators accountable for initiating and maintaining cultural diversity education and for providing culturally competent care in order to improve client recovery and shorten hospital stays. The theory of Culture Care Diversity and Universality is an excellent guide for assessing, caring for, and assisting people from diverse cultures. It is an excellent framework toward developing understanding about the client's cultural or holistic worldview and to ensure that culturally competent care is being provided in healthcare facilities. It is fortunate that nearly 45 books and almost 400 articles (many research based) are available for clinical staff to learn about transcultural nursing. The 2002 book by Leininger and McFarland offers fundamental concepts and principles, and includes many examples of cultural care based on five decades of cultural care research. Leininger's short culturalogical assessment guide incorporates six steps to providing culturally congruent care and ways to use Culture Care Theory in clinical practice (Leininger 1978, 1995, 2002). These resources are essential to help nurses provide and maintain culturally congruent care. It is imperative that clients and families from diverse cultures are treated with dignity, respect, and compassion. Cultural hatred and discrimination must be eradicated in healthcare institutions through transcultural nursing education because they can and do lead to destructive and nontherapeutic practices.

As Leininger states, "Where there is hatred, fear, prejudice, racism, or violence, there is a need to help nurses and others to lessen or remove these barriers through the use of transcultural caring knowledge and skills" (Leininger, 1999). Government officials and healthcare providers, administrators, and clinical staff need to be held accountable to practice culturally congruent care. Culturally specific transcultural nursing knowledge and research is essential to guide nurses and other healthcare workers to make appropriate and safe clinical decisions and to be respectful and skilled in meeting the cultural care needs of diverse clients in every clinical setting.

References

American Health Consultants. (2001). Rooting out health care discrimination: It's not just the right thing to do. *Healthcare Benchmarks, 8*(4), 37–44.

Barton, G. M. (1999). Personal harassment creates liability. *Healthcare Benchmarks, 3*, 35–39.

Cater, R., and Spence, M. (1996). Cultural diversity process improves organizational community in urban teaching medical center. *Journal of Cultural Diversity, 3*(2), 35–39.

Curren, D. (2003). [Curren cultural competency guide]. Unpublished guide.

Ehrmin, J.T. (2002). Family violence and culture care with African and Euro-American cultures in the United States. In M. Leininger, & M. McFarland (Eds.), *Transcultural nursing: Concepts, theories, research and practice* (3rd ed., pp. 343–345). New York: McGraw-Hill.

Galanti, G. (2003). The Hispanic family and male-female relationships: An overview. *Journal of Transcultural Nursing, 14*(3), 180–185.

Jamieson, D., & O'Mara, J. (1991). *Managing workforce 2000: Gaining the diversity advantage.* San Francisco: Jossey-Bass.

Lawrence, P., & Rozmus, C. (2001). Culturally sensitive care of the Muslim patient. *Journal of Transcultural Nursing, 13*(3), 228–233.

Leininger, M. M. (1978). *Transcultural nursing: Concepts, theories, and practices.* New York: John Wiley & Sons.

Leininger, M. (1991). Culture care diversity and universality: A theory of nursing. New York: National League for Nursing Press.

Leininger, M. (1995). *Transcultural nursing: Concepts, theories, research, and practices*. New York: McGraw-Hill.

Leininger, M. (1997). Cultural pain. *Images of nursing*. Summer, 19–20.

Leininger, M. (1999). *Transcultural nurse's prayer*. (Advanced Transcultural Nursing Seminar). Omaha, NE: University of Nebraska, Department of Nursing.

Leininger, M. (2002a). Essential transcultural nursing care concepts, principles, examples and policy statements. In M. Leininger, & M. McFarland (Eds.), *Transcultural nursing: Concepts, theories, research and practice* (3rd ed., pp. 129–130). New York: McGraw-Hill.

Leininger, M. (2002b). Phillipine Americans and culture care. In M. Leininger, & M. McFarland (Eds.), *Transcultural nursing: Concepts, theories, research and practice* (3rd ed., pp. 381–382). New York: McGraw-Hill.

Leininger, M. (2002c). The future of transcultural nursing: A global perspective. In M. Leininger, & M. McFarland (Eds.), *Transcultural nursing: Concepts, theories, research and practice*, (3rd ed., pp. 585–586). New York: McGraw-Hill.

Leininger, M. (2003). Sunrise Enabler. *Transcultural Nursing Society*. Retrieved July 2003, from http://www.tcns.org.

Leininger, M., & McFarland, MR. (2002). *Transcultural nursing: Concepts, theories, research and practice*. NY: McGraw-Hill.

Leuning, C., Swiggum, P., Wiegert, H., & Zander, K. (2002). Proposed standards for transcultural nursing. *Journal of Transcultural Nursing, 13*(1), 40–46

Lipson, J., Dibble, S., & Minarik, P. (1996). *Culture and nursing care: A pocket guide*. San Francisco: UCSF Nursing Press.

Nydell, M. (1996). *Understanding Arabs: A guide for westerners*. Yarmouth, ME: Intercultural Press.

Spinks, V., Andrews, M., & Boyle, J. (2000). Providing health care for lesbian clients. *Journal of Transcultural Nursing, 11*(2), 137–143.

Stolberg, S. (2002, March 21). Race gap seen in health care of equally insured patients. *New York Times*. Retrieved March 20, 2004, from www.nytimes.com

Tullmann, D. (1992). Cultural diversity in nursing education: Does it affect racism in the nursing profession? *Journal of Nursing Education, 31*(1), 321–324.

United States Department of Health and Human Services, Office of Minority Health. (2001). *National standards for culturally and linguistically appropriate services in health care*. Rockville, MD: Author.

United States Department of Health and Human Services, Health Resources and Services Administration. (2001). The registered nurse population: National sample survey of registered nurses. Retrieved February 18, 2001, from http://www.ASK.hrsa.gov/index.cfm.

Vaughn, J. (1997). Is there really racism in nursing? *Journal of Nursing Education, 36*(3), 135–139.

CHAPTER SIX

Culture Care of German American Elders in a Nursing Home Context

Marilyn R. McFarland, PhD, RN, CTN

Norma Zehnder, RN, PhD, APRN-BC

Introduction

The number of Anglo American elders living in nursing homes has increased dramatically since the 1960s (Kemper & Murtaugh, 1991). The dramatic increase in nursing home admissions has been due to the increasing numbers of dependent elderly people and the corresponding reduction in the pool of potential family caregivers as a result of women working outside the home. Anglo American families were reported to be as reluctant to place their elderly relatives in nursing homes (West, Illsley, & Kelman, 1984) as the elders were to agree to live in such settings (Biedenharn & Normoyle, 1991). Anglo American families have not abandoned their relatives in institutions but many have chosen a shared care pattern between themselves and a long-term care facility. The research literature has confirmed that when an Anglo American elder enters a nursing home, retirement home, or other special residential setting, families desire to share care responsibilities with the staff (Montgomery, 1983; Schmidt, 1987; Shuttlesworth, Rubin, & Duffy, 1982; Wiener & Kayser-Jones, 1990).

Purpose of Study and Domain of Inquiry

The purpose of this ethnonursing research ministudy was to discover, describe, and systematically analyze the care expressions, practices, and patterns of elderly German Americans living in a nursing home setting in a small city in the Midwestern United States. The domain of inquiry (DOI) was the cultural care of elderly German American residents within the environmental context of a nursing home. The study was guided by Leininger's Culture Care Theory, and the ethnonursing research method was used. The research focus was to enter and discover the elders' world in an institutional environmental context and systematically examine the experiences, practices, and patterns of care.

Ethnohistory, Language, and Environmental Context

An ethnohistory of present day German American elders is offered to
provide a background of information about their culture and is presented to facilitate understanding of their past and present environmental contexts. A brief review of German American history is provided
relevant to the nursing home and the German American community
where this study took place.

Ethnohistory

German Americans number approximately 43 million people in the
United States or one-sixth of all citizens in the Midwestern state where
this study was conducted who can trace their ancestry, at least in part,
to German roots (US Census, 2000). Little has been written about
German Americans who are usually recognized as *White* on application
forms, in surveys, and in research studies. This 'grouping together' of
data limits the availability of culturally specific information. Differences
in worldview, cultural beliefs, and healthcare practices among White
ethnic groups hold important implications for nurses and other healthcare providers. Therefore more cultural specific information about
German Americans has been needed.

According to historians, German immigration to America occurred
primarily in three waves with the largest group of approximately six million German people arriving between 1890 and 1920. Overall, immigration was largely the result of economic, religious, and political unrest in
Europe. Early US history indicates that a small group of settlers in
Jamestown were purportedly German. However, the 'official' onset of
German immigration to early America is generally believed to be the
founding of Deutschstadt (Germantown), Pennsylvania, in 1683
(Lassiter, 1995; Winawer & Wetzel, 1996). This group of Germans was
seeking religious freedom. According to Daniels (1990), however, large
scale German immigration did not occur for another 25 years following
the settlement of Germantown. At that time, the influx of German
immigrants to America was primarily due to economic, social, and political reasons such as overpopulation, poverty, and heavy taxation in the
German areas of Northern Europe (Daniels).

Similarly, an 82-year-old resident at the nursing home research site
explained that her grandparents came to America to ". . . find a better
life. Life was hard in Germany." In contrast, a second generation
German American 82-year-old resident, when asked why his ancestors
had migrated to the United States, said, "That's a good question. I really

don't know." Finally, because of further political and territorial adversity following World War I and preceding World War II, the last significant German immigration occurred in the 1930s and 1940s as refugees attempted to flee the Nazi Holocaust (Daniels, 1990).

Many German immigrant men initially worked in agriculture but were later employed as artisans and skilled laborers. In contrast, women were attracted to work in the service sectors as bakers, domestic workers, nurses, laundry workers, janitors, tailors, and saloonkeepers (Daniels, 1990; Lassiter, 1995). In particular, domestic work for women not only provided economically for the family but also exposed them to the home life of middle class American families. This in turn promoted the assimilation and acculturation of German immigrant women into American society.

Farming was a dominant occupation for the early settlers in the Midwestern small city where this study was conducted. An 82-year-old resident of the nursing home explained:

> Although two of my grandfather's brothers entered the ministry, my grandfather remained on the family farm. My dad was born on the farm and eventually bought it from his father. The family farm is where my four brothers and sister were raised.

Similar accounts were frequently heard from other German American residents of the nursing home. The rate and depth of assimilation differed among the various waves of immigrants. During Colonial times, assimilation occurred more slowly as early immigrants were largely agrarian, settling primarily in Eastern seaboard colonies. Their interest centered mainly on religious tolerance and equitable land distribution rather than transplanting their German heritage (Steckler, 2003). During the mid nineteenth century, immigrants focused more on transferring their German culture to American society as evidenced by speaking the German language in their schools and churches, joining their own orchestras and singing groups, and publishing German newspapers (Steckler, 2003).

This trend was particularly true in the Midwestern city where this study was conducted, as German was the dominant language spoken in the church, school, and home well past the 1930s. According to Krafft (1994), German was the official language of the church in this community from its inception in 1845 into the 1930s. Since 1998, dwindling attendance and difficulty finding a German-speaking pastor had reduced the number of German services from weekly to once a month. Nonetheless, these German services are videotaped so that residents of the nursing home may watch them, which many do.

School, in this community, was conducted in German until the mid 1930s, and in the the late 1920s and early 1930s, English was not introduced until the seventh and eighth grades (Bernthal, 1997). One 82-year-old resident explained, "We had so much to memorize . . . both in German and English." Further, he said that German was the dominant language spoken at home as well. However, he stated, "I decided when I was about six or seven I wasn't speaking German at home anymore. It was time to speak English." Regardless, German remained the language of choice spoken between his parents. He added, "It took the rural families considerably more time to convert to speaking English than those who lived in town."

One of the authors of the study, who is German American and from the local community where this study was conducted, explained her experience:

> My parents generally spoke German between themselves but always English with me. Their philosophy was that it was important to learn the English language well since we were living in the United States. Fortunately, I was able to learn enough of the German language to both read and understand [it] by listening to my parents and relatives converse. Speaking the language, however, was more difficult for me.
>
> By the mid 1940s, German was no longer taught in the [local] parochial school. About 1950, an endeavor was again made at teaching the language in school. However, that was short lived and no further attempt was made until about 1980. German has been taught in the parochial school at varying levels since. It has been taught consistently at kindergarten through eighth grade levels since 1997. In addition, German has also been offered as a language in the community high school for many years.

The third wave of German immigrants arriving in the US in the 1930s and early 1940s included well educated professionals such as physicians, architects, scientists, mathematicians, and artists (Steckler, 2003). After witnessing the horrors of Nazism, this group made no overt efforts to maintain their culture in America. They were quickly assimilated, thereby enriching American culture in the areas of mathematics, science, music, and psychology. One of the researchers distinctly recalls her mother telling her during World War II that a subtle stigma existed in surrounding communities because of the German heritage of the local area. Continuing stigma existed in the mind of one nursing home resident who remarked quietly, ". . . my name is German but I don't want to sound as if I favor Hitler."

Regardless of assimilation or enculturation, several cultural characteristics and values remained intact in succeeding German American generations. For example, a strong work ethic focused on thoroughness, orderliness, solid craftsmanship, industriousness, diligence, and attention to detail continues to be manifested among present day German Americans (Winawer & Wetzel, 1996). Several elderly residents commented on their need to have ". . . everything in its place, my possessions in order, and activities and events to start on time."

In addition, the strong emphasis on education by Germans had a profound influence on American society with many lasting contributions made to education, such as the introduction of kindergarten, use of the blackboard, and German pedagogical theories. An 82-year-old resident stated that in the local community:

> Education was always considered important even though my grandfather could not see the need for it. Grandpa felt it was useless for boys to go to school beyond the eighth grade; none of his children [had] indulged themselves that way. Fortunately, my dad supported my interest in continuing to high school and I was glad since I had already made up my mind not to be a farmer.

Family life continues to be valued as a source of mutual support and strength in times of crisis with extended family systems remaining strong and well organized (Winawer & Wetzel, 1996). This finding was supported by the large number of family photos and visitors observed in the residents' rooms by the two researchers. When questioned about family visitation, several residents remarked that their sons or daughters visited on a regular basis and they also enjoyed frequent family outings. The researchers observed many of the residents' spouses visited daily.

A commitment in service to the Lutheran Church was a continuing manifestation of their spirituality and strong work ethic. Many residents attended the weekly chapel services available at the nursing home with several denominations offering services. One resident explained that ". . . church is very important to me . . . I'm so glad we have services here because it means a lot to me." A particular fondness for the Lutheran chaplain was also found in comments such as ". . . He's a wonderful man with such a good sense of humor . . . He really makes the service interesting . . . Besides, he's a [Detroit baseball] Tiger fan!"

German immigration from Bavaria to the small city in the Midwestern United States where this study was conducted was for the purpose of establishing a mission outreach to the Chippewa Indians. Although the Indian mission effort proved relatively unsuccessful, the establishment of a local Lutheran church to serve the growing community was successful and led to a membership of 4900 people by the end of the year 2000 (St. Lorenz, 2000). In addition to the church, a Lutheran school was established in 1845 to teach the immigrant and Indian children. In 1999–2000, the present school had an enrollment of 589 students with programs ranging from preschool through eighth grade (St. Lorenz, 2000).

A further outreach of the church occurred in 1893 when representatives of Detroit Lutheran Churches and surrounding communities proposed establishing the first Lutheran Home for the Aged in southeastern Michigan. This outreach was reflected in the Mission Statement of the nursing home which states that the mission and ministry of the homes owned and operated by the Lutheran Church-Missouri Synod are focused on the care of elderly people with an emphasis on their spiritual, emotional, social, and physical needs. In 1962 the Board of Directors voted to establish a second home in the community where this study took place.

Review of Literature

German American Studies

In a thorough search for nursing research studies of German Americans in the literature, none were found. A descriptive book chapter entitled *Transcultural Health Care: German Americans* by Jessica Steckler, found in the supplement to Purnell & Paulanka's (2003) *Transcultural Health Care*, was the only reference specifically related to German American health care discovered. The author reported that German American elders unable to live alone move in with children or often move into retirement or nursing homes.

Transcultural Studies of Elder Care

In a study of the culture care of Polish American elders living in their own homes or the homes of their children, McFarland (1995) discovered that elders wanted to maintain their traditional generic lifeways and that families caring for them enhanced their health and lifeways. McFarland (1997) also conducted an ethnonursing study guided by the Culture Care Theory in a long-term care facility and discovered that Anglo and African American elders desired generic or folk care to maintain their preadmission generic lifeways and to maintain their health in an institutional setting. Elderly residents from both cultures wanted their families and nursing staff to combine generic and professional care, which led to the discovery of culturally congruent care. In addition, Leuning (Leininger & McFarland, 2002) discovered that Namibian elders in Africa who were cared for at home by their families combined generic and professional nursing care to provide culturally congruent community based nursing care.

Theoretical Framework

The Theory of Culture Care Diversity and Universality (Leininger, 1991a) was chosen as the framework for this study. This nursing theory was selected because of the researchers' own interests in using the Culture Care Theory to discover cultural lifeways and related nursing actions and decisions for culturally congruent care for elders of diverse cultures. Leininger took the idea of *culture* from anthropology and the concept of *care* from nursing and put these two ideas together to develop the Culture Care Theory. The theory has directed nurses to discover what was *universal* (or common) and what was *diverse* (or different) about human care in wellness, illness, disability, and human conditions. Thus, culture care knowledge was held to be central to transcultural nursing and to explain, interpret, and predict nursing care practice.

With the theoretical framework, the Sunrise Enabler was used as a cognitive map to focus the research study on the influencing dimensions and major constructs of the theory (Leininger, 1991a). The Sunrise Enabler was developed by Leininger (Leininger & McFarland, 2002) to help visualize different dimensions of the Culture Care Theory. An assumption or 'given' in Leininger's theory is that worldview, social structures, factors such as religion, economics, education, technology, politics, kinship, family, ethnohistory, environmental context, language, and generic and professional care factors influence care meanings, expressions, patterns, values, and practices in different cultures. These dimensions influence how individuals or groups view professional nursing care. Leininger has held that all cultures have generic, folk, or lay care practices that predate professional health care including professional nursing care. Many researchers who have used her theory have discovered that clients prefer generic or folk care to be combined with professional nursing care services which has led to care congruent with their cultural beliefs and values, and has lead to health and wellbeing (Leininger & McFarland, 2002).

Research Questions

For this study, the following research questions were developed:

1. What are the culture care expressions, patterns, and practices of German American elderly residents living in a nursing home context?

2. In what ways do worldview, social structure factors, and environmental context influence culture care expressions, patterns, and practices for German American residents of a nursing home?
3. In what ways do culture care expressions, patterns, and practices influence the health and wellbeing of elderly German Americans?

Orientational Definitions

Definitions were developed to provide a broad orientational research focus to discover the cultural care of German American elders within the environmental context of a nursing home. The definitions were not used rigidly but rather as ways to approach the domain of inquiry to generate the *emic* (insiders') views as well as the *etic* (outsiders' or professionals') meanings of the nursing phenomena under study.

1. Culture Care: Refers to the subjectively and objectively learned and transmitted values, beliefs, and patterned lifeways that assist, support, facilitate or enable another individual or group to maintain their wellbeing, health, or to improve their human condition and lifeway, or to deal with illness, handicap, or death (derived from Leininger, 1991a, p. 46).
2. Professional Care: Refers to the cognitive and formally learned, assistive, supportive, and facilitative phenomena offered to elderly residents within the nursing care context (derived from Leininger, 1991a, p. 48).
3. Environmental Context: Refers to the totality of the experience of living in an institution that includes the physical setting of the residents' rooms, the entirety of the institution including its organizational factors, social factors, physical layout, and the cultural backgrounds of the residents.
4. Health: Refers to a state of culturally defined wellbeing which reflects the ability to perform daily role activities (derived from Leininger, 1991a, p. 48).
5. German American Elderly Resident: Refers to a person aged 70 years or older living in a nursing home who identifies herself or himself as having German heritage, values, beliefs, and lifeways, and as having been born in the United States.
6. Nursing Home Context: Refers to an institutional setting where elderly people receive long-term care services often paid by commercial and-or government health or welfare programs.
7. Assisted Living Context: Refers to a section of the nursing home where residents live in a semi-independent setting with a lower ratio of staff compared to the standard nursing home; such services are not covered by government programs.

Assumptive Premises of the Research

The following assumptions for this study were derived from the work of Leininger (1991a):

1. Culture care for elders in a nursing home is for health, wellbeing, growth, survival, and to face hardships and death.
2. Culture care views, meanings, and expressions of German American elders can be identified within the nursing home setting and reflect similarities and differences among the residents.
3. The elderly German Americans' worldview, social structure, and environmental context influence care and their health, wellbeing, and satisfaction with care practices.

Method

The ethnonursing method was used to examine the expressions, patterns, and practices of care as lived by elderly German American residents in a nursing home setting. Leininger (1991b) has defined ethnonursing as ". . . a qualitative research method using naturalistic, open discovery, and largely inductively derived *emic* modes and process with diverse strategies, techniques, and enabling tools to document, describe, understand, and interpret the peoples' meanings, experiences, symbols, and other related aspects bearing on actual or potential nursing phenomena" (p. 79).

Data Collection Procedure

The observation-participation-reflection (OPR) process as described by Leininger (1991b) was an essential part of this ethnonursing study conducted over a period of 18 months. The first phase, *observation* and *active listening*, gave the researchers the opportunity to be observers and become aware of the nursing home environmental context prior to becoming full participants in ongoing activities. The second phase, *observation and limited participation*, included mainly observing but some limited participation in institutional activities such as programs or meetings that were in progress when the researchers happened to be on site. The third phase, *participation*, focused mainly on *preplanned and intensive participation* in ongoing activities such as care conferences, resident meetings, and *scheduled interviews* which included a series of open ended queries (Appendix 6-A). The fourth phase, *reflection and confirmation*, allowed for a period of time toward the end of the study to recheck the findings and reconfirm them with elderly resident informants.

Informants were carefully and purposefully selected by the researchers with the assistance of the residents and staff of the institution based on who might be most knowledgeable about the domain of inquiry. Leininger (1991b) generally recommends 12 to 15 key informants and 24 to 30 general informants for a maxi-ethnonursing study; for a mini-ethnonursing study, approximately half the numbers are recommended. Five key and ten general informants participated in this study. Key informants were those knowledgeable about the domain of inquiry and general informants were less knowledgeable but could offer reflective comments. The criteria for the selection of informants are presented in Table 6-1.

Human Subject Considerations

A verbal and written explanation was given to each informant. Details of the study, risks, and benefits of participation, right to withdraw, protection from harm, and assurance of confidentiality were discussed with each informant. Some informants requested that they sign the consent document only after it was reviewed by a relative, usually an adult child; this request was always granted. Authorization for the research was also obtained from the nursing home administration and the Investigational Review Board of the sponsoring university.

Data Analysis and Criteria for Substantiating–Confirming the Research

The data in this study were analyzed using Leininger's four phases of data analysis (Leininger & McFarland, 2002). The analysis began with collection and documentation of raw data from observations and interviews including descriptors or direct quotes from elders (first phase), then categorizing and coding the descriptors and raw data such as observations (second phase). In the third phase, recurrent patterns were identified from continually comparing codes and categories. Lastly, themes were abstracted from the patterns identified.

Trustworthiness of the study was demonstrated by using the qualitative evaluation criteria (Leininger, 1991b; Leininger & McFarland, 2002) of credibility, confirmability, meaning in context, recurrent patterning, saturation, and transferability. The 'truth' and accuracy of the findings were mutually established between the researchers and the informants. Credible findings were supported through persistent observations and prolonged and direct participation activities with the residents in the nursing home by the researchers. Credibility was established through the informants' interpretation and explanation of

TABLE 6-1 Criteria for the Selection of Informants

Key Informants	General Informants
Knowledgeable about the DOI	Less knowledgeable about the DOI
Male or female who identifies self as German American	Male or female who identifies self as German American
70 years of age or older	70 years of age or older
Born in USA	Born in USA
Able to relate or reveal major aspects of current and past life	Able to relate or reveal major aspects of current and past life
Willing to give verbal consent to participate in study	Willing to give verbal consent to participate in study

the researchers' findings. The experiences of informants became meaningful in context as all data were collected through observation, interview, and participation in activities which took place within the total context of the nursing home during the course of the research study. Repeated care patterns of German American elderly residents were used to establish the criteria of recurrent patterning. Saturation occurred when the same or similar information was obtained in duplicate words. The researchers considered whether transferability would aid in the discovery of findings that would have similar meanings in other contexts such as in other institutions where there are elderly residents with similar cultures and lifeways.

An indepth description of the ethnonursing method and use of the phases of data analysis may be found in the first and second chapters of this book by Dr. Leininger and in other culture care studies.

Findings with Discussion

The domain of inquiry for this study was the culture care of German American elders living in a nursing home context. The presentation of the findings is centered on the abstracted care patterns and themes discovered in the study. The findings revealed two universal or commonly prevailing themes and one diverse theme supported by both universal and diverse patterns. Some examples of descriptors and other raw data from interviews and observations are presented to support the themes and patterns discovered.

Universal Theme 1

German American residents viewed, expressed, and lived generic or folk care to maintain their preadmission lifeways and to maintain their health in the nursing home.

This universal theme was derived from the German American elders' cultural care expressions, patterns, and practices within the context of the nursing home setting. The generic care patterns that supported this theme were *care as 'doing for' others through individual and collective care, care as families helping elderly family members, care as spiritual or religious helping, care as living the German American lifeways and traditions, and care as having the home clean and orderly.* This theme revealed universal values which were supported by the commonalities in care patterns identified.

Care Pattern

Care as doing for others through individual and collective care.

This universal care pattern of residents helping or caring for others was viewed as essential to the beneficial and satisfying lifeways of elders by all five key informants and seven general informants. Care as doing for others was a pattern derived from the residents' worldview and social structure factors of kinship and religion. Researcher observations and participant descriptors revealed the worldview of residents not only focused inward on their daily lifeways but also outward toward the community where the nursing home was located and where most of the residents had lived much of their lives before entering the nursing home. The care pattern of doing for others was also buttressed by their kinship and religious beliefs which had encouraged the elders to care for their families, fellow church members, and others in the community. The Lutheran pastor at the nursing home related that it had always been a tradition of the Lutheran Church to reach out to people who were in need whether they were Lutherans or not.

Individual Care

Doing for others through individual care was a generic care pattern derived from observations and descriptors which fit with the spiritual beliefs of residents, revealing that elders cared for other residents in many ways. One key informant explained:

> There are three people seated at my table in the dining room at every meal and several residents who eat in the dining room are confused and not quite right . . . This is very difficult and I feel badly for them and try to help them when they say things like 'Where am I?' or 'Where should I go?' . . . I always try to help them out but sometimes it is hard to share your life with people who are confused. But it is my Christian duty to help those people.

Collective Care

Elderly residents also provided *collective care* or care that benefited many residents of the home. One key informant explained:

> . . . The bazaar we had last Friday was a huge success and we made $600 or $700 . . . the residents' council decided to spend some money [since] we had quite a cash surplus in our account . . . [The council] decided to buy flowers to plant in the outdoor courtyard . . . we also decided that since we raised so much money we would make a donation to the Salvation Army and Lutheran Hospice.

Elderly residents felt these donations were a way to do something not only for their fellow residents but also for the community as a whole. The collective care construct fit with the residents' worldview which was to focus not only inward on their lifeways in the nursing home but also on life outside the nursing home toward the community where they had spent most of their lives and where many of their family members lived. There were many other informant descriptors that confirmed this care pattern. One general informant commented:

> . . . Some of the residents are taking care of the flower beds . . . this is something most of us enjoyed doing in our own yards at home . . . and I take care of the cat here [resident feline at nursing home] . . . sometimes I get tired of it, but we all have to make a contribution for others while we are here . . .

Care Pattern

Care as families helping their elderly family members.

The generic care pattern of family help or assistance enhanced the lives of elderly residents and was grounded in their established lifeways within the German American culture. German American elderly residents received care from their spouses and adult children. Descriptors came from elders such as, ". . . my daughter comes often and takes care of my finances . . . [even though] she does have four children at home." Another resident commented, ". . . my daughter came last Sunday and took me home . . . my grandchild was confirmed that day . . . and I enjoyed my daughter's homecooking." Another elderly man explained that his wife still lives in their home in the neighborhood, and that ". . . she walks over every day and usually brings me lunch or dinner." German American family members did not abandon their elderly relatives when they entered the nursing home, but continued to visit and provide care for elders reflecting a shared care pattern between families and nursing home staff.

Care Pattern

Care as spiritual or religious helping.

The generic care pattern of spiritual or religious care was universal for all German American informants and was deeply rooted in their German American Lutheran culture. Most German American informants were members of the Lutheran church and most belonged to the local church in the community. German American residents received spiritual or religious care from the German American Lutheran pastor who served both as pastor in the nursing home and as an assistant minister at the local community church. One key informant explained, ". . . I go to the German church service which is held here every week . . . and this is a Christian place . . . the pastor is very kind and he will joke with you and talk seriously with you." A general informant confirmed the care pattern of spiritual care when he stated, ". . . the pastor mixes a lot with the old people and he is very helpful to residents and talks to them . . .". He explained further: ". . . The lady next door to me died this week and the pastor came down to talk to us and it was very helpful."

Four key and seven general informants related that the religious affiliation and activities offered as a part of the care at the nursing home helped them get through each day. One general informant, an elderly woman, said, ". . . God has helped me and I talk with Him every day . . . I ask Him to guide me . . . I live with God." Another general informant explained, ". . . the Lutheran connection and the chapel [in the nursing home] were the two reasons I came to this nursing home . . . I believe the care is affected by the church and influenced by the church."

Care Pattern

Care as living the German American traditions and lifeways.

This care pattern was reflected in the comments made by all key and six general informants about the activities and food offered in the nursing home. One key informant described a 'joyride' offered at the nursing home every spring and fall.

> They [the staff] take us in a bus or van for a ride in the countryside . . . and look at the flowers and crops being put in . . . many of the men here were farmers and we like to go out in the country and see what is happening in the fields . . . they make a big effort to take people even if they are a bit confused or in wheelchairs.

One general informant explained his frustration with confused residents, ". . . I'd like to go and see the crops coming up but I just can't go with people I can't talk to."

Several residents spoke about the activities available to them as part of the care at the nursing home. Residents mentioned how important it was for them to keep busy. One elderly woman, a key informant, explained that there were lots of things to do in the nursing home. She mentioned the garden club, sewing items for the bazaars, ice cream socials at noon, chapel services, trips to the local Lutheran church, sing-a-longs, crafts, popcorn parties, as well as meeting with other residents, the pastor, and with friends and family. She said, ". . . at the nursing home there is a lot of German pride . . . a lot of the residents here really worked hard in the past so now we need to keep busy at something so we go to all the activities." 'Keeping busy' was firmly rooted in the traditional German cultural value of hard work and always being occupied at 'something'. Another general informant commented:

> . . . It is a good place . . . there are things to do . . . cooking, crafts, and sewing . . . the entertainment's good . . . happy hour with wine and good beer starts about a half hour after lunch . . . it is really pleasant and is held in the main dining room . . . there is sometimes Karaoke or a professional entertainment and the staff try to get the residents to take part.

One former German American farmer and a general informant commented, ". . . we have dinner at noon and a light supper at night here. . . . City people eat their big meal at night but farmers eat their big meal at noon and we continue that here." Another general informant commented that he enjoyed the once a week outside barbecue with bratwursts and German beer held during the summer months. One general informant who had lived for several years in the nursing home commented:

> . . . the food is fair . . . lots of meat and potatoes like we were raised, but . . . they don't do much home cooking anymore . . . canned foods like vegetables are not as good as fresh.

Another general informant complained that the soup was no longer homemade. She explained, " . . . the home does not make their own soup and it does not have any flavor."

German American elderly residents were attached to the German language and most informants had learned to speak and write German at the local parochial schools, and spoke it at home as children. One key informant commented:

> . . . I go every Wednesday to the church service in the chapel . . . it is in German and many residents here attend that service . . . many of these residents are people I knew when I was young and we learned German at school and spoke it at home.

Care Pattern

Care as having the home clean and orderly.

A fifth generic care pattern reflected the value of having the nursing home clean and orderly without offensive odors. Several residents commented on how they appreciated the cleanliness of the nursing home. One key informant, an elderly woman, commented, ". . . there is no smell of urine here as there is in other nursing homes." This pattern was congruent with the way she had been raised in a German American home where cleanliness and order were always valued.

Diverse Theme 2

Nursing home care patterns and expressions were viewed within the daily and nightly environmental context as a continuous life experience but with differences between lifeways in the 'assisted living' rooms and the traditional nursing home rooms.

Care Pattern

The nursing home environment was less satisfying as a context for care than the 'assisted living' section.

All elderly informants found life more satisfactory and more congruent with their traditional and previous lifeways in the 'assisted living' section of the nursing home than in the standard nursing home rooms where skilled and basic nursing care services were provided. Many residents in the standard nursing home rooms had initially lived in the 'assisted living' section and had eventually moved to their present location within the nursing home.

The physical setting of the nursing home rooms offered little space for personal possessions. Hence, most personal possessions could not be secured and there was little privacy. This reflected the care pattern that the nursing home environment was less satisfying as a care context than the 'assisted living' area. One key informant explained:

> . . . I live in assisted living . . . and when I came here I could only bring six changes of clothing . . . and my roommate and I both have wheelchairs and walkers and at night I have a commode brought in and you can barely move around in our room . . . but, there is more room here than on the nursing home floors . . . I am now 92 . . . and I will run out of money in a couple of years . . . that means I must go on Medicaid and move out of assisted living . . . I will have even less space there.

When residents are enrolled in Medicaid, a government welfare program, care in assisted living is not a covered benefit but care in a nursing home room with higher levels of staffing *is* covered. An elderly general informant described his frustration with living in a nursing home:

. . . People have a problem with things missing from their rooms and there is a woman on this floor who does take things. She is very confused and the nurses try to find our things but this makes life hard. My daughter just bought me a new belt but it went missing . . . I did get it back but they found it in somebody else's room.

Care Pattern
Social factors affected the residents' satisfaction with their lifeways in the nursing home.

Frustration and lack of satisfaction with their lifeways within the nursing home setting was reflected in the comments from key and general informants that described how difficult it was to live with confused residents. One key informant and elderly resident who had been required to move from assisted living to the nursing home for financial reasons commented:

I can't sleep . . . the man in the next room hollers all night and you can hear him now. My money ran out and I had to move here. People are spitting and wiping their noses and spitting food back onto their plates and it makes me sick to eat here.

Another elderly resident of the nursing home commented:

. . . I don't like to go to the dining room early because so many people do not know what they are talking about. Why do they have to put the good ones [alert residents] in with the bad ones [confused residents]? Is there a law they have to do that?

The German American values of privacy and security for material possessions, and being financially able to pay for their own care were preserved more in the assisted living section than in the traditional nursing home rooms. All informants living in the nursing home rooms found life less congruent with their traditional lifeways than residents of the assisted living area. Those residents who lived in assisted living dreaded being transferred to the nursing home rooms and those who had been transferred to such rooms described life as "a struggle" and "difficult."

Universal Theme 3
German American elders universally viewed good health as being active, busy, and informed.

Care Pattern
Care as receiving assistance to move around the nursing home and into the community.

This care pattern was valued by five key and eight informants. One 96-year-old key informant said:

. . . People often tell me I look good . . . they say that a lot. I get around
and I'm active even if it is in a wheelchair . . . I take an interest and do
things. . . . I have a telephone and keep in touch with my son out east.
It is my link with the outside world.

Another informant described a planned walk outside organized by
the staff. He said:

. . . We are going to take a wheelchair walk to the church. Volunteers
are all lined up and they are going to push everyone who can't walk in
a wheelchair down to the church about four blocks away. You just go
crazy if you don't get out of here. I feel better if I can get some fresh air.

Another resident commented:

. . . The courtyard is a nice place to sit and some of the residents have
planted flowers . . . I think people would feel better if they would come
out here more, especially when the weather is nice.

Care pattern
Care as having opportunities for activities, events, and entertainment.
This care pattern was viewed as contributing to the residents' good
health and to satisfactory lifeways within the nursing home setting. One
resident commented, ". . . I take part in all the activities . . . as many as
I am able to get to . . . . My granddaughter is getting married and I am
going to the service and to the reception!"
Another elderly general informant commented:

. . . I do a lot of sewing here for the bazaar . . . I used to work for the
Singer Sewing Machine Company and I enjoy sewing because it keeps
me busy . . . you need to be busy and . . . one of the problems here with
some of these people is that they don't have enough to do. It is sad to
see people just sitting . . . if I keep myself busy I feel better and my
health is better.

Another general informant commented, ". . . They have a lot of
entertainment here and I like to get dressed up and put on good clothes
. . . in order to keep my health I walk, read a lot, and keep myself going."
Another general informant, an elderly woman who has Parkinson's disease, high blood pressure, and thyroid problems, stated, ". . . I'm in good
health because I can do what I want to do . . . I'm walking and my legs
are strong . . . I even go on walks by myself in the neighborhood."
Another key informant who viewed herself in good health said, ". . . I
never smoked, I have also been busy, and worked hard . . . that's why I
have lived so long . . . keeping busy does you good." Another resident
commented, ". . . I keep as active as I can because as soon as I stop moving around that's going to be it!"

Care Pattern

Care as being kept informed, discussing current events, and knowing 'what is going on.'

Descriptors given by elderly residents reflecting the care pattern were, ". . . health means keeping up on what is going on around you . . . having a good memory . . . and being alert." One elderly general informant was 102 years old and had not been able to walk for 5 years. She explained how she kept informed about local community events, " . . . I keep my radio in bed right next to me so I can tune the dial to the two local stations in town . . . it keeps me on track with what is going on." Another informant explained she really felt better when:

> . . . I sit in front of my window and look out on the street and see traffic go by, so there is always something going on outside . . . I watch the flowers bloom and the grass is green and the trees are budding with the rain we had in the last two days. . .

Health as being active, busy, and informed was rooted in the elderly German American residents' cultural values of being able to get around and to go to work, which was often discussed by the residents. If elderly residents could get to activities, keep busy, and keep up on what was happening both within the nursing home and in the surrounding community, they considered themselves healthy in spite of multiple diagnosed medical diseases such as arthritis, hypertension, and diabetes.

Discoveries for Culture-Specific Clinical Nursing Care

Leininger (1991a) predicted that specific culture care knowledge gained from using the Culture Care Theory would constitute a substantive knowledge base to guide nursing judgments, decisions, and actions in assisting people under diverse circumstances. The goal of the Culture Care Theory is to make nursing care decisions and take actions that are culturally congruent with the beliefs, practices, and values of the lifeways of people. The care decisions and subsequent actions presented herein focus on the three modes of care which are *culture care preservation and-or maintenance, culture care accommodation and-or negotiation,* and *culture care restructuring and-or repatterning.*

The Culture Care Theory and research findings were drawn upon to systematically identify the action and decision modes. The findings from this study confirmed by the elderly key and general informants revealed the following care modes which describe ways that enhance or would enhance the health and lifeways of the elderly German American residents.

Culture Care Preservation and-or Maintenance

German American religious beliefs and practices were essential to maintain the residents' health and satisfying lifeways. All informants wished to preserve the Lutheran religious services offered in German at the home every week. The Lutheran pastor assigned to the nursing home was viewed as essential to preserve the spiritual care offered to elders. Family involvement in the care of elderly residents was also valued by them as a culture-specific care practice that should be preserved. German American elderly residents valued *caring for others* and often gave care individually and collectively to other residents. They enjoyed working on projects that benefited all the residents of the home, thereby demonstrating that care for others or *collective care* was important to them. It is important for nurses to preserve and support this care practice. One resident commented, ". . . we all have to make a contribution for others while we are here."

Culture Care Accommodation and-or Negotiation

German American residents valued care and an environmental context for care that was like receiving care in their own homes. German American elders selectively supported and embraced professional nursing care provided at the home but preferred linking professional care practices with their own generic care lifeways. One resident explained that he really enjoyed the bus rides organized by the activity director out into the countryside to check on the crops. He explained that a lot of residents were farmers and this activity had been very popular at the home.

In addition, elders preferred involvement of their families in their care and were most satisfied when family members and many staff communicated about, cooperated, and shared care responsibilities. For instance, family members participated in care conferences with the resident and staff, attended social functions with elderly residents, and assisted elderly relatives with financial affairs and sometimes even shared some of the physical hands-on care such as assisting family members with eating and bathing. Many family members not only visited elderly relatives but took them home for holidays and special occasions, or attended holiday celebrations organized by the staff at the nursing home.

An important finding in this study was that the lifeways in the traditional nursing home rooms were much less satisfactory than in the assisted living section of the home and that the care was much less congruent with the German American elders' lifeways before they came to live in the nursing home. Nurses and residents made numerous efforts to negotiate making changes to adapt care routines and the environmental context for care in the nursing home rooms to fit more closely with care in the assisted living rooms or even like care in the residents' previous homes. Residents in the nursing home were encouraged to bring in small personal items and the nursing staff continually made great efforts to protect and secure these personal belongings but were only partially successful in this regard. However, residents recognized that nursing staff members were attempting to accommodate the residents' desire to keep and secure their clothing, knickknacks, and other personal items.

Culture Care Repatterning and-or Restructuring

German American elders proposed changes in care routines, privacy issues, and room designs. Culture care repatterning for German American elders living in the nursing home could include restructuring room designs for resident rooms, perhaps even private rooms, and providing a quieter environment—in general, repatterning the environmental context in which care is provided. One elder explained, "I used to talk farming to my roommate but now he is confused." Sharing a room with a roommate and eating in the dining room with disruptive, confused residents were viewed as the most difficult aspects of living in a nursing home for German American elders. This concern needs to be addressed by professional nurses.

The care mode of restructuring or repatterning requires nurses to have extensive transcultural nursing knowledge and to use that knowledge to influence the provision of culturally congruent care in long-term care settings such as nursing homes or assisted living settings. Culture care restructuring also requires coparticipation between nurses, clients, and their families with state and federal governmental agencies and legislative bodies where rules and regulations are made and the reimbursement levels are set for long-term care for elders. Nurses need to move beyond the individual care focus to a level where they can restructure long-term care on institutional, state, and federal levels.

Conclusion

With the number of elderly increasing worldwide, the importance of generic elder care or folk care specific to each cultural group will be increasingly important to transcultural nurses who practice in long-term care institutions. A universal finding from this study was that generic elder care in a nursing home was found to be essential for the residents' health and beneficial lifeways, which meant that cultural care was grounded in the traditional culture of the elders. Culturally congruent care is often contingent upon nurses being sensitive to elderly generic care and using these dimensions in professional care. The *universal* theme of generic or family care being essential for elders to maintain healthy and beneficial lifeways supports the assumptive premise of the Culture Care Theory that states, ". . . Care is essential for well-being, health, healing, growth, survival, and to face hardships or death." A *diverse* aspect of care for German American elders also supporting this premise was that the assisted living context and care practices were more culturally congruent with pre-admission lifeways and family care than what was found in the nursing home environment.

Today, nurses are faced with the care needs of increasing numbers of elders from diverse cultural groups admitted to nursing homes in the United States and other industrialized countries such as Japan, Northern European countries, Australia, and Canada, as previously discussed by McFarland (1997, 1995). Transcultural nurses need to study and discover new models and creative systems of care for the elderly in institutional settings related to culture care. For instance, this research study revealed that German American residents in a long-term care setting care for each other in many ways. The generic or folk pattern of *caring for others* or *other care* was grounded in the elders' traditional German American cultural lifeways and maintained in the nursing home setting which enhanced the residents' health and wellbeing. More importantly, generic care needs to be incorporated into professional care to make elder care acceptable and beneficial. Transcultural nursing care is imperative to meet the needs of a growing population of elders from diverse cultures (in the last phase of their lives) who strongly reaffirm their long held cultural identities.

Appendix 6-A   Resident Open Inquiry Guide

Ethnodemographics

Name:

Religious affiliation:

Informant #:

Years of formal education:

Sex:

Cultural background:

Age:

Previous occupation:

Place of residence in institution:

Dates of contact:

Years in the home:

Languages spoken:

Care Questions

1. I am interested in learning from you about the *care* here from your own experiences at this place. What does *care* mean to you from your own experiences here?
2. Did you come to this place because you needed care? If so, tell me about the care that you needed as you entered and have been here over time. How does your care meet your expectations?
3. Tell me about the care you receive here on a typical day and night.
4. What statement, words, or ideas describe the care in this home?
5. For you, then, *care* means _____.
6. Prior to coming to this setting, your mother, father, or other relative may have provided care in your home; tell me about this.
7. How would you describe a caring person? Give an example of the most caring staff person you know here. Do you find the nurses to be caring persons? How would you describe a caring nurse?
8. In your experience, tell me some stories about a caring nurse or staff member.
9. As a resident, do you at times give care to others?

Dedication

This chapter is dedicated to the memory of Leona M. Geyer (1901–1999), a German American woman who valued her cultural and spiritual traditions and lifeways. She was the mother of Dr. Norma Zehnder, and as a resident of the nursing home where the research took place, served as the inspiration for this study.

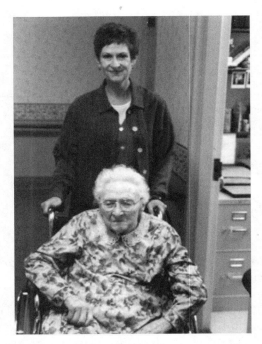

Figure 6-1 German American Mother and Daughter.

This study was funded in part through Sigma Theta Tau International, *Theta Chi* chapter.

References

Adams, W. P. (1993). *The German Americans: An ethnic experience.* Bloomington, IN: Indiana University Printing Services.

Bernthal, W. F. (1997). Growing up in Frankenmuth and other Michigan memories. The Evangelical Lutheran Church of St. Lorenz (2000). Annual report. Frankenmuth, MI: Author.

Krafft, N. A. (1994). *Beloved brother: Bootleg and bounty: Frankenmuth and the 1930s.* Frankenmuth, MI: Author.

Lassiter, S. M. (1995). German Americans. In *Multicultural events: A professional handbook for health care providers and social workers* (pp. 89–99). Westport, CT: Greenwood Press.

Leininger, M. (1991a). The theory of culture care diversity and universality. In M Leininger (Ed.), *Culture care diversity and universality: A theory of nursing.* Boston: Jones and Bartlett/National League for Nursing.

Leininger, M. (1991b). Ethnonursing: A research method with enablers to study the theory of culture care. In M. Leininger (Ed.), *Culture care diversity and universality: A theory of nursing.* Boston: Jones and Bartlett/National League for Nursing.

Leininger, M., & McFarland, M. R. (Eds.). (2002). *Transcultural nursing: Concepts, theories, research, & practice.* (3rd ed.). New York: McGraw-Hill.

McFarland, M. (1995). Culture care theory and elderly Polish Americans. In M. Leininger (Ed.), *Transcultural nursing: Concepts, theories, research, and practices.* New York: McGraw-Hill.

McFarland, M. (1997). Use of culture care theory with Anglo and African American elders in a long-term care setting. *Nursing Science Quarterly, 10*(4), 186–192.

Steckler, J. A. (2003). People of German heritage. In L. D. Purnell, & B. J. Paulanka (Eds.), *Transcultural health care: A culturally competent approach* (2nd ed., pp. 38–55). Philadelphia: F.A. Davis Company.

Whetstone, W. R., & Cruise, M. J. (1995). Home health care: Community partnerships: Home health care for elderly minorities. *Geriatric Nursing: American Journal of Care for the Aging, 16*(3), 139–140.

Winawer, H., & Wetzel, N. A. (1996). German families. In M. McGoldrick, J. Giordano, & J. K. Pearce (Eds.), *Ethnicity and family therapy,* (2nd ed., pp. 496–516). New York: The Guilford Press.

CHAPTER SEVEN

Culture Care of the Potawatomi Native Americans Who Have Experienced Family Violence

Linda S. Farrell, PhD, RN

Native Americans have experienced cultural violence in many forms since the Europeans came to America. This study explored the meanings and expressions of caring and their relationship to violence within the culture of Potawatomi Native Americans living in a rural environment in the Midwestern United States. Transcultural nursing research based care that reflects the experiences, values, beliefs, meanings, expressions, and practices of this culture was of great importance. It was essential that nurses become knowledgeable about this Native American culture to help nurses provide meaningful, culturally congruent care and to advance the discipline of nursing.

This culture care study of the Potawatomi Native Americans was conceptualized using the tenets of Leininger's theory of Culture Care Diversity and Universality. The visually conceptual Sunrise Enabler was adapted to incorporate precepts of the Native American spirituality of the Potawatomi, which is circular, holistic, and pluralistic (Allen, 1992; Crow 1993).

Domain of Inquiry

The researcher found support in the current literature on human care, family violence, and Native American traditions for an ethnonursing qualitative study designed to discover the *emic* views of caring and noncaring of rural Potawatomi Native Americans who have experienced family violence.

The domain of inquiry (DOI) for this transcultural nursing research study was the cultural care beliefs, values, meanings, expressions of caring within the lifeways of the Potawatomi Native Americans who had experienced violence within their family. The researcher focused on discovering culture care knowledge related to the presence or absence of family violence as a consideration in the provision of culturally congruent care for these rural Potawatomi people. While employed in a large acute medical care center in a rural Anglo European Michigan community where professional nursing and healthcare services seldom were used, the researcher often reflected on the Native American lifeways. It was readily apparent that those Native Americans who did seek help were extremely ill and used resources such as the emergency department as a last resort. Issues such as access to and use of professional care services by the Potawatomi and violence within their families became of interest and concern to the researcher. Lack of knowledge about and understanding of the Potawatomi care values, beliefs, expressions, meanings, and practices by health care professionals was clearly evident. Institutional professional care and practices were foreign to these rural Native Americans, and hospital staff did not understand culture-specific Potawatomi care needs. Culturally congruent and culture-specific care as the primary goals of the Culture Care Theory are stated, ". . . to improve and to provide culturally congruent care to people that is beneficial, will fit with, and be useful to the client, family, or culture group healthy lifeways" (Leininger 1991b, p. 39). Violence among Native Americans was often known or discovered by nurses and other health personnel, and it was important to discover where and how it existed and how it related to culture and care.

The researcher speculated that if culture care was provided to the Potawatmi in a sensitive manner congruent with their lifeways, their current health and wellbeing could be maintained or improved, and family violence could be reduced through professional caring actions and acceptance of their lifeways. Leininger (1991b) postulated that, ". . . clients who experience nursing care that fails to be reasonably congruent with the client's beliefs, values, and caring lifeways will show signs of cultural conflicts, noncompliance, stresses, and ethical or moral concerns" (p. 45). This researcher predicted the potential for cultural violence would exist if caring actions and expressions were not evident within families and in the community. Knowledge of cultural values, lifeways, religion, kinship, and social factors within this culture and their interrelationships to the existence of family violence was predicted to lead to understanding the healthcare needs of the Potawatomi. These postulated culture expressions related to violence were congruent with another premise of the theory, that ". . . cultural care values, beliefs, and practices are influenced by and tend to be embedded in the worldview, language, religious (or spiritual), kinship (social), political (legal), educational, economic, technological, ethnohistorical, and environmental context of a particular group" (Leininger, 1991b, p. 45).

Native Americans value their history, language, and ceremonial traditions as influencers on care and care outcomes. Historically, Native Americans have passed on their history through narrative accounts, storytelling, songs, symbols, and ceremonies. These ethnohistorical traditions were predicted to provide rich data about the epistemic and ontological aspects of the Potawatomi Native Americans studied regarding their environmental context in relation to family violence and cultural conflicts, experiences of cultural imposition, and nonadherence or resistance to professional care practices (Clifton, 1984; Horn, 1993; McGaa, 1990).

The researcher predicted that if nursing care was culturally congruent with Potawatomi cultural values and beliefs, then it could be satisfying, beneficial, health promoting, and could also reduce violence. New insights about caring within the Potawatomi culture could be used to identify care constructs to integrate into nursing care actions and decisions to facilitate the provision of high-quality culturally congruent care that was helpful to and accepted by the people. The researcher also believed it was central to the theory tenets to search for differences (diversities) and similarities (universalities) among the people studied. The Culture Care Theory was the theoretical framework used to discover generic [emic] and professional [etic] knowledge and cultural viewpoints. Culture Care Theory states, ". . . transmitted values, beliefs, and patterned lifeways of cultures need to be studied systematically to discover ways to assist, support, facilitate, or enable clients to maintain their health and wellbeing, to improve their human condition and lifeway, or to deal with illness, handicaps, or death" (Leininger, 1991b, p. 47). Other care constructs among Native Americans in America had not been widely explored except for Leininger's work (Leininger, 1991a/b). Care studies of the Potawatomi Native Americans similar or related to the domain of inquiry of this study were not found.

The following research questions were used to guide the open discovery process of learning the cultural needs and lifeways of the Potawatomi, the cultural meanings of care and caring, and the interrelationship of violence within the family to these meanings:

1. What are the culture care expressions of rural Potawatomi Native Americans?
2. In what ways do the Potawatomi Native American spiritual, social structure factors, environmental context, language, and ethnohistorical dimensions influence the health and wellbeing of tribal members?
3. What are the culture care needs of the rural Potawatomi Native Americans who experienced violence?

4. In what ways might nurses use Leininger's three modes of action
and decision to provide care that is meaningful and congruent
with the culture care needs of Potawatomi Native Americans?

Theoretical Framework

The theory of Culture Care Diversity and Universality (Leininger,
1991b) was chosen as it enabled the researcher to discover multiple
holistic factors that influenced the cultural care and health outcomes of
the Potawatomi Native Americans. A holistic approach was critical for
grasping the world of Potawatomi culture. The Culture Care Theory
(Leininger, 1991b) also was developed for the discovery of indepth
worldview, social structure factors, environmental context, and ethnohistorical values and beliefs within the cultural meanings and expressions of caring. Most importantly, the theory focuses on discovering the
diversities and universalities related to care and health outcomes. This
care knowledge would be helpful to nurses to use in providing care to
clients, families, and community groups.

The theorist also held and predicted that all cultures have forms,
patterns, expressions, and structures of care that could be discovered,
known, explained, and used to predict the health or wellbeing of cultures (Leininger, 1991a). This was a powerful idea that interested the
researcher in seeking to discover generic and professional healthcare
practices that influenced access to and the quality of care provided to
Potawatomi people as individuals and the influences of these practices
upon healthcare outcomes. The patterns, expressions, and structures of
culture care needed to be discovered with the Potawatomi in order to
know their culture care needs to the fullest dimension, which had not
been studied previously from a transcultural nursing perspective. The
theorist also held that care is the essence of and a central dominant
focus for the discipline of nursing and for transcultural nursing care
(Leininger 1991b). Hence, the researcher believed the Culture Care
Theory was appropriate for the discovery of culture care phenomena
with this Native American culture, and to obtain previously unknown
knowledge for use by nurses and other health professionals in providing
culturally congruent care.

The Sunrise Enabler (see Chapter 1, page 25) was modified to incorporate fully diverse elements of Native American spirituality. The
Potawatomi culture views spirituality as circular, holistic, and pluralistic
(Allen, 1992: Crow, 1993). The enabler was used as an important cognitive guide in conducting this transcultural research study as conceptualized using the culture care theoretical framework. The tenets and

structure factors of theory guided the researcher in discovering the cultural care values from the worldview, with specific social structure factors (religion, kinship, technology, economics, and education), philosophical values, and other specific cultural factors of the Potawatomi people. These factoral influences on the culture care practices of this Native American tribe were of central interest to the researcher.

Orientational Definitions

Orientational definitions (Leininger, 1991a/b) provided a broad research base to guide in the discovery of meanings within the informants' beliefs, values, worldview, and lifeways. The following orientational definitions were used with an open inquiry approach toward discovery:

1. Caring—Actions or activities of an individual that are perceived by another individual as supportive during times of need to maintain one's state of being (Leininger 1991b, p. 46)
2. Cultural violence—Any behavior taken against another person within the same cultural community that when carried out leads to harm or unfavorable consequences
3. Culture—Learned and shared values, beliefs, norms, and lifeways of the Native American that are passed on from one generation to the next (Leininger, 1991b, p. 47)
4. Environmental context—The totality of an event, situation, or particular experience that gives meaning to human expressions, interpretations, and social interactions in particular physical, ecological, sociopolitical, and-or cultural settings (Leininger, 1991b, p. 48)
5. Health—A state of wellbeing that is culturally defined, valued, and practiced by individuals of the Native American culture (Leininger, 1991b, p. 48)
6. Culture care—Refers to the learned values, beliefs, and lifeway patterns of the Native Americans that facilitate wellbeing or lead to illness (Leininger, 1991b, p. 47)
7. Cultural congruent (nursing) care—Supportive, preventive, and-or caring acts or decisions that fit with individual, group, or institutional cultural values, beliefs, and lifeways to provide meaningful and satisfying health care or wellbeing services (Leininger, 1991b, p. 49)
8. Potawatomi Native Americans—People of Native American origin belonging to the Potawatomi tribe of the Three Fires Alliance, specifically the Pokagon Band of Potawatomi (www.pokagon.com)

Review of the Literature

A growing body of care theory and research has documented the importance of discovering the nature of culturally relevant care and ways to
provide this care (Leininger, 1984; Rosenbaum, 1991; Wenger, 1991a/b).
However, only one article was found that used Leininger's Culture Care
Theory with Native Americans. Huttlinger and Tanner (1994) used the
theory to develop and implement a plan of care with a Navajo man with
aphasia. Leininger's culture care meanings and action modes served as
guides for enabling the client to use the peyote ceremony of the Native
American Church, a ceremony used for healing various physical, mental,
and spiritual conditions. The article illustrated the importance of incorporating traditional healing practices into nursing and collaborative care
for individuals from diverse cultural backgrounds. Two other studies
with Native Americans were also found: one addressed Navajo child
health beliefs and rearing practices (Phillips & Lobar, 1990), and the
other addressed middle ear disease in the North American Indian
(Wuest, 1991). The authors of these studies conceptualized care within a
transcultural nursing perspective, but did not use the Culture Care
Theory or the ethnonursing research method. Leininger's (1991a/b)
accounts of Native Americans provided general nursing data about
Native Americans, and there are other studies by Canadian nurses in
texts on care, but none explored violence using Culture Care Theory.

There were few studies that addressed violence in the Native
American culture (Blum, Harmon, Harris, Bergeisen & Resnik, 1992;
Durst, 1991). The review of literature revealed an abundance of articles
on alcohol and substance abuse among Native Americans (Booth, Blow,
Cook, Bunn, & Fortney, 1992; Dinges & Quand, 1992; Elia & Jacobs,
1992; Lange, 1988; Moncher, Holden, & Trimble, 1990; Van Breda,
1989). Hughes and Dodder (1984) suggested that drinking among Native
Americans may have a positive function in that it replaced lost social
institutions. Several authors (Beauvois, Oetting, & Edwards, 1985;
Schinke, Botvin, Trimble, Orlandi, Gilchrist & Locklear, 1988; Walker &
Kiulaham, 1984) suggested that drinking could be an escapist response
to acculturational stress. Grobsmith's (1989) study of 102 incarcerated
Native Americans showed between 91% to 100% of the offenses committed were alcohol and-or drug related, and that over one third of these
offenders had suffered physical abuse by parents or legal guardians.

Hasting and Hamberger (1988) identified alcohol abuse as one personality characteristic of Native Americans spousal abusers. Alcohol
consumption among the Native Americans had often led to physiologi-
cal and psychological changes that increased the probability of aggres-

sion under certain conditions and was frequently implicated in the occurrence of family violence (Campbell & Humpherys, 1993; Venn, 1988). Blum et al. (1992) in their study of 13,454 seventh through twelfth grade American Indian-Alaska Native youths found weekly or more frequent use of alcohol, starting at junior high age for both males and females. In the same group, 10% of all youths experienced physical abuse and 13% experienced sexual abuse; among the females, nearly 24% reported physical abuse and 21.6% reported sexual abuse.

Ethnohistory and Social Structure of the Potawatomi

The ethnohistory and social structure factors of the Potawatomi Native Americans of Michigan were essential areas of knowledge for understanding their cultural lifeways and care needs and for enabling their survival, health care, and wellbeing as a people. The ethnohistory of the Potawatomi of Michigan was derived primarily from the Ojibwa, Odawa, and Potawatomi tribes, whose ancestors originally came from the Algonquian tribes that clustered around the Great Lakes of Huron, Michigan, and Superior. These three tribes formed the *Three Fires Alliance* and had social and political organizations that were less complex or elaborate than the Western tribes. Tribal unity was based on a common language, kinship, and clan membership (Claspy, 1966; Clifton, 1984; Kiniets 1965; McClurken, 1991).

During the 1700s and early 1800s leaders of the United States believed they had acquired clear legal title to all lands from the Atlantic Ocean to the Mississippi River by right of conquest. A treaty of peace recognized the sovereignty of the United States and led to land cession agreements which diminished the autonomy of the Native American tribes (Claspy, 1966; Clifton 1984). In 1833 the Treaty of Chicago brought about US cession of the remaining Potawatomi lands and exile of the people to land west of the Mississippi. Later, the Pokagon Band was removed to Northern Michigan to the Ojibwa and Odawa territories. No monies had been allocated for or given to the Potawatomi for this purpose, and appropriate relocation lands in northern Michigan were not available, preventing resettlement there (Claspy, 1966; Clifton, 1984). The tribe remained in southwestern Michigan where they purchased land for farming while hunting and fishing on public domain. Given these circumstances, the Potawatomi became assimilated into other tribes and among the dominant culture of the general population. These changes necessitated many legal, social, political, economic, and religious cultural adjustments in order for the Pokagon Band of Potawatomi to remain an organized group (Clifton, 1984). It was not until September 1994 that the tribe was once again recognized as a legitimate band of the Potawatomi Indians and was given tribal status as the Potawatomi Nations of Indians, Inc. (www.pokagon.com).

Native American spirituality is an important element of their culture and cultural values, and was best described in the words of Chief Seattle of the Suwanish tribe in his letter to President Franklin Pierce in 1854 (McGaa, 1990):

> . . . How can you buy or sell the sky, the warmth of the land? The idea is strange to us. We do not own the fresh air and the sparkle of the water, how can you buy them? Every part of this earth is sacred to my people. Every shining pine needle, every sandy shore, every mist in the dark woods, every clearing and every humming insect is holy in the memory and experience of my people. The sap which courses through the trees carries the memories of the red man. So, when the Great Chief of Washington sends words that he wishes to buy our land, he asks much of us . . . Whatever befalls the earth befalls the sons of the earth. Man did not weave the web of life, he is merely a strand in it . . .

From the early 1900s to present day, individuals, families, and organized communities of the Pokagon Band of Potawatomi have devoted their energies toward attainable and realistic objectives. They have endeavored to improve their lives and to strengthen their position through work by the elected band council and leaders. They remain largely a rural culture, residing in Cass, Van Buren, and Berrien counties of Michigan (Clifton, 1984). They have sought better education for tribal members and encouraged careers in such areas as teaching, architecture, law, and accounting. What was essential to being *Neshnabek* (Potawatomi for *Indian*; translated means 'True Human') remains a defining characteristic among the Potawatomi. An old Potawatomi ethos, *Matehimadzhen*, refers to their integral relationship with the universe, the world, one another, and with their ancestors. This ethos remains important to the Potawatomi today (Clifton, 1984).

Current living conditions of Michigan's Potawatomi Native Americans demonstrate that this culture is living on the edge of survival within a dominant society. They are described as the ". . . poorest of the poor" and ". . . struggling for economic survival as a community of people" (Chapleski, 1993). They are a community with great self determination and a strong desire for long term improvement of their social and health conditions (Churchill, 1994; Clifton, 1984).

Research Method

The ethnonursing qualitative research method designed for the theory of Culture Care provided an open, flexible mode of inquiry for the discovery of largely unknown aspects of people's cultural lifeways within their naturalistic or familiar environments (Leininger, 1990, 1991a). The ethnonursing research method had several philosophical and research features that fit the Culture Care Theory. Philosophically, ethnonursing was designed to be grounded *with the people* as *knowers* in the discovery of people truths within their local environmental or *cultural context* (Leininger, 1985, 1991a). The ethnonursing research method had been developed to explicate the tenets of Culture Care Theory and required the researcher to explore differences and similarities from the domain of inquiry with focus on the cultural meanings, expressions, and lifeways of people. The method enabled the researcher to discover human care needs and cultural expressions related specifically to nursing phenomena.

Ethnonursing provided a means for explicating the epistemic and ontological knowledge of nursing related to transcultural nursing phenomena. The term *ethnonursing* was purposefully coined by Leininger (1991a) to reflect the importance of both *emic* [insiders or local people's view] and *etic* [nonlocal or outsider views] data to obtain an accurate view of the people and for discovery of their care needs.

Leininger's (1991a) general ethnonursing principles served as guides for the discovery of indepth meanings and ideas related to the researcher's specific domain of inquiry. These research principles included: a) ". . . to maintain an open discovery, active listening, and a genuine learning attitude in working with informants in the total context in which the study is conducted (Leininger, 1991a, p. 106); b) ". . . to maintain an active and curious posture about the 'why' of whatever is seen, heard, or experienced, and with appreciation of whatever informants share with you" (Leininger 1991a, p. 107); c) ". . . to record whatever is shared by informants in a careful and conscientious way for full meanings, explanations, or interpretations to preserve informant ideas" (Leininger, 1991a, p. 108); d) ". . . to seek a mentor who has experience with the ethnonursing research method to act as a guide (or reflector)" (Leininger, 1991a, p. 108); and, e) ". . . to clarify the purposes of additional qualitative research methods if they are combined with the ethnonursing method such as combining life histories, ethnography, phenomenology, or ethnoscience" (Leininger, 1991a, p. 109).

Ethnomethod enablers designed by the theorist were used throughout the research process to help explicate or tease out data that were often sensitive or difficult to know immediately (Leininger, 1991a). The Observation-Participation-Reflection (OPR) Enabler (see Chapter 2, page

52) was primarily used as the researcher entered the Potawatomi community. This enabler helped the researcher to "... enter and remain with the people while studying their lifeways, and in relation to nursing care phenomena in a systematic and reflective way" (Leininger, 1991b, p. 83). The OPR Enabler greatly facilitated entrance into the Potawatomi community through active observation and listening to informants before the researcher became a participant in the lifeways of the people. Reflection and reconfirmation were essential throughout the study to compare researcher and informant views and to confirm findings with informants. The data were continually assessed using the qualitative criteria of credibility, confirmability, recurrence, and reliability (Leininger, 1991a).

Leininger's (1991a) Acculturation Enabler (see Chapter 2, page 64) was also used to assess the extent of traditional or nontraditional orientation in the values and lifeways of the Potawatomi studied. Several dimensions of acculturation were assessed such as social structure, worldview, values, and human care practices. This guide also was invaluable for identifying cultural variabilities or diversities among the people.

The Stranger to Friend Enabler (see Chapter 2, page 51) developed by Leininger (1991a) was a very important guide in gauging the researcher's movement from stranger stage to friend stage when obtaining information from the Potawatomi informants. Difficulty in developing trust with the Potawatomi was anticipated, and required several months to occur. Thoughtful consideration of and respect for the Potawatomi was essential for becoming a trusted research friend. It was in this stage where embedded *emic* knowledge and the worldview of Potawatomi were discovered through confirmation of care meanings with informants. Each of the enablers helped to reaffirm data and to support the qualitative research criteria as previously stated.

The initial gatekeeper of the research setting congruent with the ethnonursing research method of Leininger (1985) was the director of the Potawatomi Indian Health Services. The researcher's first interview with her met with many roadblocks as she did not believe the elders would approve the study and therefore she was not willing to assist in presenting the study to the Elders' Council. Another avenue of approach for entering and remaining with the people needed to be identified. Through access provided by a mutual Potawatomi friend, the researcher was able to develop trust and acceptance by participation in volunteer work with the elders at their bimonthly luncheon meetings over a period of two years.

The initial entry into the Potawatomi community at the Elders' Hall was that of a distrusted stranger. The people at the gathering did not speak to this researcher. They watched and allowed me to serve them coffee and to clear the tables. The elder in the kitchen did not provide any instructions as to what help was needed. After several weeks of serving and clearing, she began to talk to me and explain what was occurring in the meetings. By this time, this researcher had realized the luncheons were potluck and had begun to bring a dish to pass also. The elders were guarded and careful with what information they would share with this distrusted stranger. This behavior of was congruent with Leininger's (1991b) OPR and Stranger to Trusted Friend Enablers. After approximately three months, the researcher was asked to join in with their luncheons, the 50/50 raffles, bingo games, and auctions, and thus began to learn about and from the elders. These Native Americans were interested in the study and expressed their willingness to be supportive of the researcher during the study process. Access to key informants was provided through meetings with the Potawatomi elders, family members, and identified Potawatomi gatekeepers.

Informants

The Potawatomi Native Americans was the culture studied. A written, informed consent was obtained prior to the informants interviews. Data were gathered over a period of 3 years through lengthy observations and direct presence of the researcher at family gatherings and community activities such as powwows, tribal meetings, and ceremonial events and social functions. Approximately 12 key informants and 20 general informants were selected for interview. *Key* informants were selected from adults aged 18 to 80 years of age among Potawatomi people who had experienced some form of violence, were living in a rural community, and willing to participate in the study. After screening 12 informant candidates, the researcher determined that all had met the selection criteria for participation as key informants and therefore further interviews were not indicated. To protect the confidentiality of informant identity, each person was sequentially coded. Indepth interviews were conducted by the researcher in naturalistic settings with 12 key Native American informants on three to four separate occasions for approximately 1 to 2 hours apiece. *General* informants were primarily identified through key informants and included both male and female friends and family members. The ethnonursing research method and the previously identified enablers were used to obtain broad and indepth data about Potawatomi Native Americans' lifeways.

The informants lived in rural southwestern Michigan and represented a variety of men and women who were both traditional and nontraditional in their practices and lifeways. They ranged in age from 34 to 80 years of age, and the majority (90%) had a high school education or more. All but two of the informants identified themselves as Potawatomi Native Americans, and all had lived in the rural area most of their lives (20 or more years).

Data Analysis and Evaluation Criteria

The data were analyzed using Leininger's Four Phases of Ethnonursing Data Analysis Guide (see Chapter 2). This guide provided a systemic and rigorous method of analyzing large amounts of qualitative data in theory congruent categories. The researcher initiated data analysis at the outset and continued the process throughout the entire study. After raw data were collected and coded, they were entered into the Ethnograph v5.0 computer program, which was designed to facilitate the analysis of qualitative data in accordance with the theory. The systematic data analysis required the identification of descriptors, patterns, and major themes from the informants so that continuity of ideas could be identified. Each phase built upon and was supported by the previous phase. Leininger's six criteria for evaluation of qualitative research were used to analyze the study data (Leininger, 1991c). All data were analyzed with respect to credibility, confirmability, meanings-in-context, recurrent patterning, saturation, and redundancy criteria as defined by Leininger (1990, 1991b, 2002). As other studies of a culture comparable to the Potawatomi had not been conducted, the criterion of transferability was not used.

Findings

The findings of this study were congruent with those reviewed from the literature. Alcohol and drug use were found to be major contributors to the presence of both physical and sexual abuse. Similarly, instances of oppression, discrimination, and prejudice were identified as partial contributors to violent acts or behaviors. Several Potawatomi shared feelings of prejudice and discrimination when they attempted to purchase land for their tribe. Therefore, such purchases have been kept secret and were completed by a third party because of prejudiced encounters including refusals to 'sell land to the Indians' with escalation of purchase prices.

Findings from the data, OPR Enabler, and indepth interviews with Potawatomi Native American informants led to the discovery of their culture care patterns and themes in relation to the domain of inquiry. Then, the theory tenets were examined with the DOI and the research questions were addressed. Three universal themes were discovered related to care and cultural violence. In addition, one diverse care theme was identified regarding access to health care (see Table 7-1). These themes were important guides to local nurses and other health care professionals in providing culturally congruent care for the

TABLE 7-1 Universal Culture Care and Violence Themes

	Pattern 1	Pattern 2	Pattern 3	Pattern 4
Culture Care Theme 1 Respect for all things living and nonliving	Respect for age	Respect for generosity and sharing	Respect as listening, understanding, and being there	Equality
Culture Care Theme 2 Native American spirituality influencing health and wellbeing	Living and being through harmony and peace	Doing the honorable thing	Rituals and ceremonies	
Culture Noncaring Theme 1 Noncaring as oppression undermining cultural practices and identities	Alcohol and drug abuse	Violence (physical, mental, sexual)	Low self-esteem and shame	
Culture Care Diversity Theme 1 Diversity through types of professional and generic health care used to promote health and wellbeing and when illness was present	Use of traditional healers, rituals, and folk remedies	Use of Indian Health Center	Obtaining professional health care late in the process of illness or disease	

Potawatomi, and supported Leininger's theory of Culture Care. To better assist the reader in understanding the Potawatomi Native American worldview and *emic* care perspective, verbatim qualitative statements are presented for each theme.

Themes

Care Theme 1

The first universal care theme of *culture care as respect for all things, living and nonliving* was identified by all Potawatomi informants as a central care construct to their culture, which was supported by their generic care beliefs and actions. *Culture care as respect* was reflected in the care patterns of *respect for age, respect as generosity and sharing*, and *respect as listening, understanding, and being there*.

Respect for all things was essential because it was not just Man who had a spirit, *but all animals, plants, rocks, and rivers. Every element of creation is alive in its own way* (Farrell, 2001, p. 78). This theme was expressed by all 12 key informants. *Care* meant respect as a way of thinking, living, and relating to other people, nature, spirits, and Mother Nature.

Care Pattern

The pattern of culture care as *respect for age* pervaded the Potawatomi culture as in most Native American tribal cultures. Children were often brought up by grandparents because parents were busy being providers for the entire family. The elders, having lived long and full lives, had many lessons to teach the young; elders held the wisdom and the children held the future. Both the very old and the very young were believed to have special relationships with the spirit world and the Great Creator, which were seen as part of the balance of the circle of life.

> It is our elders and children. We honor and respect our elders for what they have lived and can teach us. We honor our children for they are our new life. (Participant 3)
>
> We honor elders and children. It is also important to honor our Vets. They are our warriors. Did you know that one out of four *Neshnabe* men have served in a war? (Participant 8)

Care Pattern

Care as *respect as generosity and sharing* was a cultural care pattern. A person was held in high esteem not for the wealth he had but for his generosity. The caring act of *giving* needed to be a sacrifice; to give in any other way was not viewed as honorable. Many of the gifts given were useful and cherished by the giver. Generosity and sharing were dominant cultural care values seen in the daily lifeways of the Potawatomi.

> Part of our values or caring is in our sharing and giving to others. Often one will say . . . 'he will give you the shirt off his back.' We are like that. It comes from our belief in possessions and caring. Possessions have little meaning to us. They are not ours to keep. We give them to our people who need them. (Participant 15)

The Great Creator was revealed each day in the miracles of nature's gifts which were part of the circle of life. Each person's wellbeing was dependant on the health of the whole. Not taking more than one needed was a fundamental value for maintaining balance and harmony. Material possessions were viewed as something held ready for sharing with those who were less fortunate. Seventeen of 32 informants identified not taking more than needed and lack of importance of material things as patterns of caring.

> We don't take more than we need. When we take something we offer up a prayer to the western door to release its spirit. That is what our teachings are all about, love and caring. (Participant 3)

Many of the Potawatomi homes visited were small with minimal furnishings. There were no new, fancy cars parked outside. The Potawatomi lifeway exemplified the cultural value of possessions not being important and were often criticized by the dominant culture for not '. . . moving up in the world.' Fourteen of 32 informants emphasized the minimal focus on possessions as spiritually important to them.

> Most of us have very few possessions. They are not important to us. Look at how most of us live. Our spirituality and caring for Mother Earth are more important. (Participant 5)

The researcher was able to experience first hand the caring and generosity of the Potawatomi. On several occasions sacred herbs or medicine were given to help guide her educational path; a circle of sweet grass to safely guide her journey of discovery; cedar oil (female in nature) to put on her forehead and neck to relieve stress; sage to carry to keep away negative forces; and an eagle feather. It was important to the Potawatomi and the researcher that she be guided by their spirits to maintain a clear vision of her path. These caring actions and guidances were helpful during data collection process. Furthermore, many of these care practices became incorporated into her own care practices. Today, she still carries sage with her, and uses cedar oil to relieve stress. The researcher honors her eagle feather as one of her most valued possessions.

Care Pattern

Culture care was expressed and made meaningful by *respect as listening, understanding, and being there*. This pattern was influenced by their cultural values, lifeways, and kinship. Caring went beyond sharing and generosity. It meant *being there* when you were needed. Many participants expressed the need for one to be there, to take the time out of one's busy schedule to *be there* and help.

> Caring is *being there* for others. When you give from the heart it always comes back. Our teachings are about sharing and being there for others. (Participant 6)

The Potawatomi, as in most Native American cultures, learned their ethnohistory through tribal oral traditions. Their knowledge and wisdom were *shared and learned by heart and passed down to successive generations*.

Storytelling and music were ways that wisdom was shared and learned. Stories were used to teach the young Potawatomi tribal traditions and history. It was through such stories the Great Creator spoke and it was important to listen carefully to hear these lessons in how the story was told. Informants shared stories throughout the research process to teach about and share the Potawatomi culture and caring with the researcher.

> Listening is very important. That is how we learn. Our history has been passed down through stories. When I was a young child, I would sit at my grandmother's side listening to her stories and watching her make baskets. That is how I leaned to make the baskets. The white man doesn't listen or have the patience to sit quietly to listen. It is always go, go, go. (Participant. 12)

Caring as respect for Mother Earth as *life giving* was fundamental to the Native Americans and was viewed as *listening* and *understanding*. It was important to not only *listen* to each other but also to Mother Earth and the spirits, and *observe* what was being spoken by them and the elders.

> Everything in nature has something to teach us. We must listen with our hearts to the wordless language of the spirits. It is through these spirits that answers were provided. Only the Creator decides what is right. You must listen and observe and do what your spirit tells you. (Participant 3)
>
> Dreams are a way the spirits talk to us. If you listen to . . . your dreams, you will know what the Great Spirit is telling you. (Participant 19)

Listening was important when the Potawatomi sought professional health care and it was an important caring action for them to be given time for thoughtful listening.

> The response time for Indians to process things is longer than the dominant culture. We have been taught to listen. We need more time to think about things before we respond. (Participant 1)
>
> This one emergency room doctor really cares about his patients. He listened to me when I went into the emergency room. He allowed me time to think about what he said. He sent me to a cardiologist that listens too. Most doctors don't take the time to listen. (Participant 13)

Care Theme 2

Native American spirituality as culture care had great influence on the health and wellbeing of the Potawatomi studied. Their spirituality was demonstrated through the care patterns of *living and being through harmony and peace, doing the honorable thing, rituals and ceremonies*, and *equality*.

A key component toward acquiring inner peace for the Potawatomi was to be thankful to the Great Creator for *all that is*. Prayer was another caring spiritual practice. For many key informants, their day started with a prayer and an offering to thank the Creator for a good day. One key informant saw prayer as a way to release the disharmony and imbalance of negativity. Prayer was a way to become open to the teachings of the Great Creator.

> It is living by our four graces—peace, love, harmony, and humility. We are in harmony with Mother Earth and all beings, both two legged and four legged, and winged. It is our spirituality, a way of being and living. (Participant 3)
>
> The four directions of north, south, east, and west are caring. They have the answers to a lot of our questions. Caring spirits are the center of the Universe. You look for answers to the Great Creator. Spirits are everywhere. There is balance of life, caring for self and other people, places, and things. Be a good example. Learning to live together in harmony brings more peace. (Participant 19)

Care Pattern

Native American spirituality has long been practiced as a way of *living and being through harmony and grace*. For the Potawatomi, this meant *living by their shield teachings* or *living by the four graces*. The *harmony of give and take* was an honored and practiced lifeway. *Harmony* was honored in all social relationships and ensured tribal survival. Having peace and harmony within themselves, with others, and in all aspects of live were essential components of Potawatomi spirituality and spiritual practice. One key informant viewed harmony as being responsible for one's actions:

> Like a stone thrown into a pond, the effects go beyond our actual actions. Our thoughts and actions are like those ripples in the pond. We must be responsible for them. (Participant 6)

Care Pattern

For eleven informants, *caring as spirituality* was viewed as *doing the honorable thing* (Farrell, 2001, p. 93) by living the four graces or seven virtues. The four graces were *peace, love, harmony,* and *humility.* They were part of the seven virtues; the remaining three virtues were *bravery, truth,* and *honesty.* These teachings were fundamental to the Potawatomi spirituality belief system and lifeways. Practicing these caring actions was believed to bring *peace* and *harmony* to the world.

Care Pattern

Rituals and *ceremonies* were identified as another form of caring related to spirituality, by promoting balance and teaching love. Objects used during ceremonies hold power, love, and energy to make things happen. Renewal of inner personal strength occurred through rituals and ceremonies. Ritual care practices used by the Potawatomi were smudging, laying down of tobacco, sweat lodges, vision quests, and pipe ceremonies. All of these generic care practices helped allay tendencies toward violence; the herbs used in smudging had strong spirits and were used in healing and cleansing while the smudging smoke carried away negativity.

Tobacco was one of the most sacred herbs of the Potawatomi, as it was the first gift of the Creator and was considered to have medicinal power. The *Kinnikinnick,* a combination of tobacco and other herbs, was often used in ceremonies and was either smoked, burned, or used as an offering. Tobacco was believed to bring clarity of mind and to transform negative energies into positive ones. All of the key informants discussed or exhibited the use of tobacco as an offering or used tobacco in ceremonies.

> Tobacco is one of our ceremonial herbs. It used to be made from strawberry leaves, blueberry leaves, maple leaves, and sassafras leaves. That is called 'kennieck,' pronounced 'nic-nic.' We never used it to just smoke. It was always used in pipe ceremonies and as offerings to Mother Earth. Tobacco is something that will always be important for the Indians. (Participant 16)
>
> Rituals were used as connections between the spirit world and the physical world. It was required that one be clean of alcohol for four days before any ceremony. (Participant 16)

Care rituals were used to reveal the secret wisdom within each person, uncover the deeper realities of life, and bring peace and harmony. Many different medicine tools were used during ritual ceremonies. These tools had spiritual powers and could be used in different ways. They included the use of dress or Native regalia, prayer, herbs, pipes, and feathers.

Care Pattern

Native American spirituality as culture care for the Potawatomi was also reflected in the care pattern of *equality* for everyone. The Potawatomi believed all beings came from the Great Creator and that all beings were equal and part of the whole sacred circle of life where everything was important for the *whole* and no *part* was more important than the rest. This culture care value was influenced by Native spirituality, kinship, cultural values, and lifeways. Each being may come in different forms and have different qualities, gifts, and powers, but ultimately they were all *one*, connected through that circle of life. The sacred circle of life represented the great unending circular way of the Great Creator and was the sacred root of equality.

The sacred circle was the center of Native American spirituality and was comprised of the four directions—north, south, east, and west—which extended to seven directions adding above, below, and in the center. Each direction was represented by the four colors—red, black, white, and yellow—representing the four races. Each direction also represented the four stages of life; the four seasons; and the four elements of earth, water, fire and air.

> We are all created equal and have special gifts to offer. No one is better than another. It is like our sacred circle—no beginning and no end, all equal. That is why we do things in circles. (Participant 5)

Spirituality was centered upon *being connected* through the never-ending circle where all *parts* were connected and were important for the *whole*. Interdependence was at the center of all things, with everything and everyone connected together and also connected to the Great Creator. Care as connectedness was believed to bring peace and harmony. It manifested as balance, rhythmicity, and being connected to Mother Earth. It was balance that brought forth harmony and was how they lived their lives.

> It is all a circle. Everything and everyone is connected. You can't take parts of it. If you do, the circle is broken and it no longer exists. You have to take it all, the herbs, pipes, the dreams, sweet grass, smudging, sage, tobacco, the Great Creator. (Participant 13)

Being connected to Mother Earth was important. The Potawatomi lived with the earth on a deeply spiritual plane and were intimately connected with the lifegiving and caring Mother Earth through the sacred circle. Culture care for the Potawatomi meant not elevating one's self above another and maintaining the total connectedness and equality of all races.

> Our religion holds we are all one nation. We are all connected. It is our great circle. We give thanks to the Creator above us and to Mother Earth below us and the spirits that are all around us. Our four directions represents all races that are all connected and all equal—north is yellow for the yellow man (Asian), south is black for the black man, west is white for the white man, and east is red for the red man (Indian). (Participant 10)

Connectedness was also important in seeking professional health care. Because white man's medicine did not reflect the spirits in the plants that helped heal, the Potawatomi believed that professional health care and medicine would never be effective. It was the connectedness to the plant's spirits that was healing and needed to be maintained.

> What they (white doctors) don't understand that it takes the whole plant to heal. Natural medicine does not heal the body by itself. It is our connectedness to the plants, to the spirits of the plants, to Mother Earth, and the Great Creator that heals. (Participant 8)

Noncaring Theme 1

Noncaring was viewed as the oppression suffered by Native Americans by the dominant culture that undermined their cultural practices and identities. *Noncaring* was discovered and linked to cultural patterns of *alcohol and drug use, violence,* and *low self-esteem and shame* in the Potawatomi lifeways (see Table 7-1).

Alcoholism had been identified as a major healthcare problem for the Native Americans by Elia and Jacobs (1992) and Hughes and Doddler (1984). The oppression suffered by the Native Americans had so undermined their culture and sense of self that they found it difficult to rise above and exhibit behaviors expected of them. Many Potawatomi linked *alcohol abuse* to the noncaring acts of oppression, racism, prejudices, and discrimination experienced early in life. They learned that their care values and beliefs were in conflict with those of the dominant culture, and that their culture and traditions were not valued.

> I can remember hearing at the boarding school that all Indians were drunks. The kids (white) use to think it was funny when they told us 'the only good Indian is a dead one.' You hear it enough you begin to believe it. (Particiapant 12)

While Alcoholics Anonymous (AA) has been noted for its success in helping alcohol-addicted individuals remain in recovery, some of the philosophical underpinnings of the program were not congruent with Potawatomi cultural values, beliefs, spirituality, or practices. Potawatomi recovery was rooted in Native American spirituality and a deeply felt caring commitment to bring sobriety and dignity to their Native American brothers and sisters. One key informant described his care practices:

> I struggle every day with not drinking or using. The one thing that helps me are the spiritual practices I use like sweats, prayer, vision quests. (Participant 10)

The second cultural noncaring pattern of *abuse* was discovered in relation to and associated with the use of alcohol and drugs—physical, verbal, and sexual abuse. In the Potawatomi culture, *noncaring* was experienced *as physical, mental, or sexual abuses within families* and was related to past destruction associated with the *use of alcohol and drugs*. Abuse was confirmed as a noncaring pattern by all informants. Although personal violence was not often discussed within the Potawatomi community because it was viewed as a private matter, two key informants shared their experiences with the researcher:

> I was molested by my older brother for 6 years. It started when I was 10 years old. He was 13. Even then he was drinking. It was before my first moon time when they were always irregular. I lived in fear of being pregnant from my brother. He would threaten me that if I told anyone, he would say I wanted it. He went away to Nam when I was 16. That's when it stopped. I had such low self-esteem. My aunt told my mom that it was dad who was molesting me so she quit sleeping with him. Today my other brother says he doesn't see what the big deal is. All kids play house. (Participant 2)
>
> The violence went on there (boarding school) too. The nuns would take rulers or rubber hoses to us when we didn't toe the line. They would bend us over a desk and beat us. I was molested by one of the men there. It wasn't as bad as for some of the girls. They were raped repeatedly. (Participant 8)

The experiences of drugs, alcohol, and personal violence led to an overall sense of lost spirituality, cultural values, lifeways, and kinship within their community. The noncaring pattern of *low self-esteem* often led to more alcoholism which fostered more violence. *Shame* also emerged as a cultural noncaring pattern as a result of tribal members being associated with certain types of persons identified with the use of alcohol and drugs.

> For a long time I felt ashamed of being Indian. I drank and did a lot of drugs. It was expected of us in school. The white kids always talked about us drunk Indians. (Participant 2)

> We were always taught the Indian way was wrong. We were savages.
> We drank because we were ashamed of who we were. Alcohol brought
> us more shame. (Participant. 5)

Diverse Care Theme 1

For the Potawatomi, the theme of *culture care as diversity* was expressed
by the types of *professional and generic health care used to promote
health and wellbeing and when illness was present* (see Table 7-1).
Leininger (1990) stated, ". . . culture is dynamic, changing, and diverse"
(p. 55) and that diverse culture care patterns existed between and among
cultures. Culture care as diversity was discovered through care patterns
reflecting the of *use of traditional healers, rituals, and folk remedies; use
of the Indian Health Center*; and *obtaining professional health care late
in the process of disease or illness*. Several different combinations or single uses of traditional medicine, Indian Health Services, or professional
care emerged and were confirmed by all 32 informants, but no universal
care methods or combinations of methods were used by all informants.

Care Pattern

The first *diversity* culture care pattern was the *use of traditional healers, rituals, or folk remedies*. All key informants had used some form of
traditional medicine during their lifetime. Traditional medicine
included different herbs and teas, cleansing rituals, sweat ceremonies,
pipe ceremonies, and prayer. The use of traditional medicine was
important in Potawatomi spirituality and traditional lifeways. Five key
informants stated they had used traditional medicine, but experienced
difficulty obtaining native plants and herbs.

> Without having gathering rights it has made it difficult to gather the
> plants needed. Some we are not allowed to gather at all or we can't go
> on the lands where they grow. It makes it hard for us to practice our
> medicine. Also many don't know our traditional medicines any more.
> The white man has made it difficult for us. Sometimes there isn't a
> choice for us. (Participant 3)
> I try to stay healthy with my daily practices of prayer and ritual
> cleansing with our spiritual herbs. I will go to a doctor if I am really
> sick. Your medicine does not bring balance and harmony though.
> (Participant 7)

Care Pattern

The second diversity culture care pattern to be discovered was the *use of the Indian Health Center* for health care. Fifty percent of key informants used the Indian Health Center because they felt more confident being cared for by their own people for such services as home visits or visits to a nurse managed clinic for minor aliments. Using these professional care services was viewed as more acceptable because traditional lifeways and practices were valued there. The goal of the Potawatomi Indian Health Service was to elevate the health status of tribal members to the highest possible level. The service was operated by the Pokagon Band of Potawatomi and staffed by members from the tribe who accepted wide latitudes of individual expression and used culturally congruent creativity in providing care services.

Mistrust of the dominant culture in association with professional health care services was also discovered.

> We don't take the kids to the doctors. We either use our herbs and natural healing or we take them to our health center. Most of our people don't go to doctors unless they really need to. (Participant 10)
>
> Doctors don't understand us, and because many Indians are poor and have many health problems, they prefer to use our own services. There is less prejudice against us. Health is not about illness but living in harmony. (Participant 9)

Care Pattern

The third diversity culture care pattern discovered was that professional *health care was not obtained until late in the disease or illness* as an outcome of that mistrust and prejudice:

> Our health services goes out to check on people who are diabetic or have other problems. They would rather have us do that then go to the doctors. They [the doctors] don't value or respect our beliefs. That's not the way it is when our people go out. (Participant 14)
>
> Many won't go to the hospital or doctors until they are really sick. Even then you will see them use the home remedies along with your health care. They just won't tell you. (Participant 12)

Health policies and practices in the United States have been formulated within the context of Western scientific and cultural values (Morse, Young, & Swartz, 1991). The use of prayer, healing plants, or traditional medicine in rituals and ceremonies were discovered as important to all 20 key informants. Having access to traditional healers played a key role informants' use of traditional medicines. Informants who primarily used traditional medicine tended to be younger and less susceptible to disease. Eighteen of 20 informants blended traditional and professional healthcare practices but found cultural conflicts often resulted from differing definitions of health between traditional and Western medicine.

In summary, the dominant universal care constructs were respect, honor, and connectedness to all things. Everyone was seen as equal and important for the whole; no one was more important than the other. Noncaring was seen when traditional care practices did not prevail, such as when violence occurred due to the distrust and prejudices against native persons, their history, culture values, lifeways, and spirituality. The dominant noncaring construct of violence was related to the use of alcohol and drugs which resulted in the experiences of physical, verbal, and sexual abuse. Alcohol and drug abuse were confirmed by all 20 key informants to be a major cause of all types of violence. A major premise of Leininger's (1991a) Culture Care Theory was, ". . . Culture care concepts, meanings, expressions, patterns, processes, and structural forms of care are different and similar among all cultures of the world" (p. 45). Cultural conflicts often existed between Native American health beliefs and professional health care. For the Potawatomi Native Americans in this ethnonursing study, diversity was found in the variable use of professional care as a mode for providing health care when illness was present or care was imperative.

Discussion

The goal of Culture Care Theory has been to provide culturally congruent care (Leininger, 1991a). In transcultural nursing, it was important to provide ". . . nursing care that fits with or has beneficial meanings and health outcomes to people of different or similar cultural backgrounds" (Leininger, 1995, p. 12). Leininger postulated in her Culture Care Theory that there were three modes for guiding nursing care judgments, decisions, or actions so that nurses could provide care that was congruent with the client's culture and would benefit and hold meaning for clients. The three modes of culture care were preservation and-or maintenance; accommodation and-or negotiation; and repatterning and-or restructuring. These modes facilitated nurses' actions and decisions in helping clients to meet their healthcare needs in a culturally congruent manner (Leininger, 1991a). The findings from this study form the bases for the following culturally congruent nursing care decisions and actions for and-or with rural Potawatomi Native American informants regarding experiences, values, meanings, and beliefs about their health and wellbeing.

Theory Modes

Culture Care Preservation and-or Maintenance

For Potawatomi Native American informants in this study, the cultural care values, beliefs, meanings, and expressions that enhanced their health and wellbeing were embedded in the social structure factors of Native spirituality, cultural values, lifeways, and kinship. The findings from this study indicated several areas of generic or folk Potawatomi culture care that could help nurses preserve and maintain naturalistic folk practices. The informants identified the importance of their spirituality and living the four graces as essential to their health and wellbeing. Living the four graces should be maintained for all Potawatomi in order to preserve their health and wellbeing, and for them to live culturally congruent and satisfying lifeways. Based of the findings from this study, nurses would need to maintain the care needs of Potawatomi living in the four graces. Living each day as a "good day to die" (Farrell, 2001, p. 94) was essential for the Potawatomi. Nurses needed to have an awareness and knowledge of these values and beliefs to accommodate tribal members living these values.

Culture Care Accommodation and-or Negotiation

Findings from this study indicated the importance of nurses accommodating and negotiating with Potawatomi Native Americans when in professional healthcare settings. For many of the Potawatomi, their cultural care needs arose from noncaring and mistrustful experiences associated with the dominant white culture while receiving professional care services.

Culture care as respect for all things living and nonliving was discovered through the patterns of *respect for age, respect as generosity and sharing, respect as listening, understanding*, and *being there*. They were values and practices expressed by all key and general informants as important needs to be accommodated by nurses. Potawatomi people need sufficient time to process information before a response can be expected. Native spirituality and traditional ritual or ceremonial practices need to be understood and supported through nurses' caring acts and decisions. These key components in culture care need to be accommodated by nurses in providing culturally congruent care to the Potawatomi.

It was important for ensuring tribal members' health and wellbeing for the Potawatomi to develop open and trusting relationships with various healthcare providers. Nurses and other clinicians needed to incorporate the Native American spirituality, values, and beliefs to accommodate and-or negotiate mutually acceptable changes in the Potawatomi lifeways to promote their health and wellbeing. Accommodating and-or negotiating the ability to utilize traditional spiritual practices within the professional healthcare setting, such as smudging and pipe ceremonies, was essential for the Potawatomi to achieve balance and harmony, and to attain and maintain health and wellbeing. [Smudging in their hospital rooms and pipe ceremonies were two folk practices that were not permitted due to fire regulations.]

Because many of the participants in this ethnonursing study used both traditional and professional care services due to the severity of their illness, nurses would need to negotiate for the use of Potawatomi traditional or Native medicine. Nurses need to be familiar with the community's traditional healers and be able to assist in obtaining these services when they are desired or requested. Nurses' professional knowledge of cultural practices would allow Potawatomi Native Americans to seek professional healthcare services earlier in the course of their disease or illness with less mistrust or fear of discrimination. The Potawatomi then would be able to experience firsthand acceptance of their lifeways and spirituality by the dominant culture. This would facilitate mutual accommodation and-or negotiation when the Potawatomi next obtained care services within the professional health system.

Culture Care Repatterning and-or Restructuring

Changing lifeways and adopting new and different care patterns was difficult for the Potawatomi. For many years Native Americans have been forced to adopt the lifeways of the dominant culture. However, the Potawatomi have been able to maintain many of their cultural values and beliefs through repatterning and restructuring of their own traditional lifeways. For example, the use of alcohol and drugs has been abandoned at all ceremonies and celebrations. Alcoholics Anonymous has modified its programs to incorporate Native spiritual beliefs and practices. Smoking cessation programs were being offered by tribal members at the Elders' Hall. Children were being taught that violence in any form was not acceptable and was not congruent with traditional Native spiritual beliefs. New and different culturally congruent care patterns will continue to develop as the Potawatomi reclaim their culture care traditions and practices.

By listening, understanding, and being there, nurses and other health clinicians can assist the Potawatomi in repatterning and restructuring noncaring patterns of *alcohol and drug use, violence,* and *low self-esteem and shame* in the Potawatomi lifeways. Crucial areas where nurses could assist the Potawatomi to repattern or restructure their lifeways would be for tribal members to seek professional health care *earlier* in their illness. This would decrease the seriousness of the disease on presentation and reduce emergency room visits. Similarly, obtaining regular followup professional health care may promote better control of disease processes. Integrating generic culturally congruent nursing care actions and decisions into professional care practice would be necessary in order to successfully assist the Potawatomi in repatterning or restructuring care practices to promote health and wellbeing. An open acceptance of the Potawatomi values, beliefs, and lifeways, and working closely with tribal members and the tribal health care center would facilitate repatterning and restructuring of *non*care practices. Providing encouragement and support for tribal young adults to enter health professions was discovered to be a culturally congruent approach for providing intergenerational culturally congruent care through repatterning and restructuring. Members of the tribe who currently are or may become nurses could then further influence restructuring and repatterning of noncaring practices that are destructive to Native health and wellbeing.

Both Native and nonnative nurses prepared in transcultural nursing could influence professional care practices and services for Native Americans in organizational affairs. Although most Native Americans sought some professional health care that was unicultural and Anglo American in perspective, transcultural nurses need to develop culture-specific professional care practices for the provision of caring to Native Americans. Transcultural nurses with knowledge about culture and care with Native Americans may help the administration and staff of professional healthcare institutions to recognize and restructure care to become culturally congruent. Professional care providers grounded in principles and concepts of transcultural nursing would be able to provide culture care to promote improved Native American health and wellbeing.

Summary

This study was conceptualized within Leininger's (1991a) theory of Culture Care Diversity and Universality. It is a holistic care theory which aided this researcher to discover and learn *emic* and *etic* cultural care expressions, patterns, and practices from rural Potawatomi Native Americans. The theory was used to discover rich and indepth cultural knowledge and traditional care practices. Using the Culture Care Theory enabled the researcher to discover the universalities and diversities of human care patterns and lifeways from the worldview and culture-specific perspectives of the Potawatomi. The ethnonursing qualitative research method developed by Leininger (1991b) was used with the Culture Care Theory to guide the research process of this study. The theory and method provided the means to ". . . tease out the epistemics and ontological aspects of human caring" (Leininger, 1991b, p. 50), and also helped the researcher to ". . . envision a cultural world of different life forces or influences on human conditions which need to be considered to discover human care in its fullest way" (Leininger, 1991b, p. 50) with the Potawatomi Native Americans.

This study has contributed to the discipline of nursing by providing new and significant transcultural nursing care knowledge and by confirming the tenets of the Culture Care Theory. The findings have helped to provide professional nursing care knowledge incorporating the beliefs, practices, and values of the Potawatomi enabling them to receive culturally congruent care in therapeutic and specific ways. Such culturally congruent care may thus promote improvement in the health and wellbeing of tribal members by leading to healthier lifeways in their rural environmental context. This study contributed to the growth and evolution Leininger's Culture Care Theory through the discovery of a new body of transcultural care knowledge embedded in the Potawatomi Native American culture.

APPENDIX 7-A

Leininger's Sunrise Model Depicted Within the Native Indian's Worldview

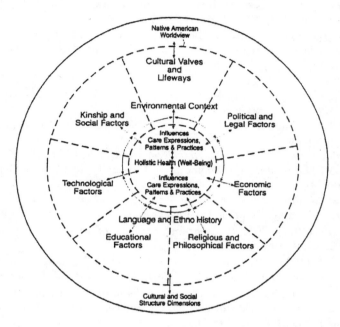

Individuals, Families, Groups, Communities, & Institutions
in
Diverse Health Systems

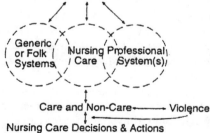

Care and Non-Care ⟵⟶ Violence

Nursing Care Decisions & Actions

Cultural Care Preservation / Maintenance
Cultural Care Accommodation / Negotiation
Cultural Care Repatterning / Restructuring

Cultural Congruent Nursing Care

Code ⟷ influences

Derived from Leininger's Sunrise Model to Depict Theory of Culture Care Diversity and Universality in Leininger, M. (1991b), *Culture care diversity and universality: A theory of nursing* (pp. 5–68). New York: National League for Nursing.

References

Allen, P. G. (1992). *The sacred hoop: Recovering the feminine in American Indian traditions*. Boston: Beacon Press.

Beauvais, F., Oetting., E., & Edwards, R. (1985). Trends in drug use in Indian adolescents living on reservations:1975–1983. *American Journal of Drug and Alcohol Abuse, 11*, 209–229.

Blum, R., Harmon, B., Harris, L., Bergeisen, L., & Resnick, M. (1992). American-Indian Alaska native youth health. *Journal of the American Medical Association, 267*, 1637–1644.

Booth, B., Blow, F., Cook, C., Bunn, J., & Fortney J. (1992). Age and ethnicity among hospitalized alcoholics: A nationwide study. *Alcoholism: Clinical and Experimental Research, 16*, 1029–1034.

Campbell, J., & Humpherys, J. (1993). *Nursing care of survivors of family violence*. St. Louis, MO: Mosby.

Chapleski, E. E. (1993). *1992 American Indian Profile State of Michigan*. Unpublished manuscript. Wayne State University, Institute of Gerontology, Detroit, MI.

Churchill, W. (1994). *Indians are us? Culture and genocide in Native North America*. Monroe: Common Courage Press.

Claspy, E. (1966). *The Potawatomi Indians of Southwestern Michigan*. Dowagiac, MI: Author.

Clifton, J. A. (1984). *The Pokagons, 1683–1983: Catholic Potawatomi Indians of the St. Joseph River Valley*. Lanhan, MD: University Press of America.

Crow, K. (1993). Multiculturalism and pluralistic thought in nursing education: Native American worldview and the nursing academic worldview. *Journal of Nursing Education, 32*, 198–204.

Dinges, N., & Quang, D. (1992). Stressful life events and occurring depression, substance abuse and suicide among American-Indian and Alaska Native adolescents. *Cultural Medicine and Psychiatry, 16*, 487–502.

Durst, D. (1991). Conjugal violence: Changing attitudes in two northern native communities. *Community Mental Health Journal, 27*, 359–373.

Elia, C., & Jacobs, D. (1992). The incidence of pathological gambling among Native-Americans treated for alcohol dependence. *International Journal of the Addictions, 28*, 659–666.

Farrell, L. (2001). Cultural care: Meanings and expressions of caring and non-caring of the Potawatomi who have experienced family violence. Doctoral dissertation, Wayne State University, Detroit, MI.

Grobsmith, E. (1989). The relationship between substance abuse and crime among Native American inmates in the Nebraska Department of Corrections. *Human Organization, 48*, 285–298.

Hastings, J., & Hamberger, L. (1988). Personality characteristics of spouse abusers: A controlled comparison. *Violence and Victims, 3*, 31–47.

Hatton, D. C. (1994). Health perceptions among older urban American Indians. *Western Journal of Nursing and Research, 16*, 392–403.

Horn, G. (1993). *Native heart: An American Indian odyssey.* San Rafael, CA: New World Library.

Huges, S., & Dodder, R. (1984). Alcohol consumption patterns among American Indian and white college students. *Journal of Studies on Alcohol, 45,* 433–439.

Huttlinger, K. W., & Tanner, D. (1994). The peyote way: Implications for culture care theory. *Journal of Transcultural Nursing, 5*(2), 5–11.

Kiniets, W. V. (1965). *The Indians of the Western Great Lakes 1615–1760.* Ann Arbor, MI: The University of Michigan Press.

Lange, B. K. (1988). Ethnographic interview: An occupational therapy needs assessment tool for American Indian and Alaska Native alcoholics. *Occupational Therapy Mental Health, 8,* 61–80.

Leininger, M. M. (1984). Care: The essence of nursing and health. In M. M. Leininger (Ed.), *Care: The essence of nursing and health* (pp. 3–15). Detroit, MI: Wayne State University Press.

Leininger, M. M. (1985). Ethnography and ethnonursing: Models and modes of qualitative data analysis. In M. M. Leininger (Ed.), *Qualitative research methods in nursing* (pp. 33–71). Orlando, FL: Grune & Stratton.

Leininger, M. M. (1990). Ethnomethods: The philosophic and epistemic bases to explicate transcultural nursing knowledge. *Journal of Transcultural Nursing, 1,* 40–51.

Leininger, M. M. (1991a). Ethnonursing: A research method with enablers to study the theory of Culture Care. In M. M. Leininger (Ed.), *Culture care diversity and universality: A theory of nursing* (pp. 391–418). Detroit, MI: Wayne State University Press.

Leininger, M. M. (1991b). The theory of culture care diversity and universality. In M. M. Leininger (Ed.), *Culture care diversity and universality: A theory of nursing* (pp. 5–68). New York: National League for Nursing.

Leininger, M. M. (1991c). Selected cultural care findings of diverse cultures using the Culture Care Theory and Ethnonursing Method. In M. M. Leininger (Ed.), *Culture care diversity and universality: A theory of nursing* (pp. 5–68). New York: National League for Nursing.

McClurken, J. (1991). *Gah-Baeh-Jhagwah-Buk: The way it happened.* Lansing, MI: Michigan State University.

McGaa, Ed. (1990). *Mother Earth spirituality.* New York: Harper Collins.

Moncher, M. S., Holden, G. W., & Trimble, J. E. (1990). Substance abuse among Native-American youth. *Journal of Consulting Clinical Psychology, 58,* 408–415.

Morse, J. M., Young, D. E., & Swartz, L. (1991). Cree Indian healing practices and Western health care: A comparative analysis. *Social Science and Medicine, 32* (12), 1261–1267.

Phillips, S., & Lobar, S. (1990). Literature summary of some Navajo child health beliefs and rearing practices within a transcultural nursing framework. *Journal of Transcultural Nursing, 1,* 13–20.

Pokagen Band of Potawatomi Indians. (1994). Information retrieved from www.pokagon.com.

Robin, R. W., Chester, B., Rasmussen, J. K., Jaransson, J. M., & Goldman, D. (1997). Factors influencing utilization of mental health and substance abuse services by American Indian men and women. *Psychiatric Services, 48*(6), 826–832.

Rosenbaum, J. (1991). Culture care theory and Greek Canadian widows. In M. M. Leininger (Ed.), *Culture care diversity and universality: A theory of nursing* (pp. 305–339). Detroit, MI: Wayne State University Press.

Schinke, S., Botvin, G., Trimble, J., Orlandi, M., Gilchrist, L., & Locklear, V. (1988). Preventing substance abuse among American-Indian adolescents: A bicultural competence skills approach. *Journal of Counseling Psychology, 35,* 87–90.

Van Breda, A. (1989). Health issues facing Native American children. *Pediatric Nurse, 16,* 575–577, 584–585.

Venn, J. (1988). MMPI profiles of Native, Mexican, and Caucasian-American male alcoholics. *Psychological Reports, 62,* 427–432.

Walker, R. D., & Kivlahan, D. R. (1984). Definitions, models, and methods in research on sociocultural factors in American Indian alcohol use. *Substance and Alcohol Actions/Misuse, 5,* 9–19.

Wenger, A. (1991). The culture care theory and the old order Amish. In M. M. Leininger (Ed.), *Culture care diversity and universality: A theory of nursing* (pp. 147–178). Detroit, MI: Wayne State University Press.

Wuest, J. (1991). Harmonizing: A North American Indian approach to management of middle ear disease with transcultural nursing implication. *Journal of Transcultural Nursing, 3*(1), 5–14.

CHAPTER EIGHT

Use of the Culture Care Theory as a Framework for the Recruitment, Engagement, and Retention of Culturally Diverse Students in a Traditionally European American Baccalaureate Nursing Program

Marilyn R. McFarland, PhD, RN, CTN

Sandra J. Mixer, MSN, RN

Averetta E. Lewis, RN, PhD, APRN-BC

Cheryl E. Easley, PhD, RN

Introduction

The challenge for the College of Nursing and Health Sciences at a medium sized public university in the Midwestern United States has been to improve access to baccalaureate nursing education for students with cultural backgrounds reflecting those of the local population. Project OPEN (Opportunities for Professional Education in Nursing) was a 3-year federally funded project focused on enabling culturally diverse students from educationally and-or financially disadvantaged backgrounds to enter and succeed in baccalaureate nursing education. Partnerships were formed between the university and community institutions such as hospitals, health departments, home care agencies, and schools to foster improved access to baccalaureate nursing education.

The Culture Care Theory together with the Sunrise Enabler (which depicts an integrated holistic view of the influencing dimensions and major concepts of the theory) provided the framework for all phases of this endeavor. A 3-phase approach for Project OPEN was used to reach the above identified student groups. During the first phase, *recruitment*, students were recruited who had not yet entered the university such as high, middle, and elementary school students, nontraditional students, those with a degree in another field, and those working as nursing assistants or licensed practical nurses. The second phase, *engagement*, facilitated prenursing students who were enrolled in prerequisite coursework preparing them for admission to the nursing program. The third phase, *retention*, involved assisting students who were in the nursing program to progress and graduate.

This chapter will present a synthesis of the creation, progression, and evaluation of Project OPEN. Several project objectives addressed increasing the number of prenursing, nursing, and graduating students from culturally diverse backgrounds. Another objective of the Project was to educate students to give culturally congruent and competent nursing care to prepare them as future nurses who will contribute to the health and wellbeing of their clients. In addition, preparation of a culturally competent nursing workforce has the potential to enhance the health and wellbeing of professional nursing practice. Health and wellbeing of students was viewed within the Project as successful progression through the program toward graduation and eventual practice as registered nurses. It was predicted that increasing the numbers of culturally diverse students would expand the worldview of prenursing and nursing students and thus have the potential to expand the worldview of the local and regional nursing workforce and the profession. One goal of the nursing program was to expand the worldview of students by challenging them to look outside the region and the university campus to the communities in which they live and work and to the world beyond.

Environmental Context of the University

Located in an agricultural and industrial region in the Midwestern United States, the university was founded approximately 40 years ago to serve a 14-county region. The region is culturally diverse (comprising African Americans, Mexican Americans, Native Americans, and economically disadvantaged residents from all of the aforementioned cultures as well as European Americans) with an environmental context reflective of small cities and remote rural areas. The region has significant numbers of people with poor educational and health outcomes (United States Census Data, 2000) making the need for professional nurses prepared to provide culturally congruent and competent health care apparent.

The 4-year baccalaureate nursing program has historically enrolled mostly young women of European American background. Students are generally admitted to the program after completing one year of prerequisite nonnursing courses such as chemistry, biology, English composition, communication, and statistics. In an effort to address the limited diversity of students in the nursing program, a nursing workforce diversity grant from the Division of Nursing, Bureau of Health Professions, Health Resources Services Administration, Department of Health and Human Services was submitted and funded for years 2001 through 2004. The target groups for this project included urban African Americans and Hispanics, rural European Americans, and older students. Students from these groups were from educationally and-or financially *disadvantaged* backgrounds and some were the first in their families to attend college.

Political and Educational Dimensions of Creating a Diverse Nursing Workforce

Examining the political and educational dimensions of creating a diverse nursing workforce was critical to development and implementation of the project. The culture of nursing embraces the shared value of a culturally diverse nursing workforce prepared to provide culturally competent nursing care for people in an increasingly multicultural world. Preliminary findings from the March 2000 national sample of registered nurses indicates that an estimated 86% of the nation's RNs are white (non-Hispanic) (U.S. Department of Health and Human Services [USDHHS], 2003). Other cultural groups are woefully underrepresented in the profession. In a group of five Midwestern states where the university is located, only 6% of registered nurses are from racial or ethnic minorities (USDHHS). A goal of the profession is to have the nursing workforce mirror the people who receive care.

The National Advisory Council on Nurse Education and Practice proposed that one of a set of federal policy goals is:

> . . . To enhance the ability of the registered nurse workforce to meet the challenges of cultural diversity in delivery of health care [and further recommends that] the federal government should support educational activities to increase the cultural sensitivity and cultural competence in nursing students. (USDHHS, 1996)

Additionally, in 1997, the American Association of Colleges of Nursing (AACN) in its Position Statement on Diversity and Equality of Opportunity stated:

. . . The objective for schools of nursing is the creation of both an educational community and a professional practice environment that incorporate the diverse perspectives of the many constituencies whom they serve. Nursing programs must provide a supportive learning environment and curriculum in which students, staff, and faculty from all walks of life and from the entire spectrum of society are full participants in the educational process. . . . As a voice for educators in baccalaureate and higher degree nursing programs, AACN believes that diversity and equality of opportunity are core values in all educational systems. . . . Despite their small numbers, minority nurses are significant contributors to the provision of health care services . . . and leaders in the development of models of care that address the unique needs of minority populations. (AACN, 2001).

In the area served by the university, the regional hospital council convened a healthcare workforce consortium in 2002 to address concerns about healthcare workforce shortages and the lack of cultural diversity of healthcare professionals (Hospital Council of East Central Michigan, 2002). Among their foci was an appeal for emphasis on cultural diversity by colleges and universities which was held ". . . to be essential for preparation of students pursuing health careers in the 21st century" (Hospital Council of East Central Michigan, 2002). Thus, for the Project, the regional challenge identified was to prepare culturally diverse residents for entrance into and academic success within baccalaureate nursing education, and thus create a nursing workforce reflecting the diversity of the region.

Universal Care Expressions, Patterns, and Practices

The Culture Care Theory depicted by the Sunrise Enabler is useful for nurses in practice, research, and education for developing educational programs, conducting research studies, or planning care for individuals, families, groups, or institutions. The critical components of the Sunrise Enabler that provided the framework for the development, implementation, and evaluation of Project OPEN are presented. The top of the Sunrise Enabler depicts the social structure dimensions and care expressions patterns and practices that needed to be considered when designing such a project. These factors were held to influence care and in turn the health of clients, and the health and success of students. Universal and diverse care expressions, patterns, and practices and related care actions and decisions (based on the three modes in the Culture Care Theory) were used with students during the development, implementation, and evaluation of project services. These factors were organized and presented to Project participants with the components of the Sunrise Enabler which together were found to be the most important influencers on care among students.

The implementation of project services related to recruitment, engagement, and retention of culturally diverse students commenced in the fall semester of 2001. Ongoing evaluation occurred throughout the project culminating in a formal qualitative student (*emic*) focused program evaluation in fall of 2003. Qualitative content analysis was used to discover culture care patterns and caring constructs from narrative data. The qualitative criteria of credibility, confirmability, meaning-in-context, recurrent patterning, saturation, and tranferability were used to evaluate these findings (Leininger & McFarland, 2002; Polit & Hungler, 1999).

An open inquiry guide was developed based on the components and major constructs of the theory and Sunrise Enabler (Leininger, 1991a/b; Leininger & McFarland, 2002). Open ended questions were used to elicit stories and reflections from the students about the Project. In consideration of the construct of care, a sample of an open ended inquiry was, ". . . I'm interested in learning about the care you received from nursing faculty, fellow students, and staff during your time here at the university." In consideration of kinship and social factors, informants were asked, ". . . Tell me about your family and friends and how they view your experience of being in school." The open inquiry guide enabler is provided in Appendix 8-A.

Of the approximately 200 prenursing and nursing Project students, 12 participated in the qualitative evaluation. These participants were purposefully selected by the evaluators to be representative of the students using Project services. Five males and seven females participated in the evaluation with ages ranging from 18 to 45 years. Six participants were from rural areas and six from urban areas; seven were European American, four were African American and one was Asian American. Four participants were prenursing students, six were nursing students, and two were recent graduates of the nursing program (within the past year).

Project OPEN faculty and staff coparticipated with prenursing and nursing students during the three years of the funded project. Along with parents and-or significant others, appropriate student-focused care actions and decisions were developed using Leininger's three modes of Culture Care Theory that were held to be important, satisfying, safe, and beneficial by these students as they transitioned through the nursing program.

Kinship and Social Factors

It was discovered that care received from families was a critical factor for students to be successful in the nursing program. Culture care from family, friends, and peers involved *listening, being there, encouraging,* and *giving direct help* such as child care or assistance with household chores. *Listening* and *being there* were reciprocal and involved frequent telephone calls and visits between the students and their families, friends, and peers. In particular, students shared that they valued family and friends visiting them on campus. Students related that they felt encouraged when spouses and other family members communicated to them a deep belief in their ability to be successful in the nursing program. A student reflected about the direct help received from her spouse, commenting that, ". . . When I needed to study, I had to exit and not deal with my daughter; my husband helped me manage my time." Some students struggled with ethnocentric bias and were challenged in relating to peers from diverse backgrounds. As students transitioned in their professional role development, they shared that peers became 'like family' and they felt connected and cared for by one another. Project faculty encouraged culture care maintenance of family and peer care, which was valued as leading to student health, wellbeing, and success in the nursing program.

Economic Factors

Students faced financial challenges related to the costs of baccalaureate education. They lacked money for tuition, books, transportation, living expenses, and for some, child care. Most of the project students needed and received financial aid. Many families expected college students to work and attend school, which has been recognized as being frequently incongruent with successful progression in the nursing program. Some student comments related to economic factors were, ". . . I worry about money constantly," ". . . The Project OPEN stipend really helps," and ". . . Financial aid is really important." Project faculty and staff used *culture care negotiation* by offering students financial aid from Project OPEN as an incentive for successful academic progression. In return, students assisted in recruitment activities geared toward future nursing students at area high school and middle schools. *Culture care restructuring* was used with parents and students to assist them in adopting positive perspectives about accepting student loans and decreasing number of hours students worked.

Many students held a family belief that one should not borrow money for education, although low-interest student loans that defer payment until after graduation were made available. Some students' employment schedules hours interfered with their studies enough that they risked failing. *Culture care restructuring* was accomplished by persuading students and their families to accept student loans which then allowed them to work fewer hours, remain in the program, and graduate in a timely manner. For students unable to decrease work hours or family responsibilities, part-time study was negotiated that permitted their continuation in the nursing program. In general, part-time students decreased their course loads by one course (or three credits) from 12 to 9 credits per semester.

Project OPEN students often had limited encouragement and opportunities to attend college, and many were the first generation in their families to pursue university education. Project faculty and staff discovered that culturally diverse students were frequently advised by school counselors to pursue vocational education or associate degree programs without giving consideration to a bachelor's degree in nursing (BSN). During high school, many area disadvantaged students were being urged to follow a vocational curriculum at a career center rather than remaining in high school to take college preparatory courses such as anatomy, physiology, human biology, and trigonometry which are recommended for success in baccalaureate nursing education.

Project faculty established a Future Nurses club at an area urban middle school to provide an opportunity for African American students to consider nursing as a viable career choice. Nursing students volunteered to accompany faculty to talk about the profession and to demonstrate practice skills (e.g., CPR and first aid). They also accompanied middle school students on field trips to local hospitals. These activities stimulated a connection between African American urban middle school students and successful nursing students.

Two activities offered to prenursing students were the opportunity to enroll in College Success Courses (in which students receive an additional credit hour of targeted instruction and tutoring) in the fall, and to participate in a project enrichment workshop in the summer prior to attending the university. This workshop was an interdisciplinary bridge program offered to high school graduates and older students entering college from educationally and-or financially disadvantaged backgrounds. The program included a series of preparatory sessions in the areas of biology, chemistry, mathematics, writing, computer technologies, and critical thinking and communication skills essential in nursing. In addition to academic instruction, the facilitation of cohort bonding within the participant group and with faculty and current nursing students promoted confidence in freshmen students, further enabling them to be successful in the university setting. That Project prenursing students greatly benefited from these activities is reflected in their overall higher grade point averages and increased retention rates when compared to their class peers who did not participate in these services (McFarland, 2004).

Tutoring was an important Project service leading to student success and graduation. A major strength of Project tutoring was the building of cohorts by prenursing students who, after being tutored in chemistry and biology, formed study groups. Peer tutoring provided the critical connections among prenursing and nursing students at various stages in the program. Nursing students provided peer tutoring to prenursing students in statistics, biology, anatomy, and physiology, and tutored sophomore and junior nursing students in nursing courses. Students viewed peer tutoring as culturally congruent care. Examples of statements they shared included: ". . . They speak our language" and ". . . They are one of us."

Another Project service was the development of a prenursing course entitled *Nursing Connections for the Future*, in which the professional nursing role was explored, covering such topics as historical foundations of nursing, current trends influencing the profession, and strategies for student success. This course expanded students' worldview of nursing and health care and introduced them to the construct of *care* as central to the practice and discipline of nursing. The course foci included collegiality as caring, connecting through mentoring and networking, recruitment, engagement, and retention for nursing, and local and global current events or trends influencing nursing. Among the comments from students taking the prenursing course were, ". . . Thank you for this class," ". . . Now I know nursing is the profession for me," and ". . . I feel like you care—thanks for the tutoring information."

Content related to culturally congruent and culturally specific care has been integrated as a Project focus throughout the nursing curriculum. Transcultural nursing concepts and principles are taught with focus on cultural assessments of individuals, families, and healthcare organizations with the ultimate goal of students providing culturally competent nursing care as registered nurses in practice.

Some Project services were found to be more widely used and congruent with student lifeways. Writing assistance was provided to students through the university writing center by a writing associate dedicated to the College of Nursing who worked with students to facilitate mastery of writing in general, assistance with specific assignments, and in developing a writing portfolio. Personal counseling for students was provided by the Project counselor. Specific services offered included personal and family counseling, time management strategies, test taking skills, study skills, goal setting, self advocacy skills, conflict resolution, and appropriate referrals for social and mental health issues. Students were encouraged to become members of the Student Nurses Association to develop professionally through networking, community outreach, university and social activities, education, and leadership. Project faculty received internal university grants allowing them to provide opportunities for students to attend international conferences (such as the Transcultural Nursing Society annual meetings) as a means of expanding their worldview and to learn the beliefs, values, and practices of the nursing profession.

Students shared that the environmental contexts of the university, the faculty, and staff were friendly, and that faculty, staff, and peers worked hard to demonstrate that they valued and embraced students' cultural traditions and practices. Student feedback revealed how critical they viewed making connections with faculty through mentoring and networking opportunities. Student descriptors of faculty care were *being there, going the extra mile, role modeling and mentoring, embracing differences, providing and coordinating services*, and *listening*. In addition, students expressed appreciation for coping assistance in dealing with their adaptation [culture shock] to the university environmental context. Project faculty and staff continued to practice culture care accommodation by making project services congruent with students' needs reflecting their cultural beliefs and values.

Political and Legal Factors

The College of Nursing and Health Sciences has taken leadership in establishing diversity initiatives on the university campus. These initiatives have included taking prenursing and nursing students from both culturally similar and diverse backgrounds to university cultural events such as the annual Martin Luther King dinner and cosponsoring a diversity workshop presented by experts from the National Coalition Building Institute International. The Project OPEN director formed a project advisory committee composed of community leaders from diverse cultural and employment backgrounds to make recommendations about future Project development and implementation.

Philosophical and Religious–Spiritual Factors

The qualitative evaluation data indicated that most students described their faith in God and use of prayer as essential components to their academic success. Students also spoke about the need to address the spiritual beliefs and values of the people for whom they provided care. Faculty and staff practiced culture care preservation by encouraging students to continue to draw on their religious beliefs and practices.

Diverse Care Expressions, Patterns, and Practices

The Culture Care Theory focuses on diverse as well as universal findings. One African American project student described racist noncaring actions demonstrated by her European American peers. Three European American rural prenursing students revealed that prior to coming to the university they had never met a person of color. These prenursing students shared that their worldview broadened once they began to develop relationships with culturally diverse peers and provide care for people from diverse cultures.

Occasionally, students who needed Project services did not access them despite the availability of these services and strong encouragement by faculty and advisory staff members to use them to promote individual student success in the nursing program. This self-noncaring pattern requires further exploration. It is predicted that services may not have been offered in a culturally congruent manner for some students. The faculty has collaboratively reflected whether approaching a faculty member may not have been culturally acceptable for some freshman college students.

Assumptive Premises Supporting the Qualitative Evaluation

Professionals and faculty provided student care and caring by using project services combined with spiritual and generic–folk family care to support and promote healthy lifeways, successful academic progression, and graduation of nursing students holding broadened worldviews. The assumptive premises derived from Leininger's Culture Care Theory supported in this qualitative evaluation were:

1. Care is the essence of nursing education and a distinct, dominant, central, and unifying focus.
2. Care is essential for student wellbeing, health, growth, successful academic progression, and graduation.
3. Culture care values, beliefs, and practices of nursing students are influenced by and tend to be embedded in their worldview, religion, kinship, social, political, legal, educational, economic, and environmental context.
4. Culture care is the broadest holistic means to know, explain, interpret, and predict student lifeways and to educate students in the delivery of culturally congruent and competent nursing care in order to prepare future nurses to contribute to the health and wellbeing of their clients (derived from Leininger, 1991a/b).

Institutionalization of Project Services

Although federal funds were used to develop a diversity retention and recruitment program, continuation of the services, strategies, and goals related to the project must become part of the culture of the institution. The mission statement of the university reflects a commitment to the recruitment and retention of a diverse student body and cadre of employees. Project services such as tutoring, prenursing coursework, prenursing advising, personal counseling, writing assistance, financial aid, and cultural enrichment experiences have been institutionalized over the course of the grant period and have been preserved as part of the College of Nursing and university culture.

Nurse educators must take into account that cultural caring values, beliefs, symbols, and lifeways of students from diverse and similar cultures are beneficial for students to have a satisfying educational experience that leads to successful academic progression and graduation. Prenursing students enter the university and college of nursing from very diverse backgrounds. Project faculty and staff endeavor to teach students ways to synthesize knowledge about the culture of the university, academic nursing program, nursing profession, and cultural knowledge of diverse groups in order for them to achieve successful academic progression and graduate.

Summary

Our challenge in the college of nursing is to continue to improve access to baccalaureate nursing education for students with backgrounds representing the diverse and similar cultures of the region. Based upon the synthesis of professional nursing knowledge, the cultural knowledge of their own focus groups, and past project surveys, these graduates have been able to provide culturally competent nursing care regionally and in their home communities. Their presence in the university setting has challenged the nursing faculty and fellow students to develop enhanced cultural sensitivity in working with clients, families, and communities from which they differ. *Preproject* target numbers met and exceeded the anticipated Project objectives. However, the ultimate goal of creating a culturally diverse nursing program and nursing workforce continues to be a *work in progress*. The nursing faculty and staff remain committed to this goal and continue to focus their efforts in reaching out to potential nursing students from culturally diverse backgrounds through focused recruitment, engagement, and retention efforts. The Culture Care Theory with the Sunrise Enabler is a framework that can be effectively used in other nursing programs, disciplines, and institutional settings to address cultural diversities and similarities related to recruitment and retention in higher education.

Project OPEN was supported by funds from the Division of Nursing, Bureau of Health Professions, Health Resources Services Administration, Department of Health and Human Services under grant number D19 HP 40362-0, titled Nursing Workforce Diversity Grants. The total amount of the reward is $523,521. The information or content and conclusions are those of the authors and should not be construed as the official position or policy of, nor should be any endorsements be inferred by, the DN, BHPR, or DHHS, or the US government.

Appendix 8-A: A Qualitative Evaluation of the Culture Care of Diverse and Similar Nursing and Prenursing Students in a Traditionally European American BSN Program

Open Inquiry Guide for Project Evaluation

Demographics

Name:

Religious Affiliation

Informant #:

Years of Formal Education:

Sex:

Cultural Background:

Age:

Prenursing or Nursing Status:

Permanent Place of Residence:

Dates of Interview:

Years at SVSU:

Languages Spoken:

Care

1. I am interested in learning about the care you have received from nursing faculty, fellow students and staff during your time here at the University.
   a. What stories, statements, words, or ideas describe the caring actions?
2. Tell me about the care you have given to your clients in practicum.
3. How would you describe a caring nurse?
4. As a nursing or prenursing student, do you sometimes give care to your peers? Give me an example.
5. Tell me some of the ways you care for yourself in school.
6. For you, then, care means _____.

This guide has been adapted from Leininger's guide entitled, "Culturalogical Care Assessment Guide," in Leininger, M. (1991a/b). "Ethnonursing: A research method with enablers to study the theory of culture care." In M. Leininger (Ed.), *Culture care diversity & universality: A theory of nursing* (pp. 73–117). New York: National League for Nursing Press.

Health (Wellbeing)

1. Tell me about care that nursing faculty, staff, or peers may have given you.
2. Tell me how this care affected your health and academic progress.
3. Tell me about your health. In your own words, tell me what health means to you.
4. What certain foods, activities, or medicines do you believe keep you healthy?
5. Tell me how your health has been while you have been in school.

Environmental Context

A. Institutional (University) Culture
   1. Describe your life. Is it different or similar since you came here?
B. Educational Factors
   1. How do you view the University nursing program? Tell me how it affects your daily life?
   2. Tell me about any of the Project OPEN services you may have used (tutoring, personal counseling, stipend, project faculty, and staff)
C. Political Factors
   1. From your experience here, tell me if you think university/state-national politics affect your progress in the nursing program. Give an example.
   2. Does the Student Nurses Association have any effect on your progress in the program? Give me an example.
D. Economic Factors
   1. Tell me about how you are financing your education.
   2. Tell me about how you are covering basic living expenses for you/your family while in school.
E. Kinship/Social Factors
   1. Tell me about your family and friends and how they view your experience of being in school.
   2. Describe your relationship with nursing faculty, staff, and peers.
F. Religious Factors
   1. Tell me what roles religion or spiritual beliefs play in your life.
   2. Describe any relationship your beliefs have with your success in the program. Tell me about this relationship. Who or what is your source of spiritual strength?

G. Technological Factors
1. How has the technology of today's university environment affected your progress in the nursing program?
2. How do you view the technology of care in the hospital?

H. Cultural Factors
1. The idea of *culture* refers to the customs and lifeways of people; tell me about your customs or cultural lifeways.
2. What traditional activities in your family are viewed as healthy or good lifeways?
3. What cultural groups are represented here among the students, faculty, staff, peers?
4. How do nursing faculty, staff, or peers view your cultural beliefs, values, or practices? Give me some examples.

Summary Questions

1. Is there anything else you want to tell me about your educational experience here? Or about the care you have received from nursing faculty, staff, peers?
2. Is there anything else you want to tell me about your health and wellbeing since you have been at the University?
3. Is there anything else you want to share with me before we close?

References

American Association of Colleges of Nursing. (2001). *Online issue bulletin: Effective strategies for increasing diversity in nursing programs.* Retrieved October, 2002, from http://www.aacn.nche.edu/Publications/issues/dec01.htm.

American Association of Colleges of Nursing. (1997). *Online position statement: Statement on diversity and equality of opportunity.* Retrieved October, 1997, from http:www.aacn.nche./edu/Pubs/diverse.htm.

Hospital Council of East Central Michigan. (2002). Newsletter.

Leininger, M. (1991a). *Culture care diversity and universality: A theory of nursing.* New York: National League for Nursing.

Leininger, M. (1991b). *Culture care diversity and universality: A theory of nursing.* New York: National League for Nursing.

Leininger, M. (2002). Part I: The theory of culture care and use of the ethnonursing method. In M. Leininger and M. R. McFarland (Eds.), *Transcultural nursing: Concepts, theories, research, and practices.* New York: McGraw-Hill.

Leininger, M., & McFarland, M. R. (Eds.). (2002). *Transcultural nursing: Concepts, theories, research, & practice*. (3rd ed.). New York: McGraw-Hill.

McFarland, M. R. (2004). [Final Report: Project OPEN (Opportunities for Professional Education in Nursing]. Unpublished raw data.

Polit, D. F., & Hungler, B. P. (1999). *Nursing research: Principles and methods* (6th ed.). Philadelphia: Lippincott.

U.S. Bureau of Census. (2000). State and County Quickfacts Web site at http://quickfacts.census.gov.

U.S. Department of Health and Human Services [USDHHS]. Health Resources and Services Administration, Bureau of Health Professions, Division of Nursing (2003). The registered nurse population: Findings from the national sample survey of registered nurses. Washington, DC: Author.

U.S. Department of Health and Human Services [USDHHS]. (1996). National Advisory Council on Nurse Education and Practice; Report to the Secretary of Health and Human Services on the Basic Registered Nurse Work Force. Washington, DC: United States Government Printing Office.

CHAPTER NINE

Culture Care Theory with Southern Sudanese of Africa

Madeleine M. Leininger, PhD, LHD, DS, CTN, RN, FAAN, FRCNA

> *Shortly after my arrival in Omaha, Nebraska, in late 1995, I began a transitional professional career. I wanted to remain active in the field of transcultural nursing that I had worked so hard to establish in the 1950s and 1960s. Shortly after settling in Omaha, I received a call from a nurse living and working in a nearby city. She said, "I am so glad you are now in the state as we have no prepared or certified trans-cultural nurses in the state or region. You are very much needed here."*

In this chapter, I present a Southern Christian Sudanese family and use the Culture Care Theory to discover and analyze their experiences. The intent is to show the context of the culture and the care needs of this large refugee family. My role was as a refugee sponsor in a large urban Midwestern city in the United States, which is discussed in this chapter. Due to space constraints, only major themes are presented.

I had already heard that the Southern Sudanese refugees from Africa had arrived in Nebraska, but I had not had any contact with them. After talking with the nurse who called me, I offered some general information to help her understand the Southern Sudanese culture. I encouraged the community nurses to maintain a friendly and caring attitude. I also suggested the nurses enroll in the transcultural nursing course I was teaching at the University of Nebraska, where I would focus on the Sudanese refugees in Omaha.

Getting Involved with the Family

A short time after this conversation, I received a call from a city social service agency asking if I would like to work with and be a sponsor for a large Sudanese family with seven children. This refugee family was from the Southern Christian Sudan region and had recently come to the city. The agency had no one to sponsor this large refugee family. By being a sponsor, one had to help the family get settled in Omaha with clothing, food, health needs, and a safe living place. It also meant helping the children to enroll in appropriate schools. After listening to the agency leader explain these responsibilities, I agreed to sponsor and help this family learn to live in the large urban Omaha community of nearly 450,000 people. Fortunately, I had been to Southern Africa (sub-Saharan) area several years ago and had stopped briefly in Sudan. As a part of my doctoral (Ph.D.) studies, I had chosen Africa as my cultural area of interest and study, along with selected Pacific Island cultures. Thus, I had some holding or background knowledge of the African cultural arena. However, I needed to be updated on current developments in Sudan, especially the terrible tribal war of recent years.

My first meeting with the family was in a large old house located in a low-income African American community. After introducing myself to the family, I explained that I was a nurse researcher interested in learning about their needs and experiences and in helping them. I also said I would be their sponsor and would help them get settled in the city and adjust to a new lifeway that was different from Southern Sudan. They were friendly and seemed very pleased someone was interested in them. I asked each of the nine family members to give their name and tell anything they wanted to share about their living in Sudan and now living in an American city. They told their stories of great interest in broken English phrases. Some cried as they spoke, but all said, "We are glad to be in America and no longer in Sudan. The war in Sudan has been terrible." The parents were about 45 years old and spoke understandable English. They were sad, restless, nervous, and cried at times as they talked. They seemed, however, eager to tell 'their story' about their life in Sudan, and the terrible tribal wars. The parents also said they were glad to be in America. But, as they told their story, both father and mother frequently cried, especially when they spoke about their horrible, frightening, and oppressive experiences in Southern Sudan. They held each other's hands and frequently wept. As I listened to them, I remained an active listener concerned about what they had experienced over several years. I used my Culture Care Theory insights to reflect on their information and to assess their holistic and critical needs. I was as compassionate as possible about what they had experienced. Their stories were of deep concern to me and I wondered how they had survived.

The Sunrise Enabler (see Figure 1-1) was an excellent guide for listening to and thinking about their situation. It was a valuable guide for doing a general cultural health care assessment (Leininger & McFarland, 2002). As the family members told their stories, I asked a few questions and they responded by telling me more about themselves. It was during the first session that the family members told about leaving Southern

Sudan and going to Egypt to come to America. They were very eager to leave the Southern Sudan as the threats of the fundamentalist Muslims made them fearful which had caused them employment problems. They told about the horrible life they had experienced in Southern Sudan for approximately five years with almost daily threats by the Muslim regime of being killed because they were Catholic. The father and mother wept and trembled as they shared their experiences. They said they were still afraid to tell what had happened for fear of retribution.

Their stories revealed a very oppressive government regime. They said they were willing to share their experiences, but it made them very sad. I gave them verbal reassurance that it was safe to tell their stories to me and that their information helped me to understand what they had experienced and their current needs. They said it was alright for me to record their stories and that they "felt safe" in telling them to me.

As they talked, it was evident this family had been terrorized with threats of being killed and they were watched daily for any minor political offenses by government officers. The parents had also been tortured and imprisoned several times mainly because they were Christians (Catholics) and unwilling to give up their faith to become Muslims. They were threatened daily that they would be killed if they did not comply with government orders. They said the government was very suspicious of them and thought they were against them (the government). The family was watched by officers day and night; whenever they left their huts, observers monitored where they went and what they did. The parents gave many accounts of how frightened they were living with the threat that they could be killed at any time. While it was difficult to fully imagine all they had experienced, nonetheless, I listened attentively and expressed my deep concerns for them with a caring attitude. I asked some clarifying questions to be sure I understood what they were telling me. I occasionally said, ". . . It must have been a horrible experience but now a great relief to be away from these people." They would always answer with a loud, "Yes!" Throughout this interview and subsequent ones, I used transcultural nursing principles to ease the communication process (Andrews & Boyle, 2003; Leininger, 1995; Leininger & McFarland, 2002).

Domain of Inquiry

After observing, listening to, and interacting with the family for several weeks in their home, the theory of Culture Care seemed appropriate to study this family. My domain of inquiry or focus of study was *the culture care needs and ways to help this immigrant–refugee Sudanese family deal with their terrible past fears and cultural oppression experiences in the Sudan with the goal to help them adjust to a different lifeway in a Midwestern American city* (Leininger, 1991; Leininger & McFarland, 2002). This domain and my sponsorship meant helping them get food, furniture, clothing, and daily necessities almost immediately as they needed help in all these areas. It also meant helping the father and mother obtain employment to meet daily living costs for a rental home, food, and other expenses. Providing for the needs of a large family of nine was a major undertaking.

Some of the major research questions related to this domain were: (1) What major fears and destructive experiences did the family want to overcome? (2) What traditional cultural care beliefs, values, and lifeways from Southern Sudan did they want to regain and retain in this new culture that would be health promoting? (3) What American culture beliefs, values, and lifeways were of interest to them; which did they want to learn about and use? (4) How might this family be helped to regain and maintain their health in a new and very different culture from what they had left in Sudan? (5) What social, cultural, religious, economic, and environmental factors seemed to influence them most while living (or existing) in Southern Sudan for cultural healing and their wellbeing? (6) How might the three modes of the Culture Care Theory be used to care for this refugee family's present needs and help heal or lessen the horrors of their past cultural experiences? (7) What could be some of the major culture care conflicts they might experience in this new environment different from Southern Sudan?

The Culture Care Theory with the ethnonursing research method and the six enablers were used to study this major domain of inquiry (DOI) (Leininger, 1990, 1991, 1997; Leininger & McFarland, 2002). I had much to learn about the past and recent Southern Sudanese lifeways and their current fears. I also needed to discover what generic family health care and wellness meant to them in their traditional Sudanese culture and what care would be congruent, acceptable, and helpful to them now. The purpose of this ethnonursing study was to discover essential indepth *emic* knowledge, to understand the family's past experiences, and to identify generic care practices that promote health and wellbeing. In this chapter, I shall refer to the family with the fictive name of 'Oto' to protect their identity.

The general health needs of this family needed early attention. All of the Oto family members were underweight, thin, and underdeveloped for their ages. The seven children were ages 6, 8, 9, 10, 13, 16, and 18. The children had no clothing except for a few old clothes they had worn traveling from Egypt to Omaha. While I could not speak their dialect language, I remained an astute observer and listener and relied on nonverbal communication. I learned common daily expressions from them but wished I knew their language. They spoke fairly good English which they had learned in Sudan. I tried to fully grasp everything they told me, and I learned many meanings and interpretations from their nonverbal and gestural expressions and affirmations. They viewed me as an 'American' willing to learn and to help them in this new country. They were always thanking me for any help I gave them. They remained eager to teach me about themselves and their Southern Sudanese culture throughout the study. A mutually trusting and friendly relationship developed.

The first urgent need was to procure clothing for all family members. This was critical as it was fall in Nebraska and cold winter weather would soon arrive. Fortunately, I was able to find some warm, clean clothing for all the family members through a local church. The family was thrilled with the clothing. They loved the bright prints of the clothes and wore them immediately.

Second, the family needed good food, as they were very hungry and the children were growing. From their accounts, they said they had not eaten any full meals or much food since they came to the United States. They also said it was hard to eat when still frightened and anxious about new experiences and living in a new country. The family often commented that they were tired, frightened, and had very limited energy to work or participate in daily activities around the home.

It was evident that this family of nine was in great need of clothing, food, and to be relieved of the cultural pain they had experienced for so long (Leininger & McFarland, 2002). They needed boots, jackets, sweaters, and underclothes as the days and nights were cold. They needed warm blankets for their beds as the old house they were living in was difficult to heat, and the landlord was not too cooperative in making the home warm. He also charged a high monthly rent for an old house, which was a major problem as the rent required a large percentage of their money. I tried several times to persuade the landlord to reduce the rent but he firmly refused. This expenditure became a critical factor in helping the family's successful transition into American culture.

To obtain clothing, bedding, furniture, and other needs, I decided to ask a large Catholic parish to which I belonged to help this family. I talked with the priest and he was very willing to help the family. The parishioners responded favorably and saw this as Christian charity. I told them about this Sudanese family and their most urgent and critical needs, and what they had experienced before coming to America. The priest and the women's guild were interested and immediately provided help for this family. I posted a notice on the parish bulletin board about the large Sudanese family and their need for clothing and basic home furnishings. I also asked for monetary contributions for the family to help with things that needed to be purchased. It was most encouraging to see the very positive response and willingness to help this Sudanese family. The parishioners gave good used clothing, bedding, and furniture. The family saw the generosity of this Catholic parish and was most grateful. At the same time, the family found it hard to believe Americans had so much to give them. They kept asking, ". . . Why do they have so much and we had so little in our Sudanese homes?" They asked, ". . . Are all Americans like this?"

Almost unbelievably, the parishioners brought big bags of used, clean clothing and many household items such as bed sheets, kitchen utensils, and many home furnishings (e.g., table lamps and small dressers) to the family. This was amazing for the family to see. They were stunned to see so many material goods. The family kept thanking the parishioners as they brought items to their home. The mother and father kept saying, ". . . Thank you, God, for taking care of us and especially for bringing us to this country."

The Oto family also knew that no refugees could remain in the United States without a sponsor. They frequently thanked me, but I said it was the Omaha people and God who gave the food and gifts. While the sponsor role was quite overwhelming and a big responsibility, one could see the benefits almost daily as this large family of nine began to feel cared for and valued again. They felt respected as human beings after being deprived and abused for so long in Sudan.

Soon the Oto family began to relax and became less tense each day. Dignity and self-respect became evident in them almost daily. Each day I was with them, I continued to learn more about their generic family lifeways and their terrible experiences in Sudan. I realized it was almost miraculous how they had survived under such lengthy persecution and continual threats. Indeed, the Oto family had learned to face hardships, threats, and daily sufferings. At the same time, they had learned to be patient and to pray for God's help. Their Catholic faith was clearly evident by their daily prayers for help as they adjusted to life in Omaha. While they remained appreciative of my help and caring assistance, they particularly wanted to thank the church members, the priest, God, and the agency for all their assistance. The kind and generous giving to the family had opened their hearts enabling them to trust strangers and start life anew in the new city. However, they still wanted to talk about their past sufferings and mental tortures by the Sudanese government officials and rebels, although this need decreased with time. They also talked about forgiveness of these terrible people "as Christ forgave others." Unquestionably, their Catholic faith had been extremely helpful to them while being tortured in Sudan and as they endured deprivation and hardship. They first asked about a Catholic church as they wanted to become members, to pray, and to thank God for His help. They wanted to thank

God, but also to receive the sacraments and to thank the priest and parishioners for their help. They told how very difficult it had been for them to attend Mass in Sudan because of the threats of being killed if they were seen practicing their faith. The government officials wanted the family to become Muslims, but they refused. So they had relinquished practicing their faith in Sudan, but they never left their faith.

The Catholic Church in Omaha (a largely Catholic city) welcomed the family and arranged refreshments for the meeting with those who had given them food and clothing. The Oto family members were overjoyed and pleased to see this response. They were excited enough to invite some of their clan members and other friends to join them at church. The occasion proved to be positive for group and family healing. Their clan groups had arrived in Omaha a few months before the Oto family came to the city. These clan members were psychologically and culturally helpful to them as they shared similar cultural interests, values, and beliefs, especially of the Sudanese traditional lifeways which the Oto family wanted to retain. Attending the Catholic church in subsequent weeks strengthened the Oto family's faith, their hopefulness, and their ability to trust strangers in their new world in America.

Initially, I visited and assessed the community where the family lived to see if it was a safe and healthy environment. I found this community had strong family and Christian oriented lifeways. It was a poor but safe community and a livable setting. In fact, some community folk gave the Oto family some tables, chairs, pots and pans, and general household supplies such as towels, sheets, silverware, cleaning supplies, lamps, and other common items as the neighborhood recognized their needs.

Each time I visited the family, they were curious about our American lifeways and how to live in a large American city. They always asked what 'acceptable behavior' was and about 'how to prevent troubles.' They began to compare life in the United States to their past life in the Southern Sudan of Africa, and talked about the differences. Material wealth, freedom to act, pray, and other areas were quickly noted. They experienced and talked about their *cultural shock* when seeing so many stores full of goods and supplies. They were perplexed about 'making choices,' particularly in choosing from so many similar items. Different choices at the food store, choices in shoes, clothing, and other items seemed extravagant to them. Learning how to make choices and what was acceptable and unacceptable were often major topics of our discussions. These discussions helped me to learn about their traditional culture, their foods, folk practices, and family ties. They also wanted to talk about the Muslim authoritarian regime and its contrast with democratic values (benefits and hindrances). I drew upon my transcultural nursing knowledge, concepts, and anthropological insights about cultural differences and similarities. I was able to use the three theory modes to help them make and enact decisions that would be congruent for or acceptable to the Oto family. They valued the joint actions and the decision-making process. Their major caring values became apparent as I moved from being a cultural stranger to a trusted American friend. It was rewarding, challenging, and meaningful to assist them in their transition from their traditional culture to the new culture. Helping them to discover new lifeways that would be meaningful to them in their new world was valued by them and facilitated their acculturation process.

Ethnohistorical Factors

From Sudanese ethnohistorical data, I learned that since 1983, the Islamic Khartoum political and religious regimes had been threatening and taking over the Southern Sudanese land and people (Hall & Ismail, 1981; Holzman, 2000; Misch, 2002). The Southern Sudanese were mainly black and white Christians living with many fundamentalist Muslims. The Khartoum regime had tried to exert its religious beliefs and *shariah* (Islamic) law. It was estimated that nearly 3000 Sudanese people had been massacred by government troops (Grace, 2003; Misch, 2002). Slavery, rape, imprisonment, public lashings, and killings had been imposed upon the Sudanese people and others who had failed to comply with governmental expectations through noncompliance or open resistance (Misch, 2002). Some have estimated that nearly two million people in Sudan have been killed and many millions more have been displaced since 1983. The Oto family often told about these terrible government practices and wondered how they ever survived.

The husband and the wife told how they were put in prison for days for false allegations of spying. However, the parents said these threats and the terrible experiences made their faith even stronger, and they depended more on their faith and God's help through prayer to survive each day. Whenever they told about these experiences, the family members would cry and hold each other's hands. They said, ". . . We also almost died due to such threats, with no food given to us and threats in our everyday living." Trying to find work and food in Sudan was very difficult, but they quickly added, it was ". . . by God's help we survived." Each time they shared these terrible experiences, there seemed to be some emotional relief to have someone genuinely interested in listening to what happened to them over a long period of time. They often thanked me for listening. Compassionate care words showing <u>concern for</u> them was an important caring mode that was beneficial (healing) to them. They often said, ". . . You are really concerned and interested in what has happened to us and care for us now. No one in Sudan or Egypt cared what happened to us."

Probably the most stressful daily experience was that the Khartoum government officers remained suspicious of them "day and night." This kept them tense and frightened that they would be killed or put in prison at any moment. The government continually accused them of 'causing problems' and spying, and would beat them or put them in prison for a few days or longer. The accusation of spying was untrue. They also used different ways to force the family to become Muslims such as giving the father a very low salary, denying them food and community benefits, or not helping them to obtain employment. However, the family said they never relinquished their goals or their Catholic faith and became a strongly unified family. The parents often said, ". . . It was our Catholic beliefs, prayers, and practices that really sustained us during these horrible threats and punishments while in Sudan. As Christ suffered, so we also must suffer and accept suffering to survive." The worst fear was that the parents would be taken from the children and the children would die alone or be killed by government officers. Both parents were sent to prison for several days and they prayed constantly for the children as their food supply was very limited. As the parents related these experiences, they would not only cry but talk about these non-Christian acts and that the officers ". . . were like the devil."

The parents told how they finally managed to leave Sudan to come to the United States via Egypt. It was a horrifying account, but they were determined to leave the threatening Muslim lifeway. The parents (especially the mother) carefully planned for quick ways to leave Sudan. They used all their small savings and left with no clothing or possessions. They frequently said, ". . . It was a miracle that we escaped and finally got to come to the United States. We are grateful to be here and alive."

Ethnonursing Research Method with Enablers

The ethnonursing research method was used in this study to obtain indepth *emic* information (Leininger, 1991, 1997, 2002). It was the desired method as I had designed it to fit the culture and research care goals of the theory. For this study, nine <u>key informants</u> were chosen. The key informants were the entire family. They were the most knowledgeable about their experiences in the Southern Sudanese culture, care experiences, and how they survived and became refugees in the

United States. These refugees had lived in Southern Sudan for eight years and had been in the United States about three years when the study began. Ten general informants were chosen, several of which were Sudanese clan relatives. They were not as fully knowledgeable as the key informants but knew Southern Sudanese lifeways. With the ethnonursing method, I systematically studied indepth and carefully documented data from the key and general informants while focused on the domain of inquiry and the tenets of the theory as presented earlier. Culture care meanings, experiences, and beliefs were documented from the informants. This ethnonursing method was comfortable and acceptable to the informants. They liked that it was a natural, casual, and humanistic way for me to talk informally with them. I listened attentively and entered their world of knowing, and then recorded their ideas. This method encouraged the informants to share ideas. They liked to share their ideas and past beliefs so than an accurate and credible account could occur. I talked with informants in a very casual, friendly, and informal manner, which is generally important with cultural strangers. All visits were usually in the informants' familiar home environment. The intent was to keep the visits and the method friendly in order to obtain accurate, reliable, and spontaneous data.

Throughout my nearly three years of visits and observations, I remained an active listener and observer. I noted differences and commonalities among the family and clan informants in accordance with the method. Identifying similarities and commonalities with contrasts in the views among the family and clan was important to the theory tenets, especially discovering the 'why' of any such differences. Culture care variations were important to discover and to use in the healing process. I encouraged the informants to share or talk out their ideas and experiences and to give examples. They were active participants in the research process from the beginning to the end. I remained an active listener and observer of the informants and noted the context in which the visits occurred, whether in church, at work, or in the home. After the first few weeks there were signs that the informants trusted me. In fact, they looked forward to my visits and to 'telling their story.' I used the Stranger to Trusted Friend Enabler, as well as transcultural nursing principles, concepts, and interview techniques described in Leininger and McFarland (2002) for research. In general, informant data of the Oto family and general informants were obtained in a nonobtrusive, thoughtful, and reflective way with these informants. They seemed to like the approach and were active contributors and eager participants. I usually talked with them in small group context within the family home setting and confirmed ideas at each session.

In keeping with the ethnonursing method, six enablers were used. I had developed them to explicate the data bearing on the theory. There were two major enablers especially used in this study. These enablers helped me to tease out covert and overt data for the domain of inquiry. The six enablers encouraged the informants to share their ideas as they knew or experienced them. The two main enablers used were: (1) Observation-Participation-Reflection Enabler (see Figure 2-2), and (2) Sunrise Enabler (see Figure 1-1). These two enablers have been fully described in Leininger and McFarland (2002, pp. 80, 90) and in Leininger's other works (1991, 1997, 2002). In addition, I watched for signs for the extent of acculturation from traditional to nontraditional lifeways. Whether the informants were more traditionally or nontraditionally oriented in their lifeways was important to document (Leininger, 1991, pp. 99–101). With the Sudanese family, this was especially important, as they had relocated and were now experiencing a new culture, namely the American culture, from the perspective of their own traditional Southern Sudanese worldview. The extent to which they were traditionally or nontraditionally oriented influenced their responses and actions. I used each enabler appropriately to obtain verbatim and observational data noting variability factors (Leininger & McFarland, 2002). The Stranger to Trusted Friend Enabler (see Figure 2-1) was a most valuable enabler to gauge my relationship with informants and to assess my influence on the informants (Leininger, 1991, p. 82; Leininger & McFarland, 2002, p. 91).

The Sudanese family with three girls and four boys remained closely united in their actions and relationships. I observed their daily activities and listened to their concerns, interests, and conflicts as they lived in the new culture. My goal was to rebuild their self-identity, self-esteem, and cultural identity, and to help them regain their health and general wellbeing through caring ways. Besides having their malnourished state alleviated, the children needed to dress appropriately to be accepted at school and to keep warm in the cold winter season. The children would generally eat the food brought to them but always preferred the Sudanese foods prepared by their mother. They especially liked beef and lamb, and they loved their mother's beef and vegetable soup, green vegetables, and fruit. The mother also made Sudanese flat bread. Unquestionably, lamb meat was their favorite food but it was expensive and not always available in Omaha. Many of our Midwestern foods were strange to them, but they were usually willing to 'try them.' They liked some fast food and especially potato chips. The Sudanese Agency gave them some food coupons, but they did not last long. The grocery store gave them new foods to try, but they always chose their favorite home-cooked foods. They learned a lot about teenage American foods and clothing at the stores, but they had limited funds to buy new foods and clothing. They liked the American jeans and wore them each day and night except for Sunday when they would 'dress up for church.'

Returning to the Sunrise Enabler, one of the first requests by the mother and father was to talk about religion. Religion was most important to them and was the first area they chose with the Sunrise Enabler. They talked about wanting to thank God for everything and especially for their survival from Africa and away from the horrible Sudanese terrorists. Each day they felt great relief from the threat of rape or the possibility of being imprisoned or killed. After six months, the family anxiety decreased, and they became more comfortable with talking to the strangers at church, in stores, and in the community. They were so pleased that the priest welcomed them to the church despite knowing what they had experienced in Southern Sudan. They were introduced to many new people at church and looked forward to Sunday Mass. They were glad to thank the parishioners who had given them food, clothing, money, and used furniture when they had arrived in Omaha. The Sunday socials at church were therapeutic and helped them to ask questions and to observe Americans in different social contexts, and to ask them about their lifeways. Taking time to pray helped them relieve their anger and past fears; they often prayed before, during, and after mass and in family evening prayers. Their Catholic faith gave them a feeling of unity within the family and church—a great comfort and consolation.

Ethnohistory and Ethnodemographics

The Sudanese have had a very long history in Africa (Pritchard, 1936). Sudan is the largest geographic nation on the African continent. It was Pritchard's (1936) anthropological study of the Neur tribe in the 1930s that helped others to learn about the Sudanese people and their complex social and cultural structure. Current books and articles on the African people and Sudanese people can be readily found. Newspaper articles on the "Lost Boys of Sudan" and a few general research African studies are helpful, but there are limited documents on the Sudanese refugees available in the United States (Grace, *World Herald*, 2003). The ethnohistory of the traditional Sudanese was essential holding knowledge for understanding the people, their cultural changes, and other transcultural nursing insights. The Sudanese are some of the oldest people in Africa, with fascinating lifeways, values, and social modes. The following brief history of Sudan is only a glimpse of a much larger history of the people and its complex social structure.

Sudan is the largest country in Africa. It is divided into two distinct regions—the North and the South. Geographically, the North is arid with limited rainfall, whereas the South is a tropical region with grasslands, swamps, and rain forests (Pritchard, 1936). Sudanese marshes and vegetation divide the two regions that are linked by the big, long Nile River. There are many tribal groups that live in the Sudan area, but the largest group is the Dinka, with the Neur next in size, and then the Shillak tribe. The Sudanese Oto family belonged to the Neur tribe; however, the mother belonged to another tribe, but they followed mainly Neur values. They mainly spoke the Neur language and followed many of their values, beliefs, and lifeways.

The Sudanese government seat is located in the northern region (Hall & Ismail, 1981; Holzman, 2000). It dominates the country and has caused many social, political, and religious problems for this family. Northern Sudan is predominantly Islamic and is also part of the Arab world. In contrast, Southern Sudan is located in the sub-Saharan region. There are many Christians in this small region due to missionaries who came into the area during the past 50 years, mainly from England. There are different religious groups but the native or traditional African religion still exists; the Oto family knew both (Holzman, 2000).

The Turkish Ottoman Empire ruled Sudan in the early 19th century. The people experienced harsh slave raids from the North until the Anglicans took over the government. Over the past several decades, the Khartoum military government imposed their Islamic laws and language onto the people. Fighting occurred between the North and South regions, and many Muslims of Southern Sudan were killed or displaced by the early 1900s. The terrible killings during the recent war, the rape of women and children, and other atrocities were frightening events that the Oto family knew and talked about (Grace, 2003). There was also severe famine in Sudan which led to the migration of Sudanese into Kenya. Some Sudanese stayed in camps there until they were refugeed to new countries before their final emigration to Canada, the United States, and Australia (Holzman, 2000).

Many refugee Neurs settled in the United States in urban and farmland communities such as Des Moines, Iowa; Omaha, Nebraska; Nashville, Tennessee; and the Twin Cities of Minnesota. To date, there are approximately 6000 Sudanese refugees in Omaha (personal communication, Sudanese Office, 2002).

The Omahan people were not knowledgeable about the Sudanese prior to their arrival. Thus, many were very frightened of them and could not understand why they came to the city. Some Omahans were afraid of these people because of their very dark skin, large body stature, language difference, and other concerns. Interestingly, the Neur have been used to migrating for years as they moved to different places in Africa to feed and water their cattle, and therefore viewed this move as one more in their cultural history. Foraging for human and animal food was a continuous activity for the Neur tribe. The Neur have been known for their strong survival and athletic abilities, as well as withstanding military regimes for many years. They have also been known as excellent hunters and runners.

In looking at other aspects of the Sunrise Enabler to get a holistic picture of the people, one finds the Southern Sudanese had very strong kinship ties with their extended and tribal families. Kinship ties had always been important for survival and to maintain their migrations and foraging activities. Such kinship ties were very strong features of the Oto family. They valued their nuclear, patriarchal, extended, and clan families. They told about maintaining strong kinship ties for protection, mutual help, and social activities while living in Sudan. Since coming to Omaha, these traditional kinship ties have been reinforced. Filial love as care among the family was readily identified among all family members, but somewhat restrained with distant clan groups. The mother and father loved their children and were very eager to care for them, and to see that they received good educational opportunities in Omaha. The mother talked about the traditional belief that wives should always obey husbands. If the wife did not obey, the husband could mildly beat her, which was an acceptable Sudanese practice. However, the Omaha people heard about Sudanese men beating their wives and had great concern about such practices. This negative information about the Sudanese was reported to the police. Mrs. Oto discussed this matter with concerned women, and the subject was dropped by the women in the community. In some U.S. cities, however, Sudanese men were arrested for beating their wives, and were charged with domestic violence.

The Neur kinship ties were linked to their clans, and to economic, political, and religious priorities, to help them survive the traditional and current lifeways (Pritchard, 1936). The Omaha people gradually saw and learned about the Sudanese kinship lifeways, and liked them. In contrast, the Neur people had many questions about American men having several wives [marriages], sexual trysts, and other overt sexual lifeways that were not acceptable to Southern Sudanese and the Oto family.

The traditional economic activity for the Neur was raising cattle. For many centuries the tribe, clans, and family identified their wealth and social status with the number of cattle they had (Holzman, 2000; Pritchard, 1936). Adolescent and adult males were kept busy tending cattle. The Sudanese lived for and strongly valued their cattle. The Neur used cattle to regulate their daily lives in accordance with their needs and relationships with others. Sudan had a cattle-based economy whose livelihoods came from milk, meat, and hides. Cattle were also used for bridewealth, in that the young woman's family received cattle from the groom's family with the marriage. Divorce rarely occurred nor was it sanctioned. If divorce did occur, the wife's family was required to return the cows or bridewealth. The Oto family was pleased to see many cattle in Nebraska even though they did not own any. It made them feel 'at home.' The Oto family recognized their kinship ties, their limited wealth, and that property (if they had any) was handled by males, especially the husband's family. Thus, the patriarchal kinship ties prevailed with the Neur and were evident within this family in Omaha.

Children are taught at an early age to value and care for land and cattle, and to respect their parents and elders. Men and women have separate labor activities and role responsibilities. Young girls learn how to cook and guide their daily lives around the cattle activities. In the traditional Sudanese culture, men spend a limited time with their wives and spend more time with other men, clans, and with their cattle. This was a sharp difference with the Omaha men and women whom they came to know. They talked a great deal about such differences. Traditionally, Sudanese men are separated from their wives during childbirth and for a period of time after the birth. Women are held responsible for children and domestic home activities. They are expected to obey their husbands and to care for their children even when the men are on cattle migrations. The parents spend time with their children whom they love and give special caring, with nurturing as a caring action.

As the Oto family became more involved in the Anglo American lifeways, they talked about the many contrasts with their traditional culture and what was questionable or missing in American lifeways. They were astute analyzers and thinkers about the differences and could find only a few similarities with American ways. Often they talked about how much freedom Americans had, especially young children, but also adults. They talked about how they believed such freedom led to difficult social and moral problems with teenagers, such as drug use and sexual problems. Such wide freedoms of choice were quite frightening to the parents. Moreover, they wanted their children to have fewer choices and to rely more on their traditional Sudanese and Christian values for good moral and ethical lifeways. The use of many technologies in health care was also frightening to them when they went to the hospital. While they were seen as 'powerful tools,' the Sudanese were afraid of them. The concept of being on time for appointments or to meet someone 'on time' was always baffling to them. They constantly asked, ". . . Why so much emphasis on 'precise time' in America?" They were also concerned about the focus and talk about sex in television programs and explicitly sexual material in newspapers and magazines. They felt sexual freedoms were far too dominant and should be curtailed and guided by moral religious values and parental input.

As a sponsor, I helped the husband and wife obtain employment in order to meet their very heavy rent and monthly food costs. Initially, the idea of the wife working outside the home was questioned by the husband, family, and clan members. However, the mother's income became essential to meet the monthly costs of rent, food, and utilities for this large family, averaging approximately $1400 per month. The husband accepted that his wife had to work, but also wanted her actively focused on home and children. Mr. Oto was never too pleased with the idea of his wife working, especially as he saw American wives working and believed this negatively influenced American social problems. Mrs. Oto finally found employment, which helped the family meet monthly bills.

Education has traditionally been highly valued by the Sudanese. The parents wanted their children to be enrolled in a Catholic parochial school, but the Omaha school system insisted they attend public schools, believing they could not speak 'good English.' The Oto children have done exceptionally well at school, receiving high marks and positive reports for two years. The children are very bright, eager to learn, and quite self-directed, as well as caring toward family, siblings, and others.

Culturally Congruent Family Care and the Meaning of Care

The phases of the ethnonursing research method were followed as presented in Leininger's work (1991, p. 105). Throughout the study, the focus was on discovering the meaning of care to the Sudanese family. Initially, the concept of *care* or *caring* was difficult to discuss as it had many meanings, and because of the cultural trauma and pain they experienced under the fundamentalist Muslim regime. Nonetheless, care was valued in their family and in the broadest sense; essentially, care meant helping or 'caring' for others who needed assistance, especially family and clan members. Caring for family members was the highest priority.

Care was closely linked to their Christian religious beliefs of helping one another. They said, ". . . Just as Christ cared for his people, so we care for ours." This statement was often given as the action meaning of *care* or *caring*. Care was best explained as ways to help one's family first as an <u>obligation</u> and <u>responsibility</u>. They said that if they had not cared for one another in Southern Sudan, they would have never been alive today. <u>Caring</u> meant <u>sharing</u> and <u>protecting one another</u>. Anything they had in the family, they shared with clan members or friends. Key and general informants demonstrated care as <u>filial love for one another and helping others in need</u>. In Omaha, they shared any extra clothing, food, and money given to them. Being kind and considerate to one another was also caring both in their traditional and present day life. They talked about care as being almost impossible to express and maintain when under the oppressive Islamic regime in Southern Sudan. However, "they still cared in order to survive." In Omaha, they talked about the church members caring for them by being generous in giving to them. They saw caring acts at school, church, and in the community, and were pleased to see this kind of care in America. They felt that maybe Americans were too generous and did not understand why they were giving so much to others. They noted that material items were readily offered to strangers such as the Oto family, but overtly loving expressions or actions seemed <u>less evident</u> within American families. Having many cars, homes, and lots of money could "ruin caring," Mrs. Oto stated. They saw donations of food, clothing, and household furnishings as a form of caring, but constantly asked, ". . . Why do they give so much away that is new and then buy similar newer items?" This practice was very hard to understand. They kept asking, ". . . Where do they get the money to buy so much?" The mode of using *culture care accommodation* in decisions and actions to their extended family members and clansmen was evident. The Oto family at times found it hard to accept so much from the church people. Occasionally they said, ". . . No, they must stop and care for their families rather than us." The many possessions of Omaha families in their homes were difficult to understand and accept when they had lived with so little in Africa. Key and general informants identified Omahans as generous and caring by their giving items or material things to their family who were true cultural strangers. They saw less caring in family and work situations and wondered about its effects.

<u>Culture Care Preservation and-or Maintenance</u> was the second major mode of caring as recognized by informants and the researcher. The Oto family members were keenly aware of how they wanted their <u>lives preserved today and in the future</u>. They knew what they valued and wanted to maintain their desired values, such as keeping the children healthy and together. That they wanted to preserve their Sudanese lifeways through caring for each other, watching, and offering <u>protective care</u> to each other whether living in Sudan or in Omaha was evident in

their daily relationships. They discussed these ideas often. The anticipation of real dangers such as war, rape, threats, dealing with a meager
food supply and maintaining their possessions were identified as preservation actions and decisions for survival. This pattern of caring by preserving and protecting what they had was crucial for the family's beliefs
and mode of survival and to maintain family closeness and love. They
spoke often about this kind of protective faith caring and that the family
was fully committed to it. They believed that practicing culture care
preservation and maintenance were essential to daily Sudanese living.
Several traditional values learned over generations became more and
more essential for their health and wellbeing. In Omaha when their food
supply ran low and there was insufficient money for monthly rent, food,
and other expenses, they were encouraged to practice care preservation
through clan sharing, and to make sacrifices each month. They knew
how to share and keep the family together in difficult, threatening, or
conflict situations in Sudan and now in Omaha. Thus, care preservation
and accommodation were dominant and prevailing care value findings
in this study.

Criteria for Evaluation and Data Analysis Mode

With the wealth of qualitative data obtained over several months,
Leininger's phases of data analysis were used as discussed in Leininger
(1991, p. 95) and in earlier parts of this book. The criteria to evaluate
this qualitative ethnonursing study were essential to confirm or refute
the theory (Leininger & McFarland, 2002, p. 95).

For the qualitative data analysis Leininger's five criteria were used:
(1) Credibility, (2) Confirmability, (3) Meaning-in-Context, (4)
Saturation, and (5) Transferability (Leininger, 1991, 1997, 2002). The
Leininger four phases of data analysis provided a systematic and rigorous
mode of data analysis using these criteria. These phases are fully
described in the above cited works.

The mode of Culture Care Repatterning and-or Restructuring was
identified as the Oto family regained their trust in a new world of people
different from the village they left in Southern Sudan. They learned to
repattern their life so as to trust new or different people who cared
about them and who would not cause them harm. This was a major and
most difficult experience due to the cultural pain and trauma they had
experienced from the Muslim government officials. They had to regain
and restructure filial ties with their extended family and clan members
as mistrust had prevailed for several months. The repatterning of these

caring relationships occurred gradually and was rewarding to witness. The family also had to repattern their concept of <u>time</u>. For example, when they went to the hospital, the staff noted that Sudanese time was not our exact American or Western time. The family was often late for appointments, which was very annoying to the staff. The Oto family's concept of time had to be repatterned to 'Omaha time' in order to receive health services and be accepted. As the Oto family <u>repatterned</u> their lifeways, they noticed that care from the hospital staff was friendly and they received less criticism. The nursing staff was grateful as the family learned hospital values and rules in receiving care, thus preventing or reducing conflicts with caregiving services. Similarly, the hospital staff had to repattern their expectations and focus on the needs of the Sudanese family and their cultural lifeways. Respecting strong kinship and clan groups was important for staff to learn as they interacted closely with the Oto family. Hence, culture care repatterning was essential and became evident over time as staff learned to repattern their approach by focusing on the <u>family</u> needs rather than placing a high emphasis on <u>individualism</u>.

The Sudanese Oto family members were eager and apt learners. They quickly adapted to Omaha practices and adjusted to accept several American norms as well as hospital norms in order to receive help from others. Amid these changes, the Oto family retained many Southern Sudanese beliefs, values, and practices recognized as different from the American cultural values in Omaha. The Oto family was willing to relearn and repattern their life to the Omaha lifeways to receive services, develop friendships, and be accepted in a new culture.

As a sponsor of the Oto family, I assisted the father and mother in their search for work to survive in a costly living environment with high rent and food costs. The Sudanese Agency and Immigration funds were very limited for feeding a large family of nine and in meeting the high cost of living in Omaha. I clarified with employers that the Sudanese were good people and able to do good work whenever potential employers were skeptical about hiring them. I gave employers examples of the Oto family strengths as hard workers who could be helpful to them. Most employers initially were reluctant to hire them as they were 'different' and sometimes feared. I also demonstrated to the parents how to negotiate when buying and selling in other crucial areas such as with the used car. As a consequence the parents learned to negotiate product sale prices and for their salaries. Initially, they did not get the highest salary on the pay scale, but as employers trusted them and saw their assets and employment reliability, they gradually paid them more over time. The parents said that <u>negotiation as caring</u> was difficult to learn as this was limitedly practiced in traditional Sudanese culture. They often talked that they were socialized to be deferent, obedient, polite, and acquiescent to others in order 'to get along' with strangers. The Oto family tried to negotiate with the landlord about their high rent for their old home. However, the American landlord would not negotiate and the family had to pay the high rent, which left them limited money for food and monthly utility bills, making it difficult for them to survive. This landlord had many cultural biases about dark-skinned people and families with many children. As a consequence, I recommended that they rent a large old home costing them less money to help them better meet their monthly expenses. They are attempting this approach but dislike leaving their home and the expenses of moving. They hope, however, to move into a Habitat for Humanity home but it will not be available for several months. They have worked hard to become eligible for this home, which they had hoped to be living in much sooner. They have been quite disappointed with the long wait given the American value for 'time' and associated expectations of promptness.

Probably the best example of negotiation for the Oto family was my ability to to negotiate for a good, used, large sized family car. The family needed a car to get to work, store, and church. However, owning a car was against immigration rules, as it was considered a luxury. In this city and in America, a car is essential for work and everyday life. I approached a Christian car dealer who saw that the Sudanese family was poor and needed a car. He negotiated with the sponsor and a used car was obtained. The Oto family saw how I negotiated with the dealer using available monies for the purchase. The direct person-to-person American style firm negotiation strategy was learned with an expression of sincere gratitude for the price reduction given in light of pressing need. After passing driving tests and getting car insurance, they found the car to be a joy as well as a necessity. The Oto family was most grateful.

In summary, the three care modes of the theory were essential and demonstrated ways to arrive at desired goals that were beneficial caring modes for this refugee family. The dominant caring modes were: <u>caring as sharing</u>, <u>care as protection</u>, and <u>care as filial kinship love</u>. These <u>dominant care modes</u> as <u>care constructs</u> for living in a new city were essential for the wellbeing of this immigrant refugee family, and would prove essential for nursing and other health care personnel to know and use in their care.

Status of the Family After Three Years

In this last section, an overview of the Oto family after three years will be shared. Undoubtedly, the reader is wondering about the current status of this immigrant refugee family. Initially, it was a very difficult struggle for the Oto family to adjust as they had many deep cultural hurts from their experiences at the hands of Sudanese government officials. They had many needs to be fulfilled as they came with nothing in the way of clothes, money, or other basic necessities. However, this immigrant family has been doing well and experiencing good health. They seem relieved of their cultural pain and the terrible emotional trauma from their experiences in Southern Sudan with the government military officers. The Oto family remains tightly united and happy to be in Omaha. They have adjusted quite well to the American urban culture. Both spouses continue to be employed, and their seven children are doing extremely well in school with top performance in their classes. In discussing the progress of the Oto family with the Sudanese Agency, they state they ". . . have been amazed that this family has done so well" and in a relatively short span of time.

In reflecting on <u>why</u> this family did well, I discussed and confirmed with the family that the following factors were important for their successful immigration and acculturation process. First, it was important to have a sponsor who was knowledgeable about traditional Sudanese (Neur) and African culture. Second, it took time and patience to gain their trust and for them to feel comfortable with an American cultural stranger as their sponsor. It was also essential to show genuine caring for the family with regard for all they had been through prior to coming to America. Recognition of their cultural pain and extended trauma was critical to their recovery from past terrible and frightening experiences while living in Southern Sudan. This transcultural and anthropological holding knowledge helped me to be alert to potential conflict areas between Sudanese values and lifeways and culture of Omaha. It was also helpful that I had studied and worked with other African people, both in Africa and in several nonWestern countries, enabling me to understand some common experiences related to poverty, famine, cultural oppression, ethnocentric or racial biases, and caring values.

Third, I worked directly with the family for nearly three years starting at the beginning of their relocation to Omaha. Being willing to enter into the Oto family's world and learn from them about their terrible past experiences in Southern Sudan was essential for understanding and helping them. My active caring manner, relying on <u>caring as listening</u>, and focusing on the family trust were essential to lessen their cultural trauma. Listening to all the traumatic experiences they wanted to share about their life in Africa seemed to be beneficial and therapeutic, as affirmed by the family. Maintaining a compassionate, caring, friendly, and authentic way of relating to and working with the family was essential for helping them to find their way and to understand and make new choices in a new land. In a way, I served as a transcultural nurse therapist in helping to ease their trauma by understanding their interests, caring values, and many concerns as they repatterned their life.

Fourth, the family was ready to share their traumatic experiences and to find someone who understood the Sudanese culture. I always called ahead for my visits to respect their wishes and available time. Focusing on all family members was also critical as the family wanted to be tightly united in the new land in whatever they did or experienced. Family unity as caring was essential for healing.

Fifth, this refugee family made favorable progress because of other factors. They had experienced very frightening and traumatic experiences in Southern Sudan for nearly five years prior to coming to America; they knew about hardships, being oppressed, discriminated against, and living with very little food and material goods for short and long periods of time. These experiences were viewed as helpful for them to adjust to and survive a new culture. The family was also eager to come to the United States to experience freedom away from political oppression, wars, and threats to their family and their children. They talked of their desire to learn American democracy but questioned many of our values that did not seem helpful to them, such as drugs, alcohol, suicide, and other problems they read or heard about from the media. They felt they would retain most of their traditional 'good' Southern Sudanese values and would not adopt several American values that appeared destructive to them or noncongruent to their traditional values and lifeways. Another factor was that the family could speak fairly good English; this facilitated their communication with strangers, enabled them in developing trust relationships, aided them in learning about new [American] ideas, and facilitated them in functioning well in their employment settings. They felt Omaha was a friendly, Christian city, but they also felt they needed to reexamine American values and to reevaluate some negative factors about raising children, especially teenagers. The Omaha culture was conservative with a 'common sense' ethos and practical 'doing' lifeway, which they liked.

Sixth, the family's caring values of being Christian and sharing filial love as caring was most valuable and congruent for immigration recovery. Maintaining their religion and praying together as a family was a vital and therapeutic care mode. Unquestionably, their religion was crucial to their survival in Sudan and for adjusting to the culture of Omaha.

They often said, their ". . . religion gave them hope and a way of coping with their past and current conflict experiences." Family love for each other was clearly observed and provided support during their adjustment to a new and different world, and to ease past traumas. In addition, the family's caring values of being kind and patient toward each other was most helpful in their interactions with strangers. These caring modes and the genuine interest of the church community in helping the family contributed to their improved health and positive immigration experience. They were grateful for what they received and waited patiently for anything they needed. This was another positive way to receive culturally congruent care from others.

In general, as their sponsor I found them to be a warm and friendly family to work with. I looked forward to visiting them. The new Sudanese Agency in Omaha was also helpful. It facilitated the family's coming to Nebraska and offered some initial financial support. The Oto family is pleased they came to America. They are hoping to move into a larger home with five bedrooms, a basement, and lower rent. They have worked to fulfill the qualifying requirements for a Habitat home. Getting a home in America is viewed as a great thrill. I believe their Catholic faith and generic Sudanese values will continue to sustain them in difficult times or should they encounter negative experiences in Sudan. They lived their faith and were united by their faith. Their religion was also helpful as a means for the family to interact with other Sudanese clan families, tribal groups, and blood relatives who had come to Omaha prior to the Oto family's arrival. They always looked forward to the visits with clan members and the opportunity to talk about their "old Sudanese friends and relatives" whom they hoped were still alive in Sudan. Lastly, the Omaha culture was friendly to them and generous in sharing their food and household items. The priest and the Catholic parishioners were deeply appreciated and valued.

As sponsor and a transcultural nurse, I found it a rewarding experience to see how this family remained open to learn and adjust to a new community after such traumatic and terrible prior experiences in Southern rural Sudan. The *resilience* of the family to *survive* was a major cultural asset. They seldom complained about difficulties except for the high rent and the landlord's cultural biases and his lack of compassion for refugees. The family's caring ways were encouraging to identify and document. Most importantly, as a transcultural nurse, I learned about a great family and how caring ways lead to survival for immigrants. Caring is a powerful healing way for oppression and traumatized immigrants. Unquestionably, my holding knowledge of the traditional Sudanese culture was essential. My theory of Culture Care was an excellent means to gain indepth knowledge and analyze data as I worked with the Sudanese family. This study reassured me that nurses and others working with immigrants and refugees need to be open to learning from immigrants and to using basic transcultural nursing principles and strategies along with a theory to guide their work. It was a good experience and I enjoyed the warm and growing friendship with the Oto family. Most assuredly, the theory of Culture Care was most valuable for discovering and organizing knowledge from the immigrant family. I believe it is mutually beneficial for immigrant families to share and use their generic caring values and beliefs in therapeutic ways in new cultural settings.

Summary

This chapter reflects a positive and successful refugee experience for a Sudanese family. I used transcultural principles and the Theory of Culture Care to discover the many hidden cultural needs of this family and to work with them to provide and maintain culturally congruent care. The fit of the theory with the ethnonursing method was valued and facilitated meaningful relationships. The Sunrise Enabler and the other enablers were all essential for this discovery and for helping the process. This chapter should be helpful as a guide to newcomers using the theory and method, and for nurses working with immigrants and refugees and other peoples of diverse cultural orientations or lifeways who need hope, understanding, and culture specific care for their health, survival, and wellbeing.

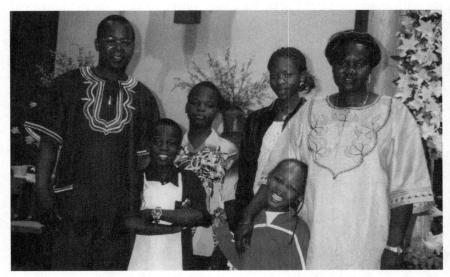

Figure 9-1   Sudanese refugee family that Dr. Leininger worked with and studied for three years in Omaha, Nebraska, USA.

References

Andrews, M. M., & Boyle, J. S. (Eds.). (2003). *Transcultural concepts in nursing care*. Philadelphia: Lippincott.

Grace, E. (2003, October 29). Bishop urges peace, aid for Sudan in visit. *World Herald*, pp. A1, A2.

Hall, M., & Ismail, B. A. (1981). *Sisters under the sun: The story of Sudanese women*. London: Longman.

Holzman, J. D. (2000). *Neur journeys, Neur lives: Sudanese refugees in Minnesota*. Boston: Allyn and Bacon.

Leininger, M. (1990). The philosophic and epistemic bases to explicate transcultural nursing knowledge. *The Journal of Transcultural Nursing, 1*(2), 40–51.

Leininger, M. (Ed.). (1991). *Culture care diversity and universality: A theory of nursing*. Sudbury, MA: Jones and Bartlett/National League for Nursing.

Leininger, M. (Ed.). (1995). *Transcultural nursing: Concepts, theories, research, and practice*. New York: McGraw-Hill.

Leininger, M. (1997). Overview of the theory of culture care with the ethnonursing research method. *The Journal of Transcultural Nursing, 8*(2), 32–51.

Leininger, M. (2002). Part I: The theory of culture care. In M. Leininger & M. R. McFarland (Eds.), *Transcultural nursing: Concepts, theories, research, and practice*. New York: McGraw-Hill.

Leininger, M., & McFarland, M. R. (2002). *Transcultural nursing: Concepts, theories, research, and practice*. New York: McGraw-Hill.

Misch, P. (2002). The lost boys of Sudan. *Saint Anthony Messenger, 10*(2), 36–42.

Prichard, E. (1936). *The Neur: An African culture*. Press unknown.

CHAPTER TEN

Selected Culture Care Findings of Diverse Cultures Using Culture Care Theory and Ethnomethods

[Revised Reprint]

Madeleine M. Leininger, PhD, LHD, DS, CTN, RN, FAAN, FRCNA

During the past three decades, the author has worked with a number of graduate students and colleagues studying Western and nonWestern cultures using the theory of Culture Care with the ethnonursing and other qualitative research methods. Presented here are sample research findings of different cultures derived from the study of worldview, social structure, environmental context, ethnohistory, and other dimensions of the theory. Unfortunately, space does not permit a full report on all cultures studied. Instead, dominant cultural care values, care meanings, and action modes will be presented to assist nurses, in part, to consider using these findings to guide their nursing practices with clients from 23 different cultures studied. These data are being shared because of frequent requests from many nurses who have heard about or seen several of these research findings and are eager to improve the quality of care to clients from the diverse cultures studied.

To use the findings reported in this chapter, the reader needs to keep in mind several facts and realities that only partial but important findings are reported about the cultures studied. Some of these realities are briefly summarized below. First, the reader needs to realize that full ethnonursing systematic studies were done with each culture often over an extended period of time (usually one to several years) by the author or another transcultural nurse researcher who was knowledgeable about the theory, the ethnonursing method, the enablers, and the data modes of analysis. Second, the primary focus of the research was on the people's *emic* knowledge (the inside culture) views, and not on the nurse's *etic* (or outsider's) views, meanings, and practices related to culture care or caring. Third, the data presented are focused on cultural values and care meanings and actions. Nonetheless, these findings offer important data to understand the culture with its *patterned* care meanings and action modes as an initial basis for nursing care. Fourth, since each culture was

282

CHAPTER TEN   Selected Culture Care Findings of Diverse Cultures
Using Culture Care Theory and Ethnomethods [Revised Reprint]

studied indepth by transcultural nurses who knew the theory of Culture Care, ethnonursing, and related qualitative methods, the findings reflect credible and accurate data for the cultures studied during the past 15 years. As researchers studied these cultures, approximately 13–18 *key* informants and usually twice that number of *general* informants (20–40) were participants in each study. Each researcher of a culture spent about three to five sessions (often 10–20 hours) with each key informant in their natural or familiar living environments (i.e., homes and communities). In keeping with the ethnonursing method, key informants were selected because they were held to be most knowledgeable about the culture and volunteered to share their lived-through insights about cultural care meanings, values, beliefs, and practices (Leininger, 1985a). Through reflection, the *general* informants participate as reflectors of the culture to help confirm some key informants' ideas and to limit highly idiosyncratic or nonrepresentative culture data. In addition, the transcultural nurse made extensive observations, interviews, and direct-participant observations of the culture and of people's lifeways. Some ethnographic data were used with the ethnonursing method. The data were analyzed with Leininger's rigorous *Four Phase Data Analysis of Ethnonursing Data*. Some methodological variability occurred with each researcher's procedure of study as is expected with qualitative investigations.

Fifth, in presenting the data on the 23 cultures, only major, recurrent, and patterned culture values and care meanings and actions are included. Thus, the reader is provided the final analysis of the care *meanings* and *modes of action*. However, there is a wealth of rich, detailed backup data to substantiate each of the care findings. These culture values and care meanings and actions can serve as a beginning guide or approach to the nursing care of clients or groups of these specific cultures to provide culturally congruent care. Users always must realize there were some cultural variations with clients due to acculturation and other factors. The reader also will note that, in keeping with the purposes of a qualitative paradigmatic study, no statistical data are presented. Instead, the goal is to understand the meanings and cultural experiences with culture care. These findings constitute the 'gold nuggets' of nursing about care and caring. They have been largely invisible or embedded in social structure factors, worldview, and other aspects of Culture Care Theory dimensions awaiting ethnonursing discovery. These care values, meanings, and modes of action can be considered the *epistemics* or root sources of people-centered care knowledge, and are essential for use in human caring processes.

Sixth, the reader needs to keep in mind that the findings revealed here were influenced significantly by the informants' ethnohistory, worldview, social structure, and environmental context. Although these dimensions were packed with information about care, they were embedded in areas which took much skill, time, and patience to explicate from informants. It seemed that the richest insights of informants were covert and deeply hidden in their thinking and experiences.

Once trust was established, informants shared their very rich data with researchers. Most importantly, these findings should not be used rigidly or as fixed absolutes to stereotype people. Instead, care themes reflect *patterns of care* that can be considered to promote positive health to individuals or groups of a particular culture. As nurses are taught how to do holistic culturalogical assessments using the Sunrise Enabler to assess an individual, group, or family to identify care variations (Leininger, 1978, 1981). In general, these findings can be used to provide specific care that *fits with* clients' cultural norms and lifeways. Culture-specific care findings can be used as ways to change unfavorable or detrimental culture practices. It is of interest that culture care values and action modes tend to remain with people over a period of time, and so these findings, which other nurses have used, remain extremely useful to understand clients and guide their care. These findings also revealed that culture values added much meaning to the care actions in all 23 cultures studied. In using these findings, however, it is well to consider them as 'holding knowledge' to guide nursing care practices until the nurse has worked with and conducted his or her own assessment of an individual, family, or group. One can *anticipate* some variabilities or diversities among clients, as well as some commonalities. To provide nursing care that is culturally congruent, nurses need 'holding knowledge.' Most encouragingly, these care findings are being used in nursing as the profession shifts from a *medical symptom–disease model* to *people-centered care.*

Finally, findings generated from the Culture Care Theory can be used to help the nurse reflect on his or her own cultural care values and lifeways to consider what is different or similar in values and expectations as the nurse works with the client from a designated culture.

Self-awareness of one's own culture is one of the 'first principles' to master in transcultural nursing. Without self-awareness, the nurse may experience culture shock and be unable to help clients. Nurses may hold very different cultural care values and practices than clients. Recognizing such differences can help the nurse to understand and explain the sources of culturally based conflicts, frustrations, and imposition practices. It also will help the nurse to understand why some nurses avoid clients because they are 'true strangers.' The nurse's professional values and practices often may be incongruent with those of the client, but awareness of care differences is essential in guiding the nurse's behavior. If the culture values of the nurse obstruct or hinder

284

CHAPTER TEN   Selected Culture Care Findings of Diverse Cultures
Using Culture Care Theory and Ethnomethods [Revised Reprint]

the recovery, cooperation, and progress of clients, this needs to be recognized and worked through with mentors in different counseling ways. Some nurses might be threatened with legal suits if they break cultural care taboos and reflect cultural care negligence or offensive behavior to some clients and families. With the rise in multiculturalism worldwide, legal cultural suits will markedly increase in the 21st century and beyond. Knowledge of culture care values and their constructs can help prevent such undesirable legal potentials.

Presentation of Culture Values and Care Meanings with Action Modes of Selected Cultures

As one studies the findings from the 23 cultures, one will note that most cultures are from the United States of America, with some from Europe, Scandinavia, and other nonWestern cultures. Some intergenerational and gender differences in each culture were documented, and remain dominant care findings within cultures. Only the *dominant emic* culture values, care meanings, and action modes are presented which were ranked by key informants of the culture. Thus, the first care construct listed was held most important by the informants and from the researcher's observations over a period of time. The informants translated the terms into English. In some cultures, *care* as a native term did not translate readily into English, and so these linguistic phrases are the closest to the meanings and action modes of care. It is extremely important to keep in mind that the linguistic terms or phrases are from the culture. They may constitute stems of a sentence or a partial sentence. Nonetheless, they are the care or essence of the value or action mode. It also is important to keep in mind that manifested care is evident repeated verbal comments and routine care actions.

Finally, the orientational definition of *culture values* and *culture care* can help the reader as stated below:

> *Culture Values* refer to the powerful, persistent, and directive forces that give meaning, order, and direction to the individual or group's thinking, actions, decisions, and lifeways, and usually over a span of time (Leininger, 1978).

> *Culture Care* refers to those assistive, supportive, facilitative, and enabling acts for or toward another individual or group to ease or ameliorate a human condition, or lifeway in order to promote or maintain wellbeing (or health), or to help clients face disabilities or death in given cultures or subcultures (Leininger, 1981, 1984).

Reflections on Research: Culture Care Research Findings

The findings from the 23 Western and nonWestern cultures represent approximately one-half of the cultures studied with the theory of Culture Care. In reflecting on the findings, the reader begins to recognize the diversities as well as similarities in culture values and care meanings among cultures. These epistemic *emic* findings from culture informants are the 'gold nuggets' and the 'holding knowledge' about care. These findings are guides to assess the clients, families, and-or specific cultures wherever the nurse functions. The nurse reflects further on these findings with other professional nurses who may have had no preparation in transcultural nursing and yet are expected to give quality care to diverse cultures.

Most importantly, these culture care findings become a *guide* to help make decisions and actions with the three theoretical modes of decision making as previously discussed in Chapter 1: culture care preservation and-or maintenance, culture care accommodation and-or negotiation, and culture care repatterning and-or restructuring. These three modes become important to consider in providing culturally congruent care to clients of the different cultures. The nurse may creatively use the culture values and care meanings and action patterns to design nursing care for the client or family of a particular culture. For example, the Greek client will value daily exercise as a care preservation mode to promote health. At the same time, the Greek client expects the nurse to provide culture care accommodation and-or negotiation to let his or her Greek kin family be with him or her for satisfying and congruent care while in the hospital and during recovery.

The challenge for the nurse is to provide care based on the client's values and care meanings, using what may be relevant or helpful from professional knowledge together with the client's generic care perspectives in order to design and arrive at congruent care practices. The nurse would study the effects of such care from both client and nurse viewpoints. In using these culture care research findings, the nurse is keenly aware not to treat everyone exactly alike, but to use *culture-specific* care values and practices as a powerful directive for nursing practices. Such an approach differs from current emphasis on using NANDA nursing diagnosis—NANDA reflecting the use of another analogous linguistic label for nursing from the medical disease model. Focusing on 'alterations,' 'deficits,' and other diagnostic terms may seriously fail to provide for the cultural care needs of clients from a specific culture. Moreover, many of the NANDA labels are culture-bound and reflect dominant Anglo-American culture and professional nursing values (Leininger, 1990). Thus, using Culture Care Theory findings provides for an entirely new and different way to serve people.

286

CHAPTER TEN   Selected Culture Care Findings of Diverse Cultures Using Culture Care Theory and Ethnomethods [Revised Reprint]

Specific culture care values, meanings, and actions of clients and nurses would remain unknown were it not for the transcultural nurse research program launched in the 1960s. Clients want their care to be culturally congruent, whether they retain more traditional values or choose to adopt new cultural values; therefore transcultural research is important. Although some clients *do* adopt a new set of permanent values, this is an infrequent practice because humans generally retain their traditional values. Nonetheless, it is encouraging to see clients respond so favorably to culture-specific care designed for them in contrast to having to accommodate to largely imposed and unknown professional practices. It is virtually impossible for a nurse to care for people effectively and successfully without the use of transcultural care values and specific care knowledge of the cultures involved.

As the nurse becomes skilled in using culture care knowledge, he or she will discover that professional skills take on new meanings; the nurse's worldview greatly expands to a deepened appreciation for human diversities and similarities. The nurse becomes aware of the subtleties that make a difference in culturally based quality care practices, and especially that clients like cultural amenities, symbols, and actions to fit their cultural ways. As the nurse's creative and professional skills grow, culture care similar to giving a 'perfect injection' may occur with the use of culture care practices. Such exquisite, assured, confident care practices will occur as the nurse knows and understands the client of a particular culture. As the nurse uses specific care values and meanings, he or she does so with open communication with the client and often with the client's family. Sometimes remaining with the client and family can be a powerful caring mode to accommodate the client's needs. *Care as presence* is often deeply valued and promotes therapeutic outcomes. As the nurse uses culture-specific care knowledge, he or she assesses client feedback and may alter care due to slight or major culture variations. The care constructs from the 23 cultures presented are being used in some clinical nurse settings, but will be used more as nurses learn about and try them. The specific care constructs need to be taught and studied further in nursing as the main knowledge base for the discipline of the future.

In general, the research findings discovered with the ethnonursing method from the 23 cultures reflect a lifelong research program of culture care studies by the author, care scholars, students, clinicians, and faculty. The findings from key and general informants are extremely valuable. It is fortunate that the theorist has focused primarily on people centered or *emic* ethnonursing findings as these provide major breakthroughs in knowledge that must continue to be discovered and updated as times and cultures change. In the meantime, transcultural nurses need to use existing knowledge with diverse cultures. The study of culture care is a tedious process and requires attention to a people's world. However, it is a most rewarding experience as one discovers some of the most meaningful ways to know, help, and understand people and their care needs.

List of Transcultural Care Constructs

During the many decades of discovering human care values, beliefs, meanings, and expressions, the author found that gently and sensitively probing informants, they were able to identify, give meaning to, and prioritize the care values and meanings held by their culture. The first care constructs discovered were with the two Gadsup village peoples of New Guinea (see Chapter 4). This experience gave the author courage to pursue study in other cultures. Graduate students and others under her mentorship helped to keep this discovery process alive for over five decades. Accordingly, there are now 175 care constructs from 58 cultures, plus additional ethnonursing care data to support the findings. In the beginning (the 1960s), the author had discovered 10 care constructs; in 1980, almost 37; in 1988, almost 100; in 1990, 173 constructs. These care constructs were largely invisible until nurse researchers probed, reflected on, and studied them indepth in their embedded 'homes' with attention to social structure factors, worldview, and culture values and opened a wealth of culture care knowledge.

The findings presented in Figure 10-24 were obtained using the ethnonursing method with primary focus on discovering the care values and meanings from adult informants aged 20 to 85 years. There were some slight intergenerational differences but the dominant care constructs prevailed. It was of interest that most informants were able to identify from four to eight care constructs dominant or central to them but no culture readily revealed all their care beliefs or values. Most informants talked about care; they wanted nurses to know about key cultural generic care meanings and viewpoints held by the people. The criteria used to select key and general informants were:

1. The informant(s) spoke English or a translator was available to help with the meanings in own native language.
2. The informant(s) identified themselves as belonging to and practicing the culture being studied about care and caring.
3. The informant(s) had been born and lived in the United States at least 15 years (the average had lived in the United States 35 years) or in their native country most of their lives (over 15 years).

288

CHAPTER TEN   Selected Culture Care Findings of Diverse Cultures Using Culture Care Theory and Ethnomethods [Revised Reprint]

4. The informant(s) volunteered and were usually interviewed in their homes or in a natural context so the researcher could also observe care practices in the natural home or work environment.

5. Culture care expressions, meanings, and patterns were studied by researchers using the Culture Care Theory with the Sunrise Model over a considerable time span (often one year).

The purpose of sharing this list of constructs is mainly to alert the reader to be aware of the great diversity of constructs used and known by the people about human care and caring. Providing this list should help the nurse realize that care has different expressions, meanings, and referents. All of these care constructs can be found in the 23 cultures presented earlier in this chapter and 35 additional cultures. The constructs also are offered to encourage nurses to do further work with these constructs with the cultures as we continue to discover the epistemic roots of care and health phenomena in many subcultures and cultures yet to be studied for care meanings and patterns within a nursing perspective.

My original question in the mid-1950s—*What is universal and diverse about human care/caring?*—has been only partially answered with the care constructs listed in Figure 10-24. These care constructs and concomitant ethnonursing research data over three decades reflects the first systematization of the epistemic and ontologic transcultural care knowledge for the discipline of nursing. It reflects the ongoing work yet to be done to discover fully the meanings, functions, and structure of transcultural care knowledge.

The author is doing a comparative synthesis of the care knowledge drawing on data from the care constructs of different cultures in light of the tenets of my theory. Hopefully, this synthesis will lead to the identification of universal and diverse care meanings, practices, and structure of care so that this knowledge can ultimately be used both for clinical practices and for curricular and teaching purposes. In time, this care knowledge will be the substantive base of nursing knowledge in schools of nursing as well as in clinical settings in the 21st century. When this occurs, it will provide a very rich and sound knowledge base for the discipline and profession of nursing.

Finally, in presenting these culture care values, linguistic meanings, and action modes, keep in mind that there was no ethical or moral judgment made of what was 'good,' 'bad,' or 'unethical.' The findings are shared to reveal the human care expressions and patterns of cultures without moral judgments, and should be understood and used with this purpose and goal in mind.

Dominant Culture Values are:	Culture Care Meanings and Action Modes are:
1. Individualism—focus on a self-reliant person	1. Stress alleviation by: • physical means • emotional means
2. Independence and freedom	
3. Competition and achievement	2. Personalized acts • Doing special things • Giving individual attention
4. Materialism (things and money)	
5. Technology dependent	
6. Instant time and actions	3. Self-reliance (individualism) by: • Reliance on self • Reliance on self (self-care) • Becoming as independent as • Reliance on technology
7. Youth and beauty	
8. Equal sex rights	
9. Leisure time highly valued possible	
10. Reliance on scientific facts and numbers	4. Health instruction • Teach us how 'to do' this care for self • Give us the 'medical' facts
11. Less respect for authority and the elderly	
12. Generosity in time of crisis	

Figure 10-1   Anglo-American Culture (Mainly U.S. Middle and Upper Class)

Dominant Culture Values are:	Culture Care Meanings and Action Modes are:
1. Extended family valued	1. Succorance (direct family aid)
2. Interdependence with kin and social activities	2. Involvement with extended family 'other care')
3. Patriarchal (machismo)	3. Filial love/loving
4. Exact time less valued	4. Respect for authority
5. High respect for authority and the elderly	5. Mother as care decision maker
6. Religion valued (many Roman Catholics)	6. Protective (external) male care
	7. Acceptance of God's will
7. Native foods for wellbeing	8. Use of folk-care practices
8. Traditional folk-care healers for folk illnesses	9. Healing with foods
9. Belief in hot-cold theory	10. Touching

Figure 10-2   Mexican-American Culture*

*These findings were from the author's transcultural nurse studies (1970, 1984) and other transcultural nurse studies in the United States during the past two decades.

290

CHAPTER TEN   Selected Culture Care Findings of Diverse Cultures
Using Culture Care Theory and Ethnomethods [Revised Reprint]

Dominant Culture Values are:	Culture Care Meanings and Action Modes are:
1. Extended family as support system	1. Involve family for support (other care)
2. Religion—God's will must prevail	2. Respect (*respecto*)
3. Reliance on folk foods and treatments	3. Trust
4. Belief in hot-cold theory	4. Succorance
5. Male decision maker and direct caregivers	5. Touching (body closeness)
6. Reliance on native language	6. Reassurance
	7. Spiritual healing
	8. Use of folk food, care rituals
	9. Avoid evil eye (*mal de ojo*) and witches (*bruja(o)*)
	10. Speak the language

Figure 10-3   Haitian-American Culture*

*These data were from Haitians living in the United States during the past decade (1981–1991).

Dominant Culture Values are:	Culture Care Meanings and Action Modes are:
1. Extended family networks	1. Concern for my "brothers and sisters"
2. Religion valued (many are Baptists)	2. Being involved with
3. Interdependence with "Blacks"	3. Giving presence (physical)
4. Daily survival	4. Family support and "get togethers"
5. Technology valued, e.g., radio, car, etc.	5. Touching appropriately
6. Folk (soul) foods	6. Reliance on folk home remedies
7. Folk healing modes	7. Rely on "Jesus to save us" with prayers and songs
8. Music and physical activities	

Figure 10-4   African-American Culture*

*These findings were from the author's study of two southern USA villages (1980–1981) and from a study of one large northern urban city (1982–1991) along with other studies by transcultural nurses.

Dominant Culture Values are:	Culture Care Meanings and Action Modes are:
1. Harmony between land, people, and environment	1. Establishing harmony between people and environment with reciprocity
2. Reciprocity with 'Mother Earth'	2. Actively listening
3. Spiritual inspiration (spirit guidance)	3. Using periods of silence ('Great Spirit' guidance)
4. Folk healers (Shamans) (The Circle & Four Directions)	4. Rhythmic timing (nature, land, and people) in harmony
5. Practice culture rituals and taboos	5. Respect for native folk healers, careers, and curers (Use of Circle)
6. Rhythmicity of life with nature	6. Maintaining reciprocity (replenish what is taken from Mother Earth)
7. Authority of tribal elders	
8. Pride in cultural heritage and 'Nations'	7. Preserving cultural rituals and taboos
9. Respect and value for children	8. Respect for elders and children

Figure 10-5 North-American Indian Culture (U.S. and Canada)*

*These findings were collected by the author and other contributors in the United States and Canada during the past three decades. Cultural variations among all nations exist, and so these data are some general commonalities about values, care meanings, and actions.

292

**CHAPTER TEN   Selected Culture Care Findings of Diverse Cultures
Using Culture Care Theory and Ethnomethods [Revised Reprint]**

Dominant Culture Values are:	Culture Care Meanings and Action Modes are:
1. Egalitarianism	1. Surveillance (to prevent sorcery)
2. Marked sex role differences	• nearby surveillance
3. Patriarchal descent recognized	• at a distance
4. Communal unity ('one vine'/'line')	2. Protection (protective male caring)
5. Prevent social accusations (sorcery)	• of Gadsups through lifecycle
6. Maintain ancestor "life-essence" and obligations	• obeying cultural taboos and rules
7. Have "good women, children, pigs, and gardens"	3. Nurturance
	• ways to help people grow and survive
	• know what they need (anticipate needs) through lifecycle
	• eat safe foods
	4. Prevention (avoid breaking cultural taboos) to:
	• prevent illness and death
	• prevent intervillage fights and conflicts
	5. Touching

Figure 10-6   Gadsup Akuna of the Eastern Highlands of New Guinea*

*This was the first transcultural care study done by the author in two villages in the early 1960s, with subsequent visits made in later years. (See Chapter 4 for a full account of these people.)

Dominant Culture Values are:	Culture Care Meanings and Action Modes are:
1. Family unity and closeness	1. Maintain smooth relationships (*Pakikisama*)
2. Respect for elder/authority	2. Save face and self-esteem (*Amor propio*); (*Hiya*—avoid shame)
3. 'Leave one-self to God' (*Bahala na*)	3. Respect for and deference to authority
4. Obligations to sociocultural ties	4. Being quiet; privacy
5. Hot-cold beliefs	5. Mutual reciprocity (*Utang Na Loob*) "the give and take" in relationships
6. Use of folk foods and practices	6. Giving comfort to others
7. Religion valued (mainly Roman Catholic)	7. Tenderness acts when ill
	8. Being as pleasant as possible

Figure 10-7   Philippine-American Culture*

*These findings were from Philippines living in the United States for at least two decades and collected by the author Z. Spangler and other transcultural nurse researchers.

Dominant Culture Values are:	Culture Care Meanings and Action Modes are:
1. Duty and obligation to kin and work group	1. Respect for family, authority, and corporate groups; family included in caring
2. Honor and national pride	
3. Patriarchal obligations and respect	2. Obligations to kin and work groups
4. Systematic group work goals	3. Concern for group with protection emphasis
5. Ambitiousness with achievements	
6. Honor and pride toward elders	4. Prolonged nurturance "care for others overtime"
7. Politeness and ritual acts	5. Control emotions and actions to "save face and prevent shame"
8. Group compliance	
9. Maintain high educational standards	6. Look to others for affection (*Arnaeru*) "save face and prevent shame"
10. Futurists with worldwide and plans	
	7. Indulgence from caregivers (young and old)
	8. Endurance to support pain and stress
	9. Respect for and attention to physical complaints
	10. Personal cleanliness
	11. Use of folk therapies (Kanpo medicine)
	12. Quietness and passivity for healing

Figure 10-8   Japanese-American Culture*

*These findings were from Japanese living and working in the United States the past two decades (1971–1991). Similar patterned findings were documented by informants in Japan, but with some recent intergenerational changes.

Dominant Culture Values are:	Culture Care Meanings and Action Modes are:
1. Harmony and balance in universe	1. Harmony and balanced caring ways
2. Extended kinship family ties (centrality of extended family)	2. Respect for elderly, family ties, cultural taboos
3. Religious and spiritual values (Buddhism and Catholicism)	3. Using natural folk-care practices and food (hot-cold theory)
4. Respect for elderly and authority	4. Spirituality in caring
5. Folk-care practices	5. Enabling others to do daily functions (other care)
6. Food and environment	6. Family-centered carings
7. Spirit healing	7. Touching to heal
	8. Hopefulness

Figure 10-9   Vietnamese-American Culture*

*These findings are mainly from Vietnamese refugees living in the United States and studied by authors and other transcultural nurses (1974–1990).

Dominant Culture Care Meanings and Action Modes are:

1. Respect extended family members
2. Involve family as responsible caregivers
3. Use of folk treatment modes
4. Avoid cultural taboos with foods and culture lifeways
5. Use spiritual caring modes
6. Males responsible for public care decisions; females for domestic (home) care
7. Respect general role differences in care and curing
8. Use limit setting with children to discipline
9. Request religious beliefs and practices

Figure 10-10   Southeast Indian American Culture*

*These findings were obtained from Southeast Indian men and women living in the United States the past two decades and collected by transcultural nurses.

Dominant Culture Care Meanings and Action Modes are:

1. Serving others (not self care)
2. Compliance with authority and elders
3. Obedience to authority, elders, and government officials (discipline children)
4. Surveillance: watching near and at distances
5. Dependence on generic folk herbs, treatment modes (acupuncture, etc.)
6. Group communal assistance to others
7. Work hard and give to the society

Figure 10-11   Chinese-American Culture*

*These findings are from Chinese living in the United States over five years. The data were collected by author and other transcultural nurse researchers (1983–1991). The author also documented similar findings in the People's Republic of China (1983).

Dominant Culture Care Meanings and Action Modes are:

1. Providing family care and support—a responsibility
2. Offering respect and privacy time for religious beliefs and prayers (five times each day)
3. Respecting and protecting gender cultural role differences
4. Knowing cultural taboos and norms (i.e., no pork, alcohol, smoking, etc.)
5. Recognize honor with obligation
6. Helping to 'save face' and preserve cultural values
7. Obligation and responsibility to visit the sick
8. Following the teaching of the Koran
9. Helping, especially children and elderly, when ill

Figure 10-12   Arab-American Muslim Culture*

*These care findings reflect several Arab-Muslims in Detroit (the largest Arab groups outside of the Middle East) and need to be viewed as common patterned expressions. While cultural variation existed among all Arab-Muslim groups, these were dominant themes supported by L. Luna's research (1989) and my work with the Arabs for over a decade (1982–1997). Many of these findings were also observed in Saudi Arabia by the author and L. Luna (1987).

Dominant Culture Values are:	Culture Care Meanings and Action Modes are:
1. "Being Amish" (in dress, frugality, and lifeways)	1. Being aware of others: needs and actions
2. Community care action	2. Ministering to others: being present in thought and action
3. Family and community care for wellbeing	3. Giving help generously: obligation and privilege
4. Non-materialism and limited technology	4. Receiving care with expectations and humility
5. Reliance on folk practices and God	5. Anticipatory care: (other care)
6. Principled pragmatism	6. Obedience to God and elders
7. Non-government community help	7. Community caring for wellbeing
	8. Using folk-care ways (spiritual healing)
	9. Limiting use of technologies in caring

Figure 10-13   Old-Order Amish-Americans*

*The author drew from A.F. Wenger's (1988) research and other researchers who studied the Old-Order Amish (1984–1990).

Dominant Culture Values are:	Culture Care Meanings and Action Modes are:
1. Keep ties with kin from the 'hollows'	1. Knowing and trusting 'true friends'
2. Personalized religion	2. Being kind to others
3. Folk practices as 'the best lifeways'	3. Being watchful of strangers or outsiders
4. Guard against 'strangers'	4. Do for others; less for self
5. Be frugal: always use home remedies	5. Keep with kin and local folks
6. Stay near home for protection	6. Use of home remedies 'first and last'
7. Mother is decision maker	7. Help from kin as needed (primary care)
8. Community interdependency	8. Help people stay away from hospitals—'the place where people die'

Figure 10-14   Appalachian Culture*

*These findings were from a study in an urban community by the author and P. Shinkel (plus other transcultural nurses) as part of a larger urban Culture Care Theory study (1984–1987).

Dominant Culture Values are:	Culture Care Meanings and Action Modes are:
1. Upholding Christian religious beliefs and practices ('pray')	1. Giving to others in need
2. Family and cultural solidarity (other care)	2. Self-sacrificing for others and God
3. Frugality as way of life	3. Being actively concerned about
4. Political activity for justice	4. Working hard at whatever one does
5. Hard work: 'Don't complain'	5. Christian love of others
6. Persistence: 'Don't give up'	6. Family concern for others
7. Maintain religious and special days	7. Eating Polish foods and folk care to stay well or recover from illness (including home remedies/spiritual healing)
8. Value folk practices	

Figure 10-15 Polish-American Culture*

*These findings are from transcultural nursing studies with midwest Polish-Americans (primarily in Detroit and Chicago—two of the largest Polish settlements in the United States) by several transcultural nurses over the past two decades.

Dominant Culture Values are:	Culture Care Meanings and Action Modes are:
1. Industriousness and being hard workers	1. Being orderly (orderliness) • things in 'proper places' • right performance • being well organized
2. Maintain order and organization	2. Being clean and neat
3. Maintain religious beliefs	3. Direct helping to others • give explicit assistance • get into action
4. Stoicism	
5. Keep environment and self clean	
6. Cautiousness	4. Watch details • follow rules • be punctual
7. Knowledge is power	
8. Controlling self and others	5. Protecting others against harm and outsiders
9. Maintain rules and norms	6. Controlling self and others
10. Scientism with logic valued	7. Eating proper foods and getting rest and fresh air
	8. Do not complain, 'grin and bear it'

Figure 10-16 German-American Culture*

*These findings are from urban and rural United States over the past three decades by author and other transcultural nurses. Similar values and care patterns also were observed and confirmed in Western Germany in past decades (1970–1980).

Dominant Culture Values are:	Culture Care Meanings and Action Modes are:
1. Extended and close family ties	1. Well being of our families
2. Patriarchialism	• "best for the family good"
3. Strong religious practices (Roman Catholic)	• keeping family active and well

4. Being socially and politically active with extended family and wider community	2. Promoting family integrity
	  • sharing among family (other care)
	  • protecting family name and status

5. Generosity and charitableness	
6. Expressive in music, art, and community service	3. Involvement with family and other Italians (being active and dealing with family affairs)
7. Responsible for Italians	4. Closeness with presence or connectedness
8. Openly express feelings (actions, music, art)	• being there; "touching a lot and hugs"
	5. Expressing oneself freely
	6. Eating fresh Italian market foods and use of wine with meals
	7. Family support (stay close to home)

Figure 10-17   Italian-American Culture*

*These findings were confirmed and substantiated by key and general informants living in a large, Italian, urban mid-central community in the United States by the author and several transcultural nursing researchers. Author worked in community project for ten years (1982–1992). While variability among Italians from the homeland was evident, the above commonalities prevailed.

Dominant Culture Values are:	Culture Care Meanings and Action Modes are:
1. Maintain Greek family ties	1. Being responsible for other Greeks as religious and social obligation
2. Preserve religious beliefs and practices	2. Assisting others as soon as possible to prevent illnesses
3. Be responsible for Greek families	3. Actively involved with Greek families
4. Strong respect for cultural heritage	4. Preventing illnesses with proper exercise; using family folk practices; avoiding hospitals; and eating 'good, healthy' Greek foods
5. Sacrificing for good of others and kin	
6. Generosity to Greek kin, the arts, and other community groups	5. Hospitality (Greeks and strangers)
7. Work with youth to help them become good adult Greeks	6. Keeping active with family and church
8. Be with other Greeks when ill (presence)	7. Reflecting on goodness of others
	8. Keeping clean and properly dressed
	9. Exercise daily
	10. Family stories of serious kin illness

Figure 10-18 Greek-American Culture*

*These care findings are from Greek families in urban United States by author's research team (1984–1999). Similar findings with other nurse–researchers (e.g., Muriel Larson), and with Greeks in Australia and Greece (1978–1990).

300

CHAPTER TEN   Selected Culture Care Findings of Diverse Cultures
Using Culture Care Theory and Ethnomethods [Revised Reprint]

Dominant Culture Values are:	Culture Care Meanings and Action Modes are:
1. Maintain respect for religious beliefs and practices (Judaism)	1. Express feelings openly
2. Keep centrality of family with patriarchal rule and mothercare	2. Get most direct and best help
	3. Accept shared sufferings
3. Support education and intellectual achievements	4. Maternal nurturance, e.g., generous feeding, permissiveness, protectiveness
4. Maintain continuity of Jewish heritage	5. Giving and helping others as social justice (*tsdokeh*)
5. Be generous and charitable to arts, music, and community service	6. Performing lifecycle (birth, marriage, and death)
6. Achieve success (financial and education)	7. Attentiveness to others
	8. Caring for own people
7. Be persistent and persuasive	9. Teaching Jewish values
8. Enjoyment of art, music, and religious rituals	

Figure 10-19   Jewish-American Culture*

*These findings are from Jewish groups living in several urban communities in the United States (1975–1991). Pattern variations were evident with orthodox, conservative, and reformed Jewish-Americans and with intergenerational differences. Several transcultural nurses contributed to findings.

Dominant Culture Values are:	Culture Care Meanings and Action Modes are:
1. Extended family closeness	1. Presence (being there)
2. Religious beliefs and prayers (Roman Catholic)	2. Helping in times of need
	3. Hospitality to others
3. Education important	4. Sharing with others (other-care)
4. Hard work and industriousness	5. Flexibility to adapt
5. Thriftiness and good use of material resources	6. Cooperation with others
6. Endurance, persistence, and suffering with economic hardships	7. Praying with others (spiritual healing)
7. Charity to others	8. Using subtle humor

Figure 10-20   Lithuanian-American Culture*

*These findings were from a large urban community in the United States. Dr. Rauda Galazis, at Wayne State University, shared her findings from two studies in the United States and from a field study in Lithuania, her parents' homeland (1986–1991).

Dominant Culture Care Meanings and Action Modes are:

1. Attention to detail
2. Self-responsibility
3. Maintaining privacy
4. Being hospitable
5. Showing orderly responsibility
6. Cleanliness: self and environment

Figure 10-21 Swedish-American Culture*

*These findings were from Swedish informants in the urban midwest collected by author and research team (1984–1991). Many of these findings also were substantiated by key and general native informants in Sweden in the 1980s.

Dominant Culture Values are:	Culture Care Meanings and Action Modes are:
1. Enduring hardships	1. Being responsible for others (*Hetios*); charity and love (*Caritas*)
2. Being frugal and watchful	
3. Being productive	2. Folk healing (saunas)
4. Maintaining neutrality	3. Listening attentively to others
5. Being nonpunitive	4. Being quiet and contemplative
6. Keeping beliefs (mainly religious)	5. Being able to suffer and obtain meaning with contemplation
7. Maintaining national pride and traditionalism	6. Being nonassertive
8. Quiet action	7. Loving others
9. Maintaining proper rituals and healing decorum	8. Protecting the vulnerable
	9. Getting sick people well
10. Belief in folk and modern healing modes	10. Taking care of self and others in their environment
	11. Communion with others

Figure 10-22 Finnish-American Culture*

*These findings were from the United States, but with support from key and general informants from Northern and Southern Finland with help from Anita von Smitten, Dr. Pirkko Merilainen, Dr. Katie Eriksson, and other Finnish authors' research associates (1989–1991).

302

CHAPTER TEN   Selected Culture Care Findings of Diverse Cultures
Using Culture Care Theory and Ethnomethods [Revised Reprint]

Dominant Culture Values are:	Culture Care Meanings and Action Modes are:
1. Egalitarianism: "All alike"; "One as good as another"	1. Treating people alike
2. Society more important than family	2. Being quiet (leave alone at times)
3. Social obligations and responsibilities	3. Giving or sharing to others
4. Nongregariousness	4. Accommodating other (ideas and needs)
5. Consensus building	5. Avoiding conflicts
6. Cultural pride in heritage	6. Maintaining societal care responsibilities
	7. Eating proper foods
	8. Daily exercise

Figure 10-23   Danish-American Culture*

*These findings were from key and general informants in Denmark and the United States with limited variability.

These *emic* (within the culture) care/caring constructs were identified in approximately 58 cultures through ethnonursing qualitative research methods(s) from 1959–2002. The cultural informants identified four or five dominant care constructs with their key meanings and action modes. None of the cultures identified more than eight major constructs. The professional nurses *etic* (or outsider) views of care are not included in this list. The findings reveal a wide diversity in the *emic* culture care meanings and action modes. All culture- or language-specific care/caring terms were documented and translated into English. This is only a small glimpse of the total care research findings.

Dominant Care and-or Caring Meanings and Action Modes:

1. Acceptance	10. Attention to/toward
2. Accommodating	11. Attitude toward
3. Accountability	12. Being nonassertive
4. Action(ing) for/about/with	13. Being aware of others
5. Adapting to	14. Being authentic (real)
6. Affection for	15. Being clean
7. Alleviation (pain/suffering)	16. Being genuine
8. Anticipation(ing)	17. Being involved
9. Assist(ing) others	18. Being kind/pleasant

Figure 10-24   List of Care/Caring (*Emic*) Constructs Derived from Leininger's Culture Care Theory Research (1959–2002)

Dominant Care and-or Caring Meanings and Action Modes:

19. Being orderly
20. Being present
21. Being watchful
22. Bribing
23. Care (caring)
24. *Caritas* (charity)
25. Cleanliness
26. Closeness to
27. Cognitively knowing
28. Comfort (ing)
29. Commitment to/for
30. Communication (ing)
31. Community awareness
32. Compassion (ate)
33. Compliance with
34. Concern for/about/with
35. Congruence with
36. Connectedness
37. Consideration of
38. Consultation (ing)
39. Controlling
40. Communion with another
41. Cooperation
42. Coordination (ing)
43. Coping with/for
44. Creative thinking/acts
45. Cultural care (ing)
46. Cure (ing)
47. Dependence
48. Direct and indirect help to others
49. Discernment
50. Doing for/with
51. Eating right foods
52. Enduring
53. Embodiment—Christian love
54. Emotional support
55. Empathy
56. Enabling
57. Engrossment in/about
58. Establishing harmony (balance)
59. Engrossment in/about
60. Experiencing with
61. Expressing feelings
62. Faith (in others)
63. Family involvement
64. Family support
65. Feeling for/about
66. Filial love
67. Generosity toward others
68. Gentle(ness) & firmness
69. Giving to others in need
70. Giving comfort to
71. Group assistance
72. Group awareness
73. Growth promoting
74. Hands on
75. Harmony with
76. Healing
77. Health instruction
78. Health (wellbeing)
79. Health maintenance
80. Helping self/others
81. Helping kin/group
82. Honor(ing)
83. Hope (fullness)
84. Hospitality
85. Improving conditions
86. Inclined toward
87. Indulgence from
88. Instruction(ing)
89. Integrity
90. Interest in/about
91. Intimacy/intimate
92. Involvement with/for
93. Kindness (being kind)
94. Knowing of culture
95. Knowing (another's reality)
96. Know cultural values/taboos
97. Limiting (set limits)
98. Listening to/about
99. Loving (love others; *caritas*)
     • Christian love
100. Maintaining harmony
101. Maintaining reciprocity

304

CHAPTER TEN   Selected Culture Care Findings of Diverse Cultures
Using Culture Care Theory and Ethnomethods [Revised Reprint]

Dominant Care and-or Caring Meanings and Action Modes:

102. Maintaining privacy
103. Ministering to others
     • filial love
104. Need fulfillment
105. Nurturance (nurture)
106. Obedience to
107. Obligation to
108. Orderliness
109. Other care(ing) nonself-care
110. Patience
111. Performing rituals
112. Permitting expressions
113. Personalized acts
114. Physical acts
115. Praying with
116. Presence (being with)
117. Preserving (preservation)
118. Prevention (ing)
119. Promoting
120. Promoting independence
121. Protecting (other/self)
122. Purging
123. Quietness
124. Reassurance
125. Receiving
126. Reciprocity (balance)
127. Reflecting goodness
128. Reflecting with/about
129. Rehabilitate
130. Regard for
131. Relatedness to
132. Respecting
133. Respect for/about lifeways
134. Respecting privacy/wishes
135. Respecting sex differences
136. Responding appropriately
137. Responding to context
138. Responsible for others

139. Restoration(ing)
140. Sacrificing
141. Saving face
142. Self-reliant (reliance)
143. Self-responsibility
144. Sensitivity to others needs
145. Serving others (*caritas*)
146. Sharing with others
147. Silence (use of)
148. Speaking the language
149. Spiritual healing
150. Spiritual relatedness
151. Stimulation (ing)
152. Stress alleviation
153. Succorance
154. Suffering with/for
155. Support (ing)
156. Surveillance (watch for)
157. Symbols (ing)
158. Sympathy
159. Taking care of environment
160. Technical skills
161. Techniques
162. Tenderness
163. Timing actions/decisions
164. Touch (ing)
165. Trust (ing)
166. Understanding
167. Use of folk foods/practices
168. Use of limit setting
169. Using nursing knowledge
170. Valuing another's ways
171. Watchfulness
172. Wellbeing (health)
173. Wellbeing (family, spiritual)
174. Wholeness approach
175. Working hard

Figure 10-24   List of Care/Caring (*Emic*) Constructs Derived from Leininger's Culture Care Theory Research (1959–2002) *(continued)*

References

Leininger, M. M. (1978). *Transcultural nursing: Concepts, theories and practices*. New York: John Wiley &. Sons.

Leininger, M. (1981). *Care: An essential human need*. Thorofare, NJ: Slack.

Leininger, M. M. (1984). Southern rural black and white American lifeways with focus on care and health phenomenon. In *Care: The essence of nursing and health*. Detroit: Wayne State University Press.

Leininger, M. M. (1985). Ethnography and ethno-nursing: Models and modes of qualitative data analysis. In M. Leininger (Ed.), *Qualitative research methods in nursing*, pp. 33–72. Orlando, FL: Grune and Stratton.

Leininger, M. M. (1991). *Culture care diversity and universality: A theory of nursing*. New York: National League for Nursing.

CHAPTER ELEVEN

Generic Care of Lebanese Muslim Women in the Midwestern USA

Hiba Wehbe-Alamah, APRN-BC, RN

Nursing as a discipline and a profession has endeavored to provide both holistic and individualistic client focused care (Erb, Kozier, & Olivieri, 1999). Incorporating culture care into the planning and implementation of nursing care actions and decisions ensures the provision of meaningful and beneficial culture specific care, prevents major transcultural conflicts, and promotes beneficial health outcomes (Leininger, 1992, 1995, 2001). Culture-specific care is an especially important concern when one takes into consideration our increasingly multicultural world and the lack of cultural diversity within the nursing workforce in the United States (Trossman, 1998).

According to the Michigan Department of Health, Arabs were the third largest minority group and the fastest growing minority population in the state of Michigan in 1988 (as cited in Connelly, Hammad, Hassoun, Kysia, & Rabah, 1999). In 1999, the Arab population in the metropolitan Detroit area alone was approximately 250,000 and included but was not limited to people from Syria, Palestine, Iraq, Yemen, and Lebanon (Connelly et al.). Arabs are not necessarily Muslims by definition, but include Christians, Jews, Kurds, and Kubts as well as Muslims. While 92% of Arabs in the world are Muslims, Arabs comprise only about 17% of the total Islamic population (Connelly et al.). According to a study conducted in 2002 by the Johnson School of Business at Cornell University, there are currently 8 million Muslims in North America—7 million in the United States and 1 million in Canada (Mohammed, 2002).

Purpose and Goal

The purpose of this study was to discover, describe, and interpret the traditional generic folk care beliefs and practices related to health and wellbeing of Lebanese Muslims from two Midwestern cities in the United States (USA). This research was inspired by the work of Luna who as a transcultural nurse specialist conducted a similar study in 1989 with Lebanese Muslim immigrants in the community and hospital contexts. The two main goals of the ethnonursing study herein were to discover the generic care practices that promote health and beneficial lifeways for Lebanese Muslims, and to explore how the three nursing care modes of Leininger's Culture Care Theory (preservation and-or maintenance; culture care accommodation and-or negotiation; and culture care repatterning and-or restructuring) could be used to provide culturally congruent care for this cultural group (Wehbe-Alamah, 1999).

Domain of Inquiry

The domain of inquiry (DOI) for this mini ethnonursing study was the generic, indigenous, or folk care meanings, beliefs, and practices related to health and illness of Lebanese Muslims living in the Midwestern USA. This domain is of major interest to nurses because of the increasing number of Lebanese Muslims living in the USA due to immigration, and the limited knowledge nurses have of the naturalistic generic folk care meanings, expressions, and practices of this immigrant culture. In addition, this study will contribute to nursing practice by discovering new knowledge to guide culturally congruent nursing actions and decisions. It was anticipated that planning professional care incorporating generic care practices would lead to meaningful and beneficial health care, and facilitate meeting the cultural health care expectations of Lebanese Muslims.

Research Questions

This study was conceptualized within Leininger's Culture Care Theory, which holds that discovered generic and professional care meanings, symbols, patterns, processes, and practices can be used explicitly to provide culturally congruent care that promotes health and wellbeing (Leininger, 1996). It was therefore predicted that knowing and combining professional nursing care practices and generic care practices of Lebanese Muslims would lead to the provision of culturally meaningful and responsible care and to the promotion of health, wellbeing, and healthy lifeways for these people.

The following research questions guided this study:

1. What are the traditional naturalistic generic (folk) care beliefs, expressions, and practices related to health and illness of Lebanese Muslims?

2. What generic health care practices promote health and wellbeing and are beneficial to the lifeways of Lebanese Muslims?
3. In what ways do worldview, cultural context, and social structure dimensions influence the Lebanese Muslims' generic care beliefs, expressions, and practices?
4. In what ways can the three nursing care modes of the Culture Care Theory facilitate the provision of culturally congruent nursing care for Lebanese Muslims?

Theoretical Framework

According to Leininger (2001) care is embedded in people's social structure, worldview, language, and environmental context. The theorist maintains that cultural differences and commonalties about human care exist among all cultures worldwide and their discovery them can be used to guide nursing care decisions and actions beneficial to clients' health (as cited in Fawcett, 1993; Leininger, 1985, 1988, 1995; Leininger & McFarland, 2002). All cultures of the world possess indigenous, folk, or naturalistic lay care systems but many have not necessarily had exposure to professional care systems. The two care systems are not always compatible with each other. Combining them can lead to people seeking and receiving culturally meaningful care, whereas disregarding either or both of them could result in a lack of health, illnesses, culture conflicts, cultural pain, and-or cultural stresses or impositions (Leininger, 2001).

The purpose of the theory of Culture Care is to discover, document, and interpret human culture care diversities and similarities as influenced by worldview, social structure, language, beliefs, values, and environmental context, and to discover new knowledge which would enable nurses to provide culturally meaningful and beneficial care practices (Leininger, 1997b, 2001, 2002). The goal of the theory is to provide culturally competent nursing care for the health and wellbeing of all people (Leininger, 1995, 1997b; Leininger & McFarland, 2002).

The theorist holds that three modes of care are used to provide culturally congruent care leading to health and wellbeing and to face death or disability (Leininger, 1996, 1997b; Leininger & McFarland, 2002). These three modes are culture care preservation and-or maintenance; culture care accommodation and-or negotiation; and culture care repatterning and-or restructuring. These modes refer to professional actions and decisions which are predicted to assist people of different cultures to retain, adapt to, and modify their lifeways to achieve beneficial health outcomes (Leininger, 1995, 2001; Leininger & McFarland, 2002). Leininger (1995, 2001) created the Sunrise Enabler as a conceptual guide and a visual map of the Culture Care Theory. This enabler was designed to depict theoretical and cultural components and conceptualizations as they influence the care and health of individuals, families, cultures, and communities, and to help nurses, researchers, and clinicians envision a holistic perspective of the many influences on culture care and the relationship between the multiple dimensions and concepts of the Culture Care Theory (Leininger, 1995, 2001).

Significance to Nursing

This study is of significance to nursing in general, and to transcultural nursing in particular, because of the high priority associated with increasing the nursing knowledge through research that investigates and describes care practices in diverse cultures. Nursing research specific to culture care emphasizes the *emic* or insider views of informants regarding health and illness as opposed to relying solely on the *etic* or outsider professional views. The American Nurses Association (ANA) Nursing Social Policy Statement (1998) advocates the provision of culturally congruent care which is primarily achieved from using new knowledge generated from transcultural nursing research. This document states that nursing is a dynamic profession that reflects the changing nature of societal needs and cultural and demographic patterns, and that ". . . the aim of nursing actions is to assist patients, families, and communities to improve, correct, or adjust to physical, emotional, spiritual, cultural, and environmental conditions for which they seek help" (p. 9). *The American Nurse* (ANA, 1998) described cultural diversity as 'a high priority' and called for strengthening cultural competency in the nursing workforce. The data from the present study was intended to provide the basis for future transcultural research with other Arab cultural groups in the USA and other countries.

Discovering and disseminating transcultural knowledge related to culturally sensitive and meaningful care is crucial to the discipline of nursing as health consumers want health care that is a combination of generic and professional care services (Leininger, 1997b). Moreover, as nursing shifts from hospital to community based care, nurses need to learn about the diverse cultures living in their communities in order to help avoid legal suits and prevent stereotyping and unfavorable consequences such as cultural clashes, cultural imposition practices, and cultural pain (Leininger, 1997b, 2002).

Ethnohistorical Dimensions

Lebanon, the Country

Lebanon is often referred to as the *Land of Alphabet*, the *Land of Art and Culture*, and the *Land of Four Seasons*. It is a little smaller than Connecticut and lies at the eastern end of the Mediterranean Sea (David M. Kennedy Center for International Studies, 1996; Government of Lebanon, 1996). The country has a total land area of 10,452 square kilometers or 4500 square miles (Fatfat, 1998) and is bordered on the north and east by Syria, by Israel and Palestine on the south, and the Mediterranean Sea on the west. The climate is similar to that of Southern California, with hot, dry summers and warm, moist winters (Sheehan, 1997).

Lebanon, the People

Lebanon's population of 3.7 million is composed of 95% Arabs, 70% of whom are Muslims. The remaining 5% non-Arabs are Kurds, Armenians, and Jews (David M. Kennedy Center for International Studies, 1996; Fatfat, 1998; Travisa Services, April 18, 1998). In 1994 the government of Lebanon estimated there were 15.4 million Lebanese immigrants worldwide with 26.1 % of these immigrants residing in the USA and 43.2 % living in Brazil (1996). The United States Immigration and Naturalization Services (INS) issued a report in 1996 stating that immigration from Lebanon to America has increased steadily over the prior 30 years. This report placed Lebanon among the 10 countries with the highest percentage of immigrants seeking to become naturalized United States citizens. More than 60% of Lebanese immigrants entering the USA between 1977 and 1991 became naturalized citizens, which was almost double the naturalization rate for other immigrant nationalities (Fatfat, 1998). In 2001, Information International estimated that 200,000 Lebanese people immigrated to America from Lebanon between 1991 and 2000, with 43,441 becoming permanent residents (Information International, 2001).

Islam, the Religion

The word *Islam* in Arabic means *peace, purity, submission*, and *obedience*. In the religious sense of the word, Islam is the act of submission to the Will of *Allah* (God) and obedience to his Law ('Abd al 'Ati, 1998). *Muslims* are practitioners of Islam, and are divided into several groups with the two major sects being the *Sunni* and the *Shiia* (Harris, 1997; Mortimer, 1982). Key Informant 3 stated:

> Islam is peace and surrender to Allah. Rab El Alameen (the Lord of the Universe) said that we are passing through this world, every human being should act for his last day. . . . Islam tells us be good, but not all Muslims do everything Allah asked us to do.

Muslims believe that the *Qur'an* is the Word of God and was revealed to prophet Muhammad through the angel Gabriel. It is considered as man's best guide to God's truth and to eternal happiness ('Abd al 'Ati, 1989; Hamid, 1996). The *Qur'an* is the highest authority for information on Islam, followed by the *Sunnah* of the Prophet. *Sunnah* refers to the words, actions, and confirmations of the Prophet in matters pertaining to the meaning and practice of Islam (Badawi, 1999).

Ethnonursing Research Method

The ethnonursing research method was developed in the early 1960s by the nursing theorist Madeleine Leininger to specifically study nursing phenomena related to her Theory of Culture Care Diversity and Universality. *Ethnonursing* refers to a qualitative nursing research method focused on naturalistic, open discoveries and largely inductive modes to document, describe, explain, and interpret informants' worldview, meanings, symbols, and life experiences as they bear upon actual or potential nursing phenomena (Leininger, 1997b). The ethnonursing research method fits well with the goal and purposes of Leininger's Culture Care Theory. The prefix *ethno* refers to people, whereas the suffix *nursing* is associated with a discipline focused on human care (Leininger, 1988). Ethnonursing research is a people-centered method that is based on data from informants' credible *emic* or insider knowledge and lifeways, and yet remains attentive to the *etic* or outsider understanding of factors that could influence data collection and interpretations (Leininger, 1996, 1997b).

Emic data were generated from a total of seven key informants (KI) and 11 general informants (GI) who were interviewed within the community context over a 2-year period for the purpose of this study. Key and general informants were purposefully selected with the help of two community gatekeepers. One gatekeeper was a Lebanese American immigrant woman who was a respected community leader and teacher of the Arabic language. Her husband, a second gatekeeper, was a spiritual leader at a local mosque. Key informants were more knowledgeable about the domain of inquiry compared to general informants who provided more general ideas about the domain and reflections on the simi-

larities and differences between their ideas and those of the key informants. Written consent in either Arabic or English language was obtained
from all informants. In one situation involving an elderly lady, the
researcher was asked to obtain the consent from her older son as well.

Data analysis was conducted through the use of Leininger's Four
Phases of Ethnonursing Analysis for Qualitative Data and a qualitative
data analysis software called Qualitative Solutions and Research for
Nonnumerical Data Indexing Searching and Theorizing (*QSR NUD*IST 4*,
1997). Leininger's qualitative criteria of credibility, confirmability, meaning-in-context, recurrent patterning, saturation, and transferability were
used for evaluation of study data (Leininger, 1997a).

Research Findings

Theme 1: Care as a Religious Duty

The worldview of Muslim Lebanese is embedded in Islam. Every aspect
of life is guided and controlled by religious teachings. Their belief in the
Hereafter, *Heaven*, and *Hell*, and their desire to please God and fulfill
His commandments motivate everyday Muslim practices. Muslims
believe God gave people life and showed them the right and wrong paths
to follow in life through His words in the *Holy Qur'an*. Believers hold
that those who choose to follow God's commandments to overcome
obstacles will earn the right and privilege of going to Heaven in the
Hereafter, and those who do otherwise will go to *Hell*. Lebanese
Muslims' reliance on the *Holy Qur'an* and the *Sunnah* of the Prophet
shapes their care beliefs, expressions, and practices. Islam *encourages*
believers to take care of the sick, including elderly parents, other relatives, strangers, neighbors, and nonMuslims, but especially *requires*
care of their elderly parents. For this reason, Lebanese people rarely
place their elderly in nursing homes; instead, they will care for them
personally and only consider a nursing home after exhausting all other
options. Lebanese Muslims use their language as a religious protective
caring practice, and consider the offering of prayers to God to heal the
ill individual as a religious duty and an obligation. The following are
emic descriptors for Theme 1 cited by key informants:

> Caring in Islam is like family, it's like when you care about someone [in
> the] Islamic way, you care about this person for the sake of Allah, you
> know because Allah ordered us to care for each other, to love each other,
> so if I care about you, and something happened to you and I helped you,
> I'm helping you 'cause I do like you but at the same time, I'm thinking in
> my head, I'm doing this for Allah too, 'cause He asked for it, so you're
> doing two favors in the same time, and you feel good about it, . . . this is
> how we take it, helping each other from Allah's order.

> There is a strong relation among family members, especially when they become elderly, there is a *Sourah* in *Qur'an* [that] means that you take care of your old parents just like they raised you when you were a child . . . Most Lebanese will take care of their elderly at home, not put them in a nursing home. Nursing homes are a last resort and sometimes a shameful thing to do when you can otherwise take care of them. (KI 2)
>
> Care is a religious duty, from a *Hadith* [saying from/about the Prophet] we learned about the story of the Jew man who used to put trash in front of the Prophet's house everyday, then the Prophet would take the trash and throw it where all trash goes, like this everyday, then one day, the Prophet, peace be upon him, did not find trash in front of his house, he got worried about the Jew, so he asked about his house, he went to his house and asked about him and about his health, the Jew was sick, and the Prophet took care of him until he got better, the Jew then became a Moslem and never put trash in front of the Prophet's house again . . . Islam says that we have to visit the sick even when we don't know them, because when they're sick, they're vulnerable psychologically.

Islam does not correlate the act of caring with a specific gender. Men and women are equally encouraged to care for each other. God does not address a specific gender when ordering believers to care for others. Six key and nine general informants described care as a religious duty. This group maintained that persons who do not value religion nor fear God are not as good in caregiving as those who *do* care about God yet may not be deeply religious. The remaining informants viewed care as a moral duty. Traditionally, women are viewed as caregivers as a reflection of cultural roles rather than a religious precept.

Theme 2: Care as a Cultural Duty

Cultural care practice patterns of Muslim Lebanese included providing care out of a cultural sense of and emphasis on *generosity* and *hospitality*. Lebanese Muslims value their cultural heritage and background and place great emphasis on transferring their legacy on to their children. The concepts of *generosity*, *hospitality*, and *helping* others are inherent to the Lebanese culture. This was evident in the way the researcher was received by all of the informants. Each time an informant's house was visited for an interview, the researcher was offered cakes, teas, fruits, juices, Turkish coffee, baklava, or other Lebanese pastries in the tradition that presenting guests with numerous offerings is believed to be a sign of caring. Refusing to accept or consume these offerings can be considered an insult to the host.

Cultural expectations exist regarding the expression and provision of care. It is a cultural duty, especially for family members, to visit the sick and offer or provide help with physical, emotional, and financial needs. Kin are expected first to offer or provide direct or indirect care followed then by friends and neighbors. The direct care role varies from visiting the sick to helping with the cooking, the housework, childcare, and, sometimes, financial needs. Praying to God for a painless and quick recovery is an indirect way of helping the ill. Failure to provide this type of culturally expected care of the sick could lead to termination of friendships and social ties. Key Informant 1 said:

> When you know someone is sick or in the hospital, it is custom that you visit, if the family does not visit in the hospital you're upset with them, so the true friend will be revealed. Usually, we expect the family members to show care . . . the family is always there, the patient will have a room full of visitors . . . the financial support comes as a secondary to the main support which is the family.

Theme 3: Men and Women are Equal but Not Identical

Men and women provide care in different but equally important ways. Women are the nurturers of the families, the persons responsible for raising the children and taking care of the sick. They play a major role in keeping the family a strongly welded social unit. Men are the breadwinners and the persons responsible for financial care. They also assist in disciplining the children. The *Qur'an* acknowledges women and men as equal in their ability to provide care and do good deeds. Men and women are considered different both in their anatomy and in their role as caregivers. While the Muslim religion does not attribute the caring role to a specific gender, sometimes the Lebanese culture does. Women usually show care in an expressive emotional and-or physical way, while men typically provide financial care. Some men consider the physical acts of caring for an ill person and helping with the housework as female roles and therefore shameful things for a man to do. The following are direct quotations from some key informants:

> To some men, it is a shame or something shameful for a man to do housework or physical work with the ill, that is for those who follow culture. Our culture contradicts our religion in some ways, for example . . . some men will not help their wives when they're sick, which is the opposite of what the prophet used to do . . .
>
> Men won't come and give you hugs and kisses like woman does, they will try to support you financially if you need it. Men try to hide their emotions, even though they care, they avoid using relaxing or emotional terms, but they try to find practical solutions and support, which also is a good strength.

The emic perspective of *care* in the worldview of Lebanese Muslim men means providing for the financial needs of the family, maintaining firm control over one's emotions so as to demonstrate strength needed in times of crisis, and finding practical solutions to problems. For Lebanese Muslim women, care meanings differ from those of men; care means engaging in acts designed to nurse a person back to health, showing and displaying emotional support, and being responsive to and fulfilling the emotional, educational, health, and sometimes financial needs of family members.

Theme 4: Changing Traditional Caregiver Roles

In the Muslim tradition, women are in charge of the family home, and responsible for child care and the provision of physical and emotional care for family members. Children express their care verbally and emotionally and through simple actions that reflect the unity and cohesion of the Muslim family such as hugging, kissing, preparing breakfast in bed for a sick parent, or helping out with home chores. Men are usually regarded as the head of the house and the breadwinner, but are also expected to assist with the discipline of the children. Men handle most of the provision of financial care. Interestingly, five key and eight general informants stated that decision making is commonly shared between the husband and wife, although the researcher did encounter informants who maintained that men have the final decision in important matters.

More Lebanese Muslim women are choosing to work outside of the home and are therefore capable of and do provide financial assistance as care to ill family members. Comparably, men are increasingly participating in providing direct 'hands on' physical care. The absence of an extended family within the immediate geographical area due to immigration away from homelands compels men to assist women (wives, mothers, sisters) in provision of direct caregiving. The acculturation process is slowly changing men's perceptions away from the more traditional view about the act of providing care that associates caring with the female gender. The contemporary belief that values cooperation and solidarity between men and women is being gradually adopted. Additional factors behind this trend include their acknowledgment of working women as productive family members and deeper understanding of the Islamic religion through the example of the Prophet. One key and one general informant offered the following comments:

> Yeah, he [husband] will help, I don't know, because I don't have any relatives here, anyone to help, but he usually do a lot of work at home, you know, like when I'm sick, he cooks, he washes dishes [chuckle],

he do everything, he gives the kids baths, he takes them to bed, you know, 'cause I don't have anybody . . .

I've seen of my husband's friends, they do help their wives, I don't know if they do that because they're religious, but I did not see that from other people, like when a person, he's a Moslem but he does not care about Islam . . . if they see their wife sleeping in her bed, they hate her, you know, they give her the attitude, you know, you shouldn't be sick, as if she's not a human being.

Maybe before [I came here] I believed what I heard from other people that the man shouldn't be responsible in helping the woman around the housework or in raising the kids, because that was what I heard from my mother and from relatives and friends . . . I think that the man should help the woman in her work, in raising up her kids, in her housework, in everything . . . and also my husband thinks the same way as I do, he helps me a lot.

The shift in the definition of the caregiving role for Lebanese Muslim men away from the clearly traditional role toward a more contemporary one seems to be related to such factors as the absence of extended family members, acculturation into the dominant society, and attempts to follow the example of Prophet Muhammad who helped his wives with housework and cooking, took care of the ill, and mended clothing. Similarly, increasing numbers of Lebanese Muslim women are taking on the traditionally held male role of financial caregiver in addition to their traditional female caregiver roles.

Theme 5: Folk Care Expressions of Islam

Lebanese Muslim folk care beliefs, expressions, and practices related to health and wellness stemmed from teachings of Islam. Islam views all aspects of life within the context of religion. The holy book of Muslims known as the *Qur'an* (also spelled *Koran*) clearly differentiates what is considered lawful or *Halal* from what is thought of as unlawful or *Haram*. Things that are believed to be *Haram* are the consumption of blood and pork products, sterilization, homosexuality, premarital sex, and artificial inseminations using the egg or sperm of a nonspouse. Therefore, most folk care practices exhibit an attempt to avoid the use of *Haram* products or the engagement in *haram* acts, and demonstrate an effort to abide by God's commands. For example, the *Qur'an* states that honey contains the cure for many diseases, that fasting cleanses the body, that cleanliness prevents illnesses, and that thinking about God and mentioning Him brings peace to the soul. This belief was exhibited by the following statements by three key and one general informant:

. . . like if the woman cannot have a baby, they will try to do her egg and her husband's only . . . if she got it from someone else, that's very *Haram*. They have here in America, they call it sperm bank, so they go borrow someone's sperm, so . . . you have a baby, how about if this baby you gonna have, the same sperm was going to another person, and this kids grow up, and then, they're gonna marry each other . . . Tubal ligation is *Haram*, if it's a man or a woman, but any other form [of birth control] that you can stop [conception] is *Halal*.

Regarding to health, anything that was prohibited by *Rab Al Alameen* (The Lord of the Universe) I stay away from it, because if it wasn't harmful, the Lord won't prohibit it.

Also, Muslims do not eat any pork, bacon, or sausage, also gelatin, because it is made from the hoofs of pigs, as it is said in the *Qur'an*: "*Hourrima alaikum dam al mayyet wa lahm al khanzeer*" (It is forbidden to you the blood of the dead and the meat of the pig) . . . Muslims are not allowed to eat pork, because it was found that there is a worm in the pork, which is not good for our health.

. . . the Prophet, peace be upon him, said: "*Soumou Tasohhou*" (Fast and you shall heal) . . . it's like when you fast, you give your stomach a rest for a few days . . . when we fast we feel humble, we feel like we are close to Allah, and then we feel like your stomach is empty then your mind is working . . . and we think of people who cannot eat everyday, so we feel with them . . . you feel like you wanna feed somebody... you invite a friend over, it's a good bond...

All general and key informants either directly linked the origin of their health care beliefs, expressions, and practices to their religion (Islam) or confirmed this theme when asked about it.

Discoveries for Culture Care and Nursing Care

Culture Care Preservation and-or Maintenance

In order to *preserve and-or maintain* the culture care of Muslim Lebanese-Arab persons, nurses and other health care providers are encouraged to ask their clients culturally focused questions to determine how they would prefer to receive care. Helping Lebanese Muslim immigrants preserve and maintain cultural practices can be achieved by respecting their cultural and religious beliefs. For example, nonMuslims need to abstain from shaking hands with persons of the opposite sex unless initiated by them first. Nonverbal cues indicating Muslims' reluctance to shake hands include putting the right hand over the heart or putting both hands behind the back.

Muslim women who wear *Hijab* (scarf covering the hair, long sleeves and dresses) typically do not wish to do so during their hospitalization, and may remove their veil for comfort. Providing the option of having a same-sex health care provider and ensuring that men do not enter their rooms without being announced first (giving the women time to cover themselves) are actions that promote culture care preservation and accommodation. When asked of single, divorced, or widowed Lebanese Muslim women, queries related to sexual practices must be phrased in a culturally sensitive manner for culture care preservation to occur. Relatives of a dead person should not be pressured to give consent for conducting an autopsy as this would be culturally offensive.

Nursing actions that promote *culture care maintenance* for Lebanese Muslim immigrants include providing *Halal* meals, if available, at the health care institution and excluding pork and its derivatives, such as gelatin, from their menus. Gelatin is normally found in Jell-O, marshmallows, certain ice cream brands (Edy's), some insulin formulations, and gelatin-encapsulated medicines. Providing privacy and a clean place to perform *Wudu'* (ablution) and prayer, knowing the North-East direction of prayer (toward the *Kaaba* in Mecca, Saudi Arabia), and not touching the *Qur'an* unless wearing clean gloves or given permission are ways of ensuring maintenance of cultural care for Lebanese Muslims. As a rule, only people who have showered since their last menstrual period or intercourse are allowed to touch the *Qur'an*.

Culture Care Accommodation and-or Negotiation

Numerous actions can be taken by nurses to *accommodate and-or negotiate* culture care with Lebanese-Arab Muslims. For example, if *Halal* meat is unavailable, nurses can request seafood or vegetarian meals for their clients, or negotiate with the appropriate hospital personnel to allow an individual's relatives to bring homecooked meals to the client. Human or bovine based insulin can be prescribed for diabetic patients instead of pork based preparations. Nurses can negotiate with the pharmacists to supply their patients with vegetable based vitamin A, D, and E (such as Solgar brand made with vegetable gelatin) which are available at health food stores, and with nongelatin-encapsulated alternatives to medicines such as liquid or tablet forms. Other changes nurses can implement include altering medication schedules from daytime to nighttime to accommodate client fasting, and when hospitalized, negotiating with the institution's kitchen staff to arrange for a light meal (*Sehour*) to be consumed by the patient shortly before sunrise. For persons wishing to have *Iftar* (breaking of the fast) evening meals with their families, appropriate private space can be arranged. It is important to keep in mind that not all Muslims will fast during Ramadan as Muslims are permitted to abstain from fasting when ill.

Lebanese Muslim patients anticipate large numbers of visitors when hospitalized and expect a family member to stay with them at night. Nurses can negotiate with the individual and his or her family about the number and frequency of visitors and the length of each visit. Arranging for a comfortable chair or extra bed in the room would be welcomed. For persons expressing their wish to keep their wedding band on or take a *Qur'an* with them into the operating room, nurses can accommodate them by covering the wedding band and-or *Qur'an* with sterile plastic wrap. For persons unable to communicate in English, nurses can request Arabic interpreters (same-sex interpreters are preferable) sworn to confidentiality as a means of accommodating linguistic needs and enhancing the communication process.

Finally, nurses can negotiate with hospital administrators to allow the friends of relatives of a deceased person access to the body to perform a special washing and body wrapping ritual using a special white garb called *Kafan*. This religious custom is traditionally carried out immediately upon death so as to hasten burial, as Islam dictates that the body of a dead person should be buried soon after death, preferably the same day, and before sunset. Washing, wrapping, and burying of the dead require the application of specific actions that are performed in an orderly fashion. Burial on the day of death or soon thereafter is viewed as a Muslim duty that protects the living from the odor or illnesses that could stem from decay of the dead body and lessens the possibility of cultural violation of the deceased.

Culture Care Repatterning and-or Restructuring

In order to *repattern and-or restructure* some of the potentially harmful health practices of Lebanese Muslims, healthcare providers are encouraged to engage in facilitative actions that help clients reorder, change, or modify harmful lifeways while respecting the clients' cultural values and beliefs. The ultimate goal when providing these nursing actions is to engage the client in a healthier mutually established lifeway. This goal can be achieved by nursing actions such as educating clients about the harmful effects of medication sharing, polypharmacy, smoking, and using lemon eyedrops to whiten the sclera and improve vision. Nurses can encourage clients to quit smoking cigarettes and water pipes by emphasizing the effect of secondhand smoke on children and adults, and by offering creative alternatives to this culturally and socially accepted practice. Nurses can educate clients who use kerosene shampoos on their children to treat head lice about the potential danger of systemic and pulmonary toxicity associated with kerosene use, and by offering access to public health resources that provide free head lice medications. By explaining the importance of consulting with a physician or nurse practitioner prior to consuming any folk or generic medications and by facilitating access to free or affordable health care through education about available resources, nurses can lessen medication sharing and improve the health behaviors of Lebanese Muslim immigrants.

Reflection

The themes from this study confirmed the earlier findings from Luna's 1989 maxistudy. Although the study by Luna was performed 10 years earlier, most of the patterns and themes first identified by Luna were rediscovered in the data analysis of the present ministudy which was completed in 1999. Luna's study pioneered research with the Lebanese Muslim culture and involved informants from community, hospital, and clinic contexts, whereas the current work was conducted solely in community settings. The purpose of Luna's study was to describe and analyze the meanings and experiences of care for Lebanese Muslims as influenced by different cultural contexts. The purpose of this study was to discover the traditional generic folk care beliefs and practices related to health and wellbeing of Lebanese Muslims, and to place emphasis on discovering generic healthcare practices. A plethora of folk care practices were shared by informants, which led to the discovery of the fourth and fifth themes as discussed. From these themes came the specific and detailed examples of culturally congruent nursing care actions using the three modes of the Culture Care Theory.

Summary

The purpose of this chapter was to discuss some of the transcultural generic health care beliefs, attitudes, and practices that are found among Lebanese Muslim immigrants in the United States. Specific guidelines pertaining to nursing actions related to Leininger's three care modes of the Culture Care Theory were described with examples of *emic* folk care practices by Lebanese Muslims (Leininger & McFarland, 2002). Nurses and healthcare providers should find this information useful as a guide to providing culturally congruent care to Lebanese Muslim and Arabic clients. The findings from this study have contributed to the growing body of transcultural nursing knowledge to guide nursing actions and descisions.

The importance of discovering worldview, cultural context, social structure dimensions, and traditional folk care beliefs, expressions, and practices of Lebanese Muslims and Arabs is essential for nurses to provide culturally sensitive, safe, congruent, and meaningful care throughout the world. Nurses must remain alert to cultural variations among individuals, but also within cultural communities and institutions.

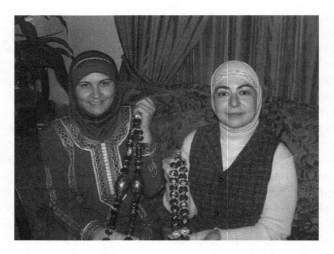

Figure 11-1   Fatme Saleh (left), a Lebanese Arab American key informant, and Hiba Wehbe-Alamah (right), displaying cultural artifacts known as masabih.

Lebanese Muslim Sunrise Enabler

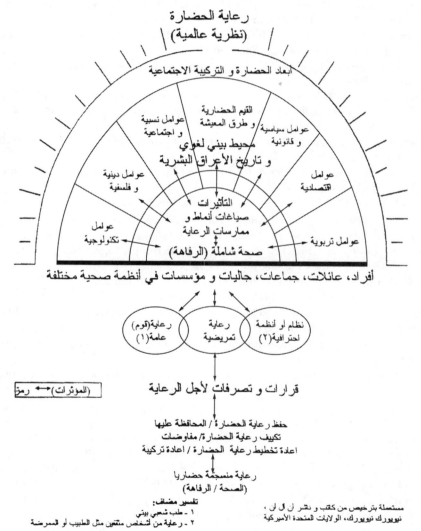

Figure 11-2 Leininger's Sunrise Enabler Model in Arabic.

References

'Abd al 'Ati, H. (1998). *Islam in focus.* Beltsville, MD: Amana.

American Nurses Association (1998). *ANA addressing cultural diversity in profession. The American Nurse, 30*(1), 25.

Badawi, J. (1999). *Gender equity in Islam.* Plainfield, IN: American Trust.

Connelly, M., Hammad, A., Hassoun, R., Kysia, R., & Rabah, R. (1999). *Guide to Arab culture: Health care delivery to the Arab American community.* Dearborn, MI: ACCESS Community Health Center.

David M. Kennedy Center for International Studies. (1996). *Culturgrams: The nations around us.* Chicago: Facts on File.

Erb, G., Kozier, B., & Olivieri, R. (1999). *Fundamentals of nursing.* Boston, MA: Addison-Wesley.

Fatfat, M. (1998). *The migration of Lebanese professionals to the U.S.: Why they left Lebanon and why they are staying in the U.S.* Unpublished doctoral dissertation, University of Pittsburgh, Pennsylvania.

Fawcett, J. (1993). *Analysis and evaluation of nursing theories.* Philadelphia: Lippincott.

Government of Lebanon. (1996). *Touristic and Cultural Map of Lebanon.* Beirut, Lebanon: Ministry of Tourism.

Hamid, A. (1996). *Islam the natural way.* London: The Cromwell Press

Harris, W. (1997). *Faces of Lebanon.* Princeton, NJ: Markus Wiener.

Information International. (2001). *Facts about Lebanese emigration (1991–2000).* Retrieved November 07, 2001, from http://www.information-international.com/pdf/immigration_report_english-1.pdf.

Leininger, M. (1985). Transcultural care diversity and universality: A theory of nursing. *Nursing and Health Care, 6*(4), 209–212.

Leininger, M. (1988). Leininger's theory of nursing: Diversity and universality. *Nursing Science Quarterly, 1*(4), 152–160.

Leininger, M. (1992). The need for transcultural nursing. *Second Opinion, 17*(4), 83–86.

Leininger, M. (1995). *Transcultural nursing: Concepts, theories, research, and practices.* Columbus, OH: McGraw-Hill College Custom Series.

Leininger, M. (1996). Culture care theory, research, and practice. *Nursing Science Quarterly, 9*(2), 71–78.

Leininger, M. (1997a). Overview of the theory of Culture Care with the ethnonursing research method. *Journal of Transcultural Nursing, 8*(2), 32–52.

Leininger, M. (1997b). Transcultural nursing research to transform nursing education and practice: 40 years. *Image, 29*(4), 341–347.

Leininger, M. (2001). *Culture care diversity and universality: A theory of nursing.* New York: National League for Nursing Press.

Leininger, M. (2002). Culture care theory: A major contribution to advance transcultural nursing knowledge and practice. *Journal of Transcultural Nursing, 13*(3) 189–192.

Leininger, M. & McFarland, M. R. (2002). *Transcultural nursing: Concepts, theories, research, and practice*. New York: McGraw-Hill.

Luna, L. (1989). *Care and cultural context of Lebanese Muslims in an urban U.S. community: An ethnographic and ethnonursing study conceptualized within Leininger's theory*. Unpublished doctoral dissertation, Wayne State University, Detroit, MI.

Mohammed, W. D. (2002). Bridges TV—Where American Muslims Come Home. *Muslim Journal, 28*(12), 1, 3.

Mortimer, E. (1982). *Faith & power: The politics of Islam*. New York: Vintage Books.

Qualitative Solutions and Research. (1997). *QSR NUD*IST 4*. Thousand Oaks, CA: Sage.

Sheehan, S. (1997). *Cultures of the world: Lebanon*. New York: Marshall Cavendish.

Travisa Services. (1998). *Welcome to Lebanon*. Retrieved April 18, 1998, from http://www.travisa.com/etravelplan/Lebanon/Lebanon.htm/.

Trossman, S. (1998). Diversity: A continuing challenge. *The American Nurse, Jan/Feb(1)*, 24–25.

Wehbe-Alamah, H. (1999). *Generic health care beliefs, expressions, and practices of Lebanese Muslims in two urban U.S. communities: A mini ethnonursing study conceptualized within Leininger's theory*. Unpublished master's thesis, Saginaw Valley State University, University Center, Michigan.

CHAPTER TWELVE

Culture Care and Health of Russian and Vietnamese Refugee Communities in the United States

Anna Frances Z. Wenger, PhD, RN, CTN, FAAN

Building healthy communities that include immigrants and refugees continues to be a major issue worldwide as population shifts increase and become more daunting in this age of globalization. DeSantis (1997) developed a construct of what constitutes a ". . . healthy community for immigrants and refugees" (p. 20) and challenged transcultural nursing to be a force in helping to build such communities.

The term *refugee* is used in the United States (USA) to determine immigration status according to the definition as set forth in the Refugee Act of 1980 (United States Department of Health and Human Services [USDHHS], Office of Refugee Resettlement, 2001). A refugee is any person who wants to immigrate to the USA because of persecution or fear of persecution due to race, religion, nationality, membership in a particular social group, or political opinion in addition to several other specific situations requiring the order of the President of the USA (US Citizen and Immigration Services, 2003).

Refugees and Acculturation

The social and political context of refugee status intensifies the cultural differences between the refugees and the persons in the dominant culture. Although previous studies (Benisovich & King, 2003; Cronkright, DeHaven, & Kraev, 1993; Frye, 1991; Gold, 1992; Korb, 1996; Lang & Torres, 1997–1998; Maltby, 1999; Muecke, 1990; Simon, 1983; Ying, 1990; Wenger, 1983, 1985) have contributed to the knowledge base about health and care beliefs and values of various refugee groups, little is known about those that influence family and community wellbeing and healthcare decision making during the process of acculturation.

In most cultures, women tend to be the bearers of health and care information that is passed on from one generation to the next (Wenger, 1988). For refugees involved in acculturation, women are often isolated from the dominant culture, interacting almost solely with persons within the refugee culture. Because their main contacts are with persons of their own culture they tend to take much longer to learn the language of the dominant culture than their husbands or sons, thus inhibiting their communication with healthcare providers. Thus, there is often limited verbal interchange with healthcare personnel concerning healthcare needs and care practices from the perspective of the refugees themselves.

During the years 2003 and 2004, the majority of refugee resettlement in the USA included persons from Africa, more so after the federal government increased quotas for Africa. However, the steady stream of refugees into the USA and other parts of the world makes the critical need for studies regarding the reciprocal interchange between healthcare providers and refugees, particularly during the acculturation process. Another trend that made this study relevant at this time was the fact that refugees were not experiencing the kind of welcome they had previously (Personal Communication, Deborah Duchon, immediate past Director of the Center for Research and Anthropology, Georgia State University, February 23, 2004). This was due in part to the slowed economy, lack of jobs, and that the concept of *refugee* had lost some of its allure. Churches and other agencies were experiencing *compassion fatigue* and some communities where refugees had resettled had been experiencing a cultural backlash. In addition, funding for refugee programs had been severely diminished, thus forcing some offices to close and others to downsize. These trends markedly increased the imperative for understanding the *emic* view regarding the meaning of health and care.

Acculturation added another dimension to culture context that made the situation even more complex. Acculturation is a dynamic process involving change in both the dominant group and the subgroup whereby certain values and practices are changed while others are retained (Teske & Nelson, 1974). Acculturation is also a multidimensional process in which at least two cultural groups came into continual firsthand contact. Therefore, the definition of *acculturation* implies that one could expect changes to occur within the healthcare system as well as within the refugee communities. This change process may generate stress for all persons involved in the acculturation process and may lead to health consequences for refugees due to altered lifeways and stress leading to increased susceptibility (Berry, 1990).

Research Parameters

Domain of Inquiry and Purpose

The domain of inquiry was the culture care and health of Russian and Vietnamese refugees and their acculturation to the USA.

The purpose was to learn about health and care beliefs, values, and practices that promote family and community wellbeing and influence healthcare decision making in two major refugee groups involved in acculturation, namely refugees to the USA from former South Vietnam and from the former Soviet Republics.

Research Program

This study was part of a research program investigating the relationship between culture context and culture care. *Cultural context* is defined as the situation or environment that is relevant to the care belief, values, and practices of a particular culture (Leininger, 1991). *Culture care* refers to the meanings and expressions that support and enhance a sense of personal, family, and community wellbeing, assisting them to improve human conditions, or face disabilities or death (Leininger, 1991). Context provides the milieu or environment in which to understand behavior and values. Care values and actions are developed and communicated within each culture in ways that promote the survival of that group. When people care for themselves and others, their cultural values about health and illness influence the caring modalities they choose (Wenger, 1988, 1991b).

A previous ethnonursing study of health and care phenomena among Russian Jewish immigrants from the former Soviet Republics now involved in the acculturation process was conducted by this author (Wenger, 1983, 1985). These informants had immigrated to a major Midwestern metropolitan city. Major conflicts for them in acculturation focused on beliefs about actions they thought were necessary in order to receive personalized health care from professionals. These actions were often misunderstood by the healthcare providers in the USA. Culture context became more evident in a subsequent study with another *high context culture*, the Old Order Amish (Wenger, 1988, 1991a, 1991b; Wenger & Wenger, 2003), in which caring practices were described and contextual themes were abstracted.

The present comparative study focused on Vietnamese and Russian refugees now living in a major Southeastern metropolitan area in the USA. In this study, informants originally from former South Vietnam were referred to as *Vietnamese* and informants from the former Soviet Republics were referred to as *Russian*. The researcher used these terms because the informants referred to themselves in this way. The Russian immigrants frequently made a distinction about their country of origin in terms of north or south USSR, but more specifically spoke in terms of the post-USSR era using the names of their homelands. All of the Russian key informants were ethnically Jewish, although many of them did not share a sense of deep personal meaning of being religiously Jewish. This sometimes became a point of puzzlement between Russian immigrants and their American Jewish sponsors.

These two cultures were chosen because they constituted two of the larger immigrant groups in the area. Two groups were chosen to add the dimension of comparison, an important perspective of ethnographic and ethnonursing research (Leininger, 1985; Simon, 1986; Torsch & Ma, 2000).

Conceptual Framework

Cultural Care Diversity and Universality Theory

The theory of Cultural Diversity and Universality (Leininger, 1991; Leininger & McFarland, 2002) and Hall's (1976) cultural context model were used for this ethnonursing study. Leininger's theory provided the cultural framework and general set of assumptions. Sociocultural factors within the historical and environmental context of the informants influenced their health beliefs, values, and practices, and their healthcare decisions. This theory is predicated on the premise that culturally congruent care is essential for the promotion of health and wellbeing of cultures (Leininger & McFarland, 2002). ". . . A meaningful and satisfactory fit of culture care beliefs, values, and practices between healthcare providers and care recipients is needed in order to preserve, maintain, or change care practices for the benefit and satisfaction of clients" (Leininger, 1991 as cited by Wenger, 1991b, p. 97). Leininger's Sunrise Enabler was used to show and predict the relationships among worldview, sociocultural dimensions, environmental context, language and ethnohistory, diverse health systems, and principles, and to guide nursing decisions and actions. These dimensions were important areas of study.

Cultural Context Model

Hall's (1976) cultural context model contributed the premise on which to search for understanding about the context dependency in the human environment interchange. According to Hall's conceptual model of high and low context cultures and communication, both Vietnamese and Russian cultures were considered as *high context*. *High context* cultures compared to *low context* cultures are characterized by having more long-term relationships, many shared life activities, less variability in cultural lifeways, more intergenerational kinship knowledge, more restricted linguistic codes, high social support and control, and insider-outsider distinctions about sociocultural boundaries. In contrast, the dominant American culture is a *low context* culture in that there were fewer long-term relationships, greater mobility, more variability in cultural lifeways, and elaborated linguistic codes. Low social control and support and limited intergenerational knowledge blur sociocultural boundaries. These general differences in high and low context cultures influenced communication patterns between the *low context* American culture and the *high context* cultures, such as the Vietnamese and Russian refugee cultures, and are indicative of the need for research to discover the meaning of health and care from refugees during their acculturation process. Hall's (1976) conceptual framework helped the researchers to define the boundaries of the study; however, it did not dictate the research process.

Method

To study the domain of inquiry of the culture care and health during acculturation of Vietnamese and Russian refugees in a metropolitan area of the Midwestern USA, some broad heuristic questions were used to guide the ethnonursing research process, the researcher's thinking, and to allow open discovery without having preestablished expectations. The following questions were used to provide an openness to fully discover the domain of inquiry.

Research Questions

1. What are the meanings and expressions of *care* and *health* for Vietnamese and Russian refugees during acculturation?
2. What social structure factors, environmental context, and cultural lifeways influence the use of folk and professional healthcare services by Vietnamese and Russian refugees?
3. What are the similarities and differences in the meanings of *care* and *health* for Vietnamese and Russian refugees?
4. What are the ethnonursing and healthcare system implications of refugee perceptions of care and health?

The goal of the Culture Care Theory is to make nursing care decisions and actions that are culturally congruent with the beliefs, practices, and values of the lifeways of the people.

Research Design

This study was conducted using Leininger's Ethnonursing Research Method in which observation-participation and informant interviewing are used to discover patterns and themes about health, care, and healthcare decision making. Observation-participation refers to the process over time of observing and participating in activities related to the domain of inquiry (Leininger, 1990). Some of the activities in this study included attending a celebration dinner for Russian refugees hosted by the Jewish Family Association, a visit with the publisher of the Russian Jewish newspaper, family visits, and attendance at various Vietnamese community events. Informant interviewing involved scheduled interviews and informal discussions with key and general informants.

Informants

Key informants referred to those informants who were members of the Russian and Vietnamese cultures knowledgeable about the cultural lifeways of the people, and able to articulate the deeply held shared values and beliefs about their culture's health and care. *General informants* were persons in the community with whom the researchers interacted, but interviewed less frequently. General informants were often used for member checking, that is, to confirm or elaborate on a specific idea or piece of information. Key informants were *intended* to be Vietnamese and Russian women who had lived in the United States between 3 and 6 years and who were between the ages of 25 and 50 years of age. The rationale for these criteria was to focus the study on the lifecycle stage when informants' children would be living in the home, and to exclude the first two years of their acculturation period as many resettlement adjustments could obscure healthcare decision making related to cultural beliefs and values (Wenger personal knowledge). Women in the childbearing and childrearing years were frequently confronted with health and care decisions for themselves and their families. However, the researchers found it impossible to adhere to these age criteria because the exact ages were not always known at the time of the interviews when the individual immigration histories were learned.

Vietnamese key informants ranged in age from 26 to 60 and had lived in the USA between 1 and 8 years. Russian refugees were older, ranging in age between 23 and 61 years, with only 3 being under 50 years. They had lived in the USA between 1 and 4 years. Total interview time with 16 key and 10 general Vietnamese informants was 51 hours conducted over time to capture the steps involved in their acculturation. For Russian informants, the total interview time was 56 hours, with 11 key and 5 general informants. Interpreters were used with informants who were more comfortable talking in their native languages. A tape recorder was used only with informant consent. The researchers kept field journals and field notes in addition to the tape recordings. The tape recordings were used as memory joggers and to capture and identify any missed or difficult to understand data. In accordance with the ethnonursing method, data were reconfirmed with informants throughout the study.

Setting

The interviews took place in naturalistic settings, such as the informants' homes, in their places of work, or at community centers. Both Vietnamese and Russian refugees settled in a section of the city that was highly multicultural, thus attracting refugees and immigrants to live in that area during their initial years of becoming acculturated to their new environment.

Research Personnel

Research personnel included the author as principal investigator and three research assistants. The principal investigator had educational preparation in transcultural nursing and qualitative research methods as well as previous experience in conducting research using the ethnonursing method. The research assistants participated in activities such as development of the interview probes, doing windshield surveys of the communities, attending community events, and meeting some healthcare professionals who provided services to refugees. Access to the communities was gained through refugee resettlement and health organizations.

Data Collection

Entry to the Field

Contact was made first with health-related organizations that assisted refugees in resettling to this urban setting. The researcher's contacts included a counselor and refugee from Jewish Family Services and refugee health professionals from Vietnam. Three informants were introduced to the researchers through the Jewish Family Services, Asian Community Services, and the Refugee Women's Association. The remaining contacts were made through referrals from other key informants. This approach provided for diversity of contacts in each refugee community.

Informant Interviewing

Two to four interviews were held with each key informant; total interview time for each informant ranged from approximately 3 to slightly more than 8 hours. One interview was conducted with each general informant from both refugee groups. During some interviews husbands, children, and friends were present. All key informants signed informed consent forms after a verbal explanation of the information was provided through translation. A set of interview probes was used to stimulate discussion about health and care phenomena during the key informant interviews. The sociocultural dimensions from the Sunrise Enabler were used as guides to develop these probes to elicit ideas about *health* and *care* phenomena from the refugees, and to discover cultural values, beliefs, and practices that influenced healthcare decision making during the acculturation process. In addition, Leininger's Acculturation Scale was used to develop acculturation profiles of the key informants.

Record Keeping

All key informant interviews were tape recorded. Field notes were also recorded and each data collector kept a reflective journal of the research process and personal responses during the period of data collection and analysis. These records became an integral part of the study documentation and were used as an audit trail for the continuous data analysis and confirmation processes.

Data Analysis

Data were analyzed using Leininger's (1990) Four Phase Data Analysis Enabler. The analysis flowed from the raw data to identification of descriptors, to selection of categories or patterns, and finally to themes that were derived inductively and were grounded in the data. *Gofer*, a text management computer program, was used to identify and search for terms and categories. Constant comparative analysis began with the first interview. Within 24 hours after each interview, the researchers recorded an extended account (Spradley, 1979) using their field notes, tape recordings, and reflective journals. As the data were entered into the computer, the researchers included preliminary comments and suggested categories. The Four Phases of Data Analysis required scrutinizing data to be used for guiding the succeeding interviews and in doing peer briefing and member checking. Patterns and themes were identified during the final phase of the analysis process, and the findings were shared with several informants in order to verify credibility and establish confirmability with the research evaluation criteria used for the study (Leininger, 1990; Lincoln & Guba, 1985).

Evaluation Criteria

Evaluation criteria specific to qualitative research methodology were used. The four major criteria were credibility, confirmability, transferability, and dependability (Leininger, 1990; Lincoln & Guba, 1985). *Credibility* was established through prolonged contact. In this study, two to four interviews were held with each key informant over a period of two to three months. Findings were shared with key and general informants so that they could reflect on and confirm the researchers' understanding and suggest changes as indicated. Member checking was used throughout the study. *Confirmability* refers to the degree to which the researcher's interpretations of the findings are supported by the informants. All raw data were recorded using a coding system so as to protect identities of the informants, were maintained in a secure place, and were used as needed for an audit trail. *Transferability* refers to the probability of the study being done similarly elsewhere. A process, data, and methods log was kept and made accessible to the research team. *Dependability* refers to accountability of the data. To ensure dependability, records were kept of any shift in the research process. For example, some key informants included in the study were refugee women older than the 25–50 year age range originally stated as an informant selection criterion. These women were involved in caring for children of younger women and therefore continued to be actively involved in healthcare decision making in the American setting.

Limitations of the Study

Given that the researcher is the instrument in ethnonursing research, it would have been highly desirable for all researchers to speak the first language of the informants, which none of the researchers did. However, German and Yiddish were used to a limited extent with a few of the Russian Jewish refugees. Experienced interpreters were obtained through references from key organizations who work with refugee resettlement. Although the researchers tried to work diligently with the interpreters, it was understood that some meaning could be lost through the processes of translation and interpretation.

Findings

Major Themes

Three themes were discovered from the four stages of analysis of the raw data and were confirmed by informants. They were: *here-there*, *health and care*, and *healthcare decision making*.

Theme 1: Here-There

Here-there is a very interesting theme; it is an *emic* term meaning the insider view as used linguistically and culturally by the people. *Here-there* refers to the cultural context within which these refugee informants thought about health and care. Most informants of both cultures put their comments into comparative statements referring to their home country and their current context in the USA whenever they expressed ideas about health and care options in America. When they talked about health and care they thought comparatively about their current situation and health care options in relation to what they had left behind, often clarifying by using the words *here* and *there*. The following descriptors, examples from the raw data, illustrate this *here-there* theme:

1. Vietnamese Descriptors
   a. *Here*: In USA, have much government health care, like Medicaid.
      There: Little government health care in Vietnam.
   b. *Here*: Can apply for aid but do not trust others as much.
      There: Children care for parents; people must help each other.
   c. *Here*: Must be careful about folk treatments being viewed as abuse.
      There: Use folk care first.
2. Russian Descriptors
   a. *Here*: Less free health care but better technology.
      There: More free government health care in Russia with low technology.
   b. *Here*: Children have more freedom, are more independent.
      There: Parents and children help to care for each other throughout life.

c. *Here*: Must ask for doctor and get little time, and they do not know home situation or home remedies.

There: Use many kinds of health care including herbs, and doctors come to the homes.

In Leininger's (1991) Data Analysis Model, patterns were identified by the researcher's categorization of descriptors. Patterns are the third level of abstraction in the analysis process. Several patterns related to the culture context theme were referred to as *here-there*. The following patterns illustrate the way *here-there* was discovered as a culture context theme in both refugee groups. The descriptors listed in Table 12-1 applied to both Vietnamese and Russians, except where indicated with V for Vietnamese and R for Russians:

The cultural context theme of *here-there* was abstracted from the patterns and descriptors that provided evidence of the way these refugee informants constructed meaning about health and care during the acculturation process. Cognitive awareness of the present seemed to be tempered by a simultaneous awareness of the past so that discussions about health and care in their current situation were almost always accompanied by a reflection on their past lives in their home countries.

Theme 2: Health and Care

The researchers tried to elicit perceptions about health and care from the informants' worldview. Many social scientists and health professionals use ethnographic approaches to learn about health-related beliefs and practices, focusing on illnesses and orthodox or traditional medical practices (Harwood, 1996; Hunt, Browner, & Jordan, 1990; Modiano, 1995). Nurse researchers, especially those who use ethnonursing methods, have been building a body of knowledge related to health and care phenomena for many years (Leininger, 1991; Luna, 1994; Lundberg, 2000; McFarland, 1997; Morgan, 1996; Pacquiao, Archeval, & Shelley, 1999; Rosenbaum, 1988; Wenger, 1985, 1991a/b; Spangler, 1992; Zoucha, 1998). It was difficult work because informants generally found it easier to describe illness or disease episodes than the meanings of *health* and *care*, which had tendencies for being less concrete. This was especially true for generic care practices, which were embedded into each culture in ways that may not have been cognitively thought about within the cultures themselves.

Although the data set contains some information related to illness perceptions, this discussion refers only to their descriptions of a healthy person and the meaning of health and care. Describing a healthy and an unhealthy person had been found to be effective in eliciting cultural meanings about health. For informants in both cultures, the meaning of health included physical, emotional, and social attributes. Descriptors of a healthy person are shown in Table 12-2.

Care Patterns

The meaning of *health* as a pattern was similar in both cultures. The Vietnamese informants referred to *health* as *the way one feels* but also as *a state of being that affects the whole community*. They used terms

TABLE 12-1   Descriptors Used to Discover Patterns of *Here-There* (Theme 1)

Here	There
Pattern: Lifestyle	Pattern: Lifestyle
Descriptors:	Descriptors:
Some family members here	Extended family support
Visit only when invited	Much visiting all the time
Must work; concerned about losing job	Worked but also took long vacations
V: Here, only one wife	V: There, men can have many wives
Pattern: Role of Government	Pattern: Role of Government
Descriptors:	Descriptors:
Government cares for you	Government doesn't care for you
Government cares for elders and child (Medicare, Medicaid)	Children care for parents
Pattern: Religion	Pattern: Religion
Descriptors:	Descriptors:
V: Not as important here	V: Buddhism very important
R: For Jews, religion is very important	R: Religion not discussed much, nor for Jews
Pattern: Healthcare Delivery System	Pattern: Healthcare Delivery System
Descriptors:	Descriptors:
DIFFICULT—must make appointments	There, do not always need appointments
Public hospitals OK here	Public hospitals do not treat you well
Can apply for government aid	
Doctors and nurses are kind	
Pattern: Trust	Pattern: Trust
Descriptors:	Descriptors:
Hard to give tips (bribes*) here	Give tips (bribes*) to nurses to ensure care
V: If no one is home, people can steal	V: Less stealing, more trust
R: Not sure when to trust health care persons; not part of government	R: Do not trust healthcare providers; they are part of government

* Note: Bribes was the term used by R (Russians); tips was the term used by V (Vietnamese).

TABLE 12-2   Healthy Person Descriptors

Vietnamese	Russian
Feel happy	Happy without problems
Exercise daily (all ages including babies)	Active according to age
Go to bed early	Work a lot
Want to go places	Smile
Feel brave	Good feelings
Gain respect of others	Helping others
	'Nerves' are good
	(Nerves cause most illness)
	Good skin color

like *wanting to go around, going to temple, family visiting, family asks about you, children showing respect,* and *wanting to work.* Russians emphasized that *health* means *having a schedule, exercising, good food, music in the home, balance,* and ". . . *work, work, work.*" One informant said it this way: ". . . Balance of food and a regular schedule for the day helps one to stay healthy and regain lost health." Although the importance of family was discussed in terms of care, when discussing the meaning of health, family was not mentioned as often by the Russians in the way it was by the Vietnamese informants.

For Vietnamese informants, the pattern of *care* was reflected by the meanings *respect, politeness, teaching children by practicing for them (role modeling),* and *paying attention to people.* One Vietnamese informant suggested that women care more than men in relation to health and illness concerns; however, others reflected this notion also in relation to women being responsible for the care and nurturance of children. Nurses in the USA were described as more professional than in Vietnam and were more caring. By this they referred to what were perceived to be caring acts like *asking about family, speaking gently,* and *giving personalized care.*

For Russian informants, the pattern of *care* was reflected by the meanings *politeness, asking about what the person prefers,* and *doing things for others like caring for the elderly.* Nurses and doctors in the USA were also perceived by the Russians as more caring than health-care professionals in their homelands because they smile more. One Russian informant said, ". . . There is good middle staff—nurses and nursing assistants who smile and make you feel good, keep the room clean, and you have a clean bath, good conditions." However, it was noted that physicians in America should ". . . think more about the whole body and not just the parts; in Russia and Europe doctors are more general." Health care in the American context was often considered to be rushed; they perceived that people in the USA were expected to get well quickly and get back to work. Both Vietnamese and Russian informants discussed the value of long vacations and health leaves to recuperate, regain strength, and relax in order to decrease feelings of stress. They discussed missing that aspect of life as when living in their homelands. One Russian informant's comment reflects the general value of care and caring, ". . . Caring comes from the heart; it is my philosophy. When you see something is wrong, don't ask—do."

Theme 3: Health Care Decision Making

During acculturation, refugees searched for healthcare services that had some familiar attributes, could be trusted, were affordable, and allowed sociocultural supports that were valued by their people. Some of the most salient considerations that were mentioned repeatedly were:

1. Vietnamese Descriptors: Use folk care first (*coining, pinching, cupping, herbs, teas*); ask friends to help; do things to keep warm when ill; consider balance in *hot* and *cold*; look for balance between internal and external winds and positive and negative emotions. *Bad winds* refers to an imbalance of internal and external winds (meaning insides and outside of the body) exacerbated by an imbalance of emotions. In the home, the mother makes healthcare decisions. When professional help is needed the husband and wife decide together. A Vietnamese doctor is preferred—or at least a doctor or nurse who explains and listens.

3. Russian Descriptors: Nearest family member finds out what is wrong first; grandmothers are consulted whenever possible; use folk remedies and sometimes consult healers. They will call a physician for the big health or illness problems and prefer a Russian doctor or at least a family doctor who explains and listens. They respect high technology and yet are fearful of it, thinking that they may not fully understand its use especially when there are language barriers. American doctors were perceived to be very good at surgery but not at medicine and healing. One Russian informant put it this way, ". . . *Here* we can't use advice; it is too far from us." This informant was referring to the difficulty in trusting healthcare decision making advice because they did not always trust the new healthcare environment and were also *reflecting* on the past as they *consider* the present. The distance between what they as refugees understood as healthcare options in the American context sometimes seemed too far removed from what they had learned to know and trust in their homeland.

Three major patterns were identified as relating to the theme of *healthcare decision making*, namely *use of folk or traditional care, persons involved in healthcare decisions*, and *relationships with professional care providers*.

Care Patterns

Both Vietnamese and Russian informants talked about how they continued to *use folk care* in the American context. The general pattern in both cultures was to continue using folk or traditional care first and to continue using both traditional and professional care simultaneously whenever possible. Vietnamese informants spoke about needing to be careful in talking with American professionals about traditional health practices such as *coining, pinching*, and *cupping* because they may be accused of abuse. This did not seem to be a concern for Russian informants as the traditional health practices they chose to use involved home remedies such as *teas, ointments*, and *leaves* that they brought with them from their homelands. Russian informants also talked about consulting with healers in their community and continued to use healers when available in the American context.

The second pattern related to *persons who are usually involved in healthcare decision making*. Vietnamese refugees mentioned that the mother was generally in charge of healthcare options in the home, but when that was not sufficient the father and mother together made the decision to obtain professional help. However, when they were in a professional setting, the husband took the lead in discussing their options with the doctor or nurse. In Russian families, the nearest family members found out what was wrong and then consulted with the grandmother if she was available. When professional help was needed the husband or nearest male relative was included in the decision making process.

The third pattern focused on the *relationships of the refugee family with heathcare professionals*. The descriptors in this third care pattern focused on healthcare preferences when the refugees chose to consult with professionals and the preferences they had for those relationships that were involved in making difficult decisions. In both cultures, refugees talked about their preference for having both husband and wife, and sometimes the grandmother, present in the professional healthcare setting to talk with doctors and nurses. Whenever possible they also preferred having a Vietnamese or Russian doctor, or at least a doctor who spoke their language. If this was not possible, then they preferred to relate to doctors and nurses who would explain and listen so that they could be involved in making healthcare decisions.

Discussion

Here-there was found to be the theme that provided the cognitive map for the informants who were refugees from Vietnam and the former Soviet Republics as they thought about health and care phenomena while becoming acculturated to living in the USA. This contrastive interplay with what they remembered from their homelands and what they encountered in their new setting regarding health and care options provided a useful context for them to think about health and care options and to make decisions that were culturally congruent for them. *Thinking about* health and care issues and options could then be given consideration, in that they, as refugees, could remain cognitively engaged with the past as they considered the present.

The relevance of ethnohistory related to health and care phenomena became apparent as the cultural context theme of *here-there* was discovered as the structure for health and care discussions with refugees. Leininger (1991; Leininger & McFarland, 2002) discussed ethnohistory as part of the environmental context that influences care expressions, patterns, and practices related to health and wellbeing. *Ethnohistory* refers to past events and experiences that help researchers to interpret cultural lifeways over a long period of time. In this sense, the ethnohistories of these refugees were important and related to their cultures' environmental context, in that *environmental context* referred to the *totality* of their situation in both past and present that gives meaning to human expressions, interpretations, and social interactions (Leininger, 1991; Leininger & McFarland, 2002). The challenge for nurses and other healthcare providers is to learn about the ethnohistories and environmental contexts of refugees and immigrants who are engaged in acculturation and to find ways to promote discussions about health and care that is culturally congruent for them.

Three Modes of Culture Care

Leininger's Sunrise Enabler (1991; Leininger & McFarland, 2002) provided three modes for nursing decisions and actions that led to culturally congruent care: *culture care preservation and-or maintenance, culture care accommodation and-or negotiation,* and *culture care repatterning and-or restructuring.* The data from this study were used to demonstrate application of these modes for nursing decisions and actions with refugees.

Culture Care Preservation and-or Maintenance

The first requisite of culturally congruent care is to preserve and-or maintain those health and care values and practices that promote health and wellbeing (Leininger, 1991). Both Vietnamese and Russian informants mentioned *politeness* as a care value. In their *here-there* context, they perceived American healthcare personnel to be more *polite* than health personnel in their homelands. They referred especially to nurses and ancillary health personnel in reflecting upon their feelings of being cared for in a personalized manner. They also talked about how *politeness* extended to caring within the family and that smiling and feeling happy was an attribute of a healthy person. This then signified a need for healthcare providers to engage in *polite* and *courteous* communication with refugees. Nurses could also encourage clients who are Vietnamese and Russian refugees to express their feelings and to be active participants in their own health care as a means of preserving and maintaining a healthy lifestyle.

Culture Care Accommodation and-or Negotiation

The second mode calls for accommodation and-or negotiation, which implies that there may need to be some change on both sides of the healthcare system-client interface. For these Vietnamese and Russian refugees, family caring was emphasized. Many times the grandmother or a *fictive* kin needed to be present during consultation or family and friends may have gathered at the clinic or hospital expecting to be present with the ill person. Each situation should be considered in terms of the culture care needs of the client and family as well as the institutional needs of the unit or hospital. Having family members present with the ill person may require some modification in institutional rules for the wellbeing of the individual and the family who *together* consider themselves as 'the client.'

Given that the refugees had been used to having many extended family members available in the home to assist with caring responsibilities, the nurse and other healthcare personnel need to assess the home situation during acculturation in relation to the presence of an effective support system for meeting the healthcare needs of the client and the family. Accommodation by the healthcare institution personnel is required to allow sufficient time for the increased work necessary within the referral system and for assessment of the home environment. It is hoped there would be a care support system available to the refugee client who is in transition and learning to understand and function within the context of a different healthcare system.

Culture Care Repatterning and-or Restructuring

Whenever change is recommended in health and care practices, the *here-there* culture context of the refugee client becomes increasingly important, because long held cultural values and beliefs are involved. Repatterning or restructuring implies that the support of culture, family, and individual beliefs were involved in the recommended change. Two important maxims should be kept in mind: build on the strengths as negotiations for change to occur and begin with a common ground of understanding.

For both Vietnamese and Russian refugees there was common ground with American healthcare providers related to an expressed desire to be healthy and to extend help to those in need. Albeit some of the folk caring practices seemed to be less accepted in the American context and some seemed to be harmful or ill advised in the American context. In those situations, culture care repatterning or restructuring was recommended. The first step was to acknowledge the common ground assets that were shared by American nurses and other healthcare providers and by the Vietnamese or Russian refugees, such as the desire to be healthy and to engage in health-promoting practices and to provide care generously for others. For the Vietnamese practices used for relieving the body of *bad wind* or other imbalances, the second step would be to learn about the ethnohistory of the harmful traditional practices, such as *coining* or oxybustion (*cupping*). The third step would be to teach the refugees how these practices were perceived in the American culture. The fourth consideration would be to determine if there were any substitute ways to respect the cultural belief about bad wind without engaging in practices that caused dermabrasion or burns. The fifth action would be to teach ways to treat these untoward symptoms based on scientific professional facts while at the same time supporting beneficial traditional caring practices. The same process applied to help Russian refugees to restructure their health and caring practices for nerves, which were believed to be the underlying cause of most physical and psychological illnesses. The essential aspect of cultural care repatterning and-or restructuring was the negotiated understanding of the underlying causes of the illnesses and the cultural acceptance of the new treatments and caring practices. Finally, in all nursing interactions it was essential to include the family's healthcare decision makers when proposing caring actions.

The following list of suggestions summarizes the proposed guidelines for nursing care actions:

1. Include the family's healthcare decision makers when planning interventions.
2. Ask about health beliefs and practices in the family, in the home country, and in their new setting in this country.
3. Discuss both folk and professional care preferences.
4. Incorporate their health and care beliefs into professional healthcare negotiations.
5. Incorporate culturally congruent strategies into healthcare system protocols and public policy.

Conclusion

This ethnonursing study of health and care phenomena compares healthcare decision making of Vietnamese and Russian refugees engaged in the process of acculturation to their new American setting in a Southeastern metropolitan area. Leininger's (1991) theory of Culture Care was used to study the domain of inquiry. Several ethnonursing enablers were used including the Sunrise Enabler, Stranger to Trusted Friend Guide, Acculturation Assessment Profile, and the Ethnonursing Data Analysis Guide (Leininger, 1995, 1997). Informant interviewing and observation-participation were used to collect data from key and general informants.

One culture context theme, an *emic* term referred to as *here-there*, was identified as the basis for informants to discuss other themes such as *health* and *care* and *healthcare decision making*. Context was not easy for the refugees to define. It involved *here-there* comparisons that included ethnohistory and family history, sometimes painful yet poignant, but always relevant. Given that acculturation implied a selective change that was multidimensional, two unanswered questions remained for the researchers:

1. In what ways can healthcare professionals become open to learning about the relevant contextual care components of refugees?
2. How could the professional healthcare system implement changes based on the study findings with these refugee or culturally different groups of people in order to provide culturally congruent care?

The findings of this research study revealed that more studies are needed with these two refugee cultures, as well as other cultures, focusing on the discovery of health and care phenomena during the refugee process of acculturation.

References

Benisovich, S. V. & King, A. C. (2003). Meaning and knowledge of health among older adult immigrants from Russia: A phenomenological study. *Health Education Research, 18*(2), 135–144.

Berry, J. W. (1990). Acculturation and adaptation: Health consequences of culture contact among circumpolar peoples. *Archives of Medical Research, 49*, 142–150.

Cronkright, P. J., DeHaven, K., & Kraev, I. A. (1993). Issues in the provision of health care to Soviet emigrants. *Archives of Family Medicine, 2*(4), 1425–428.

DeSantis, L. A. (1997). Building healthy communities with immigrants and refugees. *Journal of Transcultural Nursing, 9*(1), 20–31.

Frye, B. A. (1991). Cultural themes in healthcare decision making among Cambodian refugee women. *Journal of Community Health Nursing, 8*(1), 33–44.

Gold, S. J. (1992). *Refugee communities: A comparative field study.* Newbury Park: Sage Publications.

Hall, E. T. (1976). *Beyond culture.* Garden City, NY: Anchor Press.

Harwood, A. (1996). Sex, drugs, and the spread of HIV/AIDS in Belle Glade, Florida. *Medical Science Quarterly,(10)*1, 83–93.

Hunt, L. M., Browner, C. H., & Jordan, B. (1990). Hypoglycemia: Portrait of an illness construct in everyday use. *Medical Anthropology Quarterly, (4)*2, 190–210.

Lang, P., & Torres, M. I. (1997–1998). Vietnamese perceptions of community and health: Implications for the practice of community health education. *International Quarterly of Community Health Education, 17*(4), 389–404.

Leininger, M. M. (Ed.). (1985). *Qualitative Research Methods in Nursing.* Orlando, FL: Grune & Stratton, Inc.

Leininger, M. M. (1990). Ethnomethods: The philosophic and epistemic basis to explicate transcultural nursing knowledge. *Journal of Transcultural Nursing, 1*(2), 40–52.

Leininger, M. M. (1991). *Culture care diversity and universality: A theory of nursing.* New York: National League for Nursing.

Leininger, M. M. (1997). Overview of the theory of culture care with the ethnonursing research method. *Journal of Transcultural nursing, 8*(2), 32–52.

Leininger, M. M., & McFarland, M. R. (2002). *Transcultural nursing: Concepts, theories, research and practice* (3rd ed.). New York: McGraw-Hill Publishing.

Lincoln, Y., & Guba, E. (1985). *Naturalistic inquiry.* Thousand Oaks, CA: Sage Publications.

Luna, L. (1994). Care and cultural context of Lebanese Muslim immigrants: Using Leininger's theory. *Journal of Transcultural Nursing, 5*(2), 12–20.

Lundberg, P. C. (2000). Culture care of Thai immigrants in Uppsala: A study of transcultural nursing in Sweden. *Journal of Transcultural Nursing, 11*(4), 274–280.

Maltby, H. (1999). The common thread: Health care activities of Vietnamese and Anglo-Australian women. *Health Care for Women International, 20*(3), 291–302.

McFarland, M. R. (1997). Use of culture care theory with Anglo- and African American elders in a longterm care setting. *Nursing Science Quarterly, 10*(4), 186–192.

Modiano, M. R. (1995). Breast and cervical cancer in Hispanic women. *Medical Anthropology Quarterly, (9)*1, 75–77.

Morgan, M. (1996). Prenatal care of African American women in selected USA urban and rural contexts. *Journal of Transcultural Nursing, 7*(2), 3–9.

Muecke, M. (1990). Vietnamese refugees in the American health care system. *American Journal of Public Health, 173,* 831–838.

Muecke, M. A. (1992). New paradigms for refugee health problems. *Social Science Medicine, 35*(4), 515–523.

Pacquiao, D. F., Archeval, L., & Shelley, E. E. (1999). Transcultural nursing study of emic and etic care in the home. *Journal of Transcultural Nursing, 10*(2), 112–119.

Rosenbaum, J. N. (1988). Mental health care needs of Soviet Jewish immigrants. In M. Leininger, (Ed.), *Care: Discovery and uses in clinical and community nursing,* (pp. 107–121). Detroit: Wayne State University Press.

Simon, R. J. (1983). Refugee families' adjustment and aspirations: A comparison of Soviet Jewish and Vietnamese immigrants. *Ethnic and Racial Studies, 6*(4), 492–504.

Simon, R. J. (1986). Refugee women and their daughters: A comparision of Soviet, Vietnamese, and native born American families. In C. L. Williams and J. Westermeyer, *Refugee Mental Health in Resettlement countries,* (pp. 157–172). Washington DC: Hemisphere Publishing.

Spangler, Z. (1992). Transcultural care values and nursing practices of Philippine American nurses. *Journal of Transcultural Nursing, 4*(2), 28–37.

Spradley, J. (1979). *The ethnographic interview.* New York: Holt, Rinehart & Winston.

Teske, R. H. C., & Nelson, B. H. (1974). Acculturation and assimilation: A clarification. *American Ethnologist, 1,* 351–367.

Torsch, V. L., & Ma, X. G. (2000). Cross cultural comparisons of health perceptions, concerns and coping strategies among Asian and Pacific Islander American elders. *Qualitative Health Research, 10*(4), 471–489.

United States Citizen and Immigration Services. (2003, February 28). *The Immigration and Nationality Act* (refugee definition). Retrieved March 7, 2004, from http://uscis.gov/graphics/howdoi/refugee.htm.

United States Department of Health and Human Services, Office of Refugee Resettlement (ORR). (2001). *Annual report to Congress.* Retrieved February 20, 2004, from http://www.acf.dhhs.gov/programs/orr/policy/01arc2.htm.

Wenger, A. F. Z. (1983). *Health and care phenomena among Soviet Jewish immigrants in the acculturation process: A mini ethnonursing study.* Unpublished master's field study, Wayne State University, Detroit, Michigan.

Wenger, A. F. Z. (1985). Learning to do a mini ethnonursing research study: A doctoral student's experience. In M. Leininger, (Ed.), *Qualitative research methods in nursing*, (pp. 283–316). New York: Grune & Stratton.

Wenger, A. F. Z. (1988). The phenomenon of care in a high context culture: The Old Order Amish. (Doctoral dissertation, Wayne State University, 1989), *Dissertation Abstracts International, 50–02B*, 500.

Wenger, A. F. Z. (1991a). The culture care theory and the Old Order Amish. In M. M. Leininger, *Cultural care diversity and universality: A theory of nursing*, (pp. 147–178). New York: National League for Nursing.

Wenger, A. F. Z. (1991b). The role of context in culture specific care. In P. L. Chinn (Ed.), *Anthology of Caring*, (pp. 95–111). New York: National League for Nursing.

Wenger, A. F. Z., & Wenger, M. R. (2003). The Amish. In L. D. Purnell, & B. J. Paulanka (Eds.), *Transcultural Health Care: A culturally competent approach* (2nd ed., pp. 54–72). Philadelphia: F. A. Davis.

Ying, Y. (1990). Explanatory models of major depression and implications for help-seeking among immigrant Chinese American women. *Culture, Medicine and Psychiatry, 14*, 393–408.

Zoucha, R. D. (1998). The experiences of Mexican Americans receiving professional nursing care: An ethnonursing study. *Journal of Transcultural Nursing, 9*(2), 34–44.

The author thanks Connie Hannah, MPH, RN; Theresa Lerch, MSN, MPH, RN; and Amanda Sue Niskar, DrPH, MPH, RN, who were research assistants at the time of the study. They participated in weekly research teams' discussions and assisted with data collection and analysis.

CHAPTER THIRTEEN

Application of Culture Care Theory for Clinical Nurse Administrators and Managers

Ann O. Hubbert, PhD, RN, CTN

Introduction

There is a new era emerging for nurse administrators and managers, and it is envisioned as a new kind of role in *transcultural nursing administration* (Leininger, 1996). Since the 1950s, Madeleine Leininger, a visionary nursing leader, has predicted that societies and health care will become increasingly multicultural, and as a result, skills in cultural competence are essential for successful relationships in all aspects of human care. The relationships nurse administrators and managers face within nursing and health care are increasingly multicultural, which necessitates being able to move from a predominantly unicultural to a uniformly multicultural mode of operation (Leininger, 1996; Wenger, 1995). Leininger also emphasizes the urgency for nurses to recognize their ability to be leaders in the globalization of nursing and health care.

Nurse administrators and managers in the 21st century are directly involved in multiple areas in the globalization of health care, which impacts upon individual health care systems. In this chapter, the author discusses how direct application of Leininger's Culture Care Theory using the universal care constructs and the Sunrise Enabler guides the assessments, decisions, and action modes of nurse administrators, managers, and practitioners.

Nurse administrators and managers are providing foundations for care decisions and actions in ever changing and complex health care environments. Their skills should reflect the growing responsibilities placed upon them in response to the new dimensions of health care, including having the skills necessary for successful team building within and among organizations and their networks (Marquis & Huston, 2003).

Transcultural nursing administration expertise offers foundations for
survival, growth, satisfaction, and achievement of goals in multicultural
healthcare systems (Andrews & Boyle, 1999). The evolving roles of
nurse administrators and managers require that they have a working
transcultural knowledge base and the skills to promote advocacy and
cohesiveness between and among multicultural teams. These teams
need to be proficient in using transcultural knowledge along with
administrative skills to provide care for the expanding multicultural
client populations and their special needs.

The facilitation of successful team building contributes to cohesiveness between and among nursing and interdisciplinary teams. Wilson and
Porter-O'Grady (1999) have challenged nursing leaders to urgently
respond to the outcry for new leadership practices by expanding their
interpersonal skills to develop and manage a vast variety of relationships.
These authors advocate that nurse leaders should have the freedom and
authority to change what they do and how they do it to successfully move
forward in the change environment within health care systems. Nurse
administrators and managers need excellent interpersonal skills for working with individuals, among groups, and across groups, within multiple
cultures and-or subcultures. Transcultural knowledge increases their abilities as leaders to create and sustain new dimensions of cohesiveness and
performance among diverse cultures that exist within groups of healthcare providers, healthcare systems, and client populations.

The newly evolving nurse leader is an advocate for learning and
changing (Wilson & Porter-O'Grady, 1999). Transcultural theoretical
knowledge and skills are crucial to guide administrators and leaders in
their new relationships, decisions, and skills relevant to changing organizational structures. Transcultural nursing concepts, principles, and
research findings can be most helpful when used with care services that
recognize cultural differences in health needs and beliefs. These dimensions are equally as important as biological and psychological needs for
clients and providers (Glittenberg, 1995; Leininger & McFarland, 2002).
To effectively respond to and provide for the cultural needs of clients,
multicultural team members also need to be understood and supported
by nurse administrators and managers.

Challenges

Increasing Cultural Diversity

The United States has increasing numbers of diverse immigrants and
refugees arriving from many places in the world. Nurses are challenged
to provide culturally competent care. This means using culturally based

knowledge in creative, congruent, and meaningful ways to provide beneficial, safe, and satisfying health care in order to meet the culture care needs of rapidly changing client populations (Leininger, 1991; Leininger & McFarland, 2002). In the year 2010, minority cultures will represent 32% of the US population; by the year 2050, they will represent 50% (USDHHS Office of Minority Health, 2001). The increasingly multicultural nature of health care in American society requires that nurse administrators and managers have the ability to offer effective leadership within the context of cultural differences as well as similarities.

Expectations of Nurses

Healthcare providers are expected to respond to the Department of Health and Human Services, Office of Minority Health, CLAS (Culturally and Linguistic Appropriate Services) Standards. This agency expects healthcare service agencies to provide culturally and linguistically appropriate services as a means toward decreasing healthcare disparities (USDHHS Office of Minority Health, 2001). This requirement necessitates that nurse administrators be able to provide care services for a variety of cultures within their institutions. Fulfilling this requirement can realistically occur only when grounded in transcultural knowledge and skills. Leininger (1997a) stated that among these expected skills should be included the following: nurses can and will be culturally sensitive and competent with all clients and with other team members; nurse administrators or managers can successfully mentor nurses from various cultures; and nurse administrators or managers can orient teams about cultures.

Cultural Systems in Health Care

The American Nurses Association's Council on Cultural Diversity in Nursing Practice (1991) identified three cultural systems of health care: (1) provider culture, (2) client culture, and (3) setting culture. However, there are innumerable subcultures within each of these identified cultures that are important for nurse administrators and managers to recognize. Leininger (1995) defined nursing culture and subculture in her work.

> *Culture of nursing* refers to the learned and transmitted lifeways, values, symbols, patterns, and normative practices of members of the nursing profession of a particular society. *Subculture of nursing* refers to a group of nurses who show distinctive values and lifeways that differ from the dominant or mainstream culture of nursing (p. 208).

Nurse administrators and managers continually work between and among many cultures and subcultures. These cultures and subcultures are complex and include, in part, nursing and nursing subcultures, medicine, social work, pharmacy, and other professions and ancillary service providers in the health system, agency providers, and corporate and organizational cultures. These are in addition to the multiple cultures of clients, families, and communities. Nurse administrators and managers are expected to understand and function within this myriad of organizational, staff, and client cultures. It is these diverse, multidisciplinary cultures and subcultures that contribute to enabling the provision of culturally congruent client care especially when administrators facilitate this care (Uhl Pierce, 1999). Organizational administrators and leaders are expected to assume active roles in developing organizational cultures that are successful in providing culturally congruent care (Marquis & Huston, 2003). Managers are responsible for the ongoing assessment of the organizational culture and for facilitating care within the context of the nursing culture and subcultures. If nurse administrators and managers lack the foundational transcultural knowledge about what creates cultures and subcultures, it can greatly diminish the successful development of relationships and positive organizational outcomes. One goal identified in the literature for nurse administrators and managers is to demonstrate skills that will facilitate the development of relationships between and among themselves, staff, cultures, and subcultures in diverse communities (Wilson & Porter-O'Grady, 1999; Leininger, 1995, 1996). Relationship skills are critically important to transculturally based administrative practices so that they function successfully and competently within multicultural health care systems.

Cultural Imposition, Ethnocentrism, and Biases

Within any multicultural team, nurse administrators and managers may face a variety of cultural imposition practices (knowing *what is best*) between and among the team members (Gardenswartz & Rowe, 1998; Leininger & McFarland, 2002). Ethnocentric views of having *the best answers* and *the best decisions* of how care should be accomplished by others, especially for cultural strangers, may be evident and prevalent among team members. Such ethnocentrism poses serious ethical and quality of care concerns. It requires that nurse administrators and managers have knowledgeable use of transcultural principles, concepts, and theoretical frameworks to guide their decisions and actions. Valuing cultural sensitivity and knowledge is important as preconceived ideas about certain cultures or subcultures may lead to stereotyping and racial biases for clients, families, and staff.

Ethnocentric beliefs (the belief that our Western administrative ways are best or superior) leads to cultural imposition or imposed actions that are based on the *etic* view of *what is best* (Leininger, 1991; Leininger & McFarland, 2002). Decisions or actions made by corporate teams, nursing staff, and-or interdisciplinary team members about clients and-or families, based on consequent preconceived judgments of *what is needed* or *what is best* may result in fears or refusals to cooperate.

A serious problem is the existence of cultural bias (a firm position that one's own values and beliefs are superior to others; Leininger, 1995) between and among team members, which may lead to a lack of cooperation, cohesiveness, and-or effective care outcomes. Staff members who strongly identify with a particular culture may elicit biases from clients resulting in fears or refusals to work with or participate in care actions involving certain team members. This may be especially evident with people from a markedly different culture. These potential problems necessitate a hard look into organizational policies and practices by management and-or administrative officers. Promoting personal cultural awareness is an essential task for nurse administrators and managers. It is a wise strategy to offer healthcare members the opportunity to identify the cultures and-or subcultures (e.g., ethnicities, gender, age, marital status, political views, urban, rural, single parent, etc.) with which they strongly identify. Then healthcare teams will be able to discuss and share ways for understanding different client and staff cultures. Applying transcultural nursing insights toward developing group cultural awareness and sensitivity toward other cultures is beneficial, promotes growth, and rewards staff and team members (Leininger, 1997a; Leininger & McFarland, 2002).

Culture Care Theory

Leininger's theory of Culture Care Diversity and Universality (Culture Care Theory) was built with a scientifically sound and humanistic knowledge base (Leininger, 1991; Leininger & McFarland, 2002). The theory has become a foundation for discovering relationships for working among and between diverse cultures and subcultures. Culture Care Theory challenges nurses to discover indepth dimensions of *care* using Leininger's core tenet that care is the essence, the central premise, and dominant domain of nursing and transcultural nursing (Leininger, 1988, 1991). The author contends that this theory can be a valuable means for nurse administrators and managers to obtain fresh new knowledge about clients of diverse cultures, as well as the health care system, and the diversity of nurses and multidisciplinary team members within various caring contexts.

The use of the Culture Care Theory to discover diversities and commonalities in transcultural nursing administration has been a major breakthrough in nursing and healthcare systems. Leininger's (1991; Leininger & McFarland, 2002) Sunrise Enabler is a powerful guide to help nurse administrators to identify factors influencing staff recruitment and retention. It is also helpful in assessing fiscal management, power and politics, and strategic and operational planning. Data from these sources can be valuable for use in marketing, risk management, continuous quality care improvements, conflict management areas, and for ideas in providing beneficial client care and organizational decisions. The theory offers a strong foundation for the actions and decisions of nurse managers responsible for the daily operations of nursing units and direct client care. The theory also helps administrators to discover their own cultural beliefs and action modes.

Ethnonursing researchers have discovered both universal and diverse culture-specific care constructs valued by virtually all cultures (Leininger, 1991; Leininger & McFarland, 2002). These findings include 12 dominant care constructs discovered by transcultural nurses doing indepth studies over time in naturalistic or familiar settings (Leininger, 1998). By understanding these care constructs and their care meanings and uses, nurse administrators and managers can discover what the various cultures and subcultures desire as care from the organization, administration, and management leaders. The following are the 12 dominant universal health care constructs listed in priority ranking from Leininger's 1998 summary analysis: respect for or about [highest priority]; concern for or about; attention to; helping, assisting, and facilitative acts; active listening; giving presence (being physically present); understanding cultural beliefs, values, lifeways; being connected to or showing relatedness; protection of or for; touching; providing comfort measures; and showing filial love.

Each of these constructs has meaning, symbols, beliefs, and practices for different cultures, and are valuable to understand and should guide nurse administrators' and managers' culturally based decisions and actions.

Culture Care Constructs and Administrative Behaviors

Nyberg (1998) synthesized components of the extensive work by Leininger (1988, 1991) and Watson (1994) on the application of *care* in nursing administration, identifying two primary roles for a caring nurse administrator: a leader of a caring profession, and a facilitator of caring in a health care organization. Nyberg suggested that what nurses desire from a caring administrator can be directly correlated to the ten most frequently identified universal care constructs of the Culture Care Theory.

First, nurses want administrators-managers who love nursing, care for clients, and who promote the use of these care constructs for culturally congruent administrative practices, with the first universal care construct of *respect* as a top priority and goal. It is vital, yet may not prevail in practice. The nurse administrator who demonstrates genuine respect for nurses as individuals and the work they do provides *care to nurses* through leadership behavior and role modeling. Relative to this, nurse administrators and managers should be aware that their actions need to reveal their *concern for and about nurses*, a major care construct for providing culturally competent care. Secondly, nurses want an administrator who actively listens to them. *Active listening* is a universal care construct. Astute administrators and managers can promote creative means to assure staff that their opinions are *heard*. Third, nurses desire an administrator who does not *abandon nurses and nursing* or become less visible due to the administrative role. The universal care constructs of *giving presence* (being there physically), *helping, facilitating, providing assistive acts, being connected to*, and *providing attention to* are essential to attain and maintain the theory based goal of providing culturally congruent care. Nurse administrators who are knowledgeable about cultural care constructs and transcultural nursing principles are then able to demonstrate their use through action. Underlying all is the construct of *understanding* the nurses' own cultural beliefs and values. A nurse administrator or manager who understands his or her own cultural values and practices, and who values and is sensitive to diverse and universal care constructs will be able to demonstrate identifiable caring behaviors. Caring communication and behavior become readily evident and are appreciated by staff and colleagues.

Sunrise Enabler

Culture Care Theory with the use of the ethnonursing research method can provide a valuable guide for nurse administrators and managers to 'bring the theory into action.' The Sunrise Enabler helps nurses to discover and reflect on their decisions and actions. The Sunrise Enabler has three modes of decision and action (Leininger, 1991; Leininger & McFarland, 2002) which are creative and new ways to practice administration and to arrive at the goal of the theory, namely culturally congruent care. Nurse administrators and managers with their foundational transcultural knowledge base can apply the following three modes of action on a daily basis as they work between and among many cultures. For example:

1. Culture Care Preservation and-or Maintenance: What client or staff care assistance is wanted? How can therapeutic culture care be preserved and maintained by administrators?
2. Culture Care Accommodation and-or Negotiation: What care beliefs or practices need to be accommodated, or what needs to be negotiated with staff, clients, and others? Some *administrative* decisions and actions need to be accommodated and others negotiated to be beneficial to people in the organization. Policies and practices may need to be changed to be helpful to clients from diverse cultures.
3. Culture Care Restructuring and-or Repatterning: What practices need to be restructured, or repatterned? If needed, how can administrators actively provide these changes or practices to meet these needs?

Nursing Administration and Management Use of the Sunrise Enabler

Problem Solving and Decision Making

Problem solving, decisions, and actions of nurse administrators need to be guided by the theoretical framework to discover and understand culturally different viewpoints, values, expressions, and meanings. At the same time, they need to uphold moral, ethical, and legal rights of cultures within the framework of the Culture Care Theory (Cameron-Traub, 2002). A professional approach to problem solving, making decisions, and actions involves using a theoretical model as the basis for understanding, discovering findings, and applying critical thinking skills (Leininger & McFarland, 2002; Marquis & Huston, 2003). Leininger's Culture Care Theory and Sunrise Enabler along with five other enablers of the theory are powerful guides for gaining indepth knowledge that will help strengthen nurse administrators' and managers' professional approach to problem solving and making decisions. The theory is holistic, providing a total view of the informants involved (including staff) and the influencing social structure factors meaningful to clients (Leininger, 1991; Leininger & McFarland, 2002). The theory can be a valuable guide for nurse administrators to make creative and sound decisions in such areas as situational conflict resolution, strategic planning, interdisciplinary and collegial teams, and personnel issues.

Foreign Educated Nurse Recruitment

The USA's national nursing shortage has motivated many nurse administrators to rely on the recruitment of foreign educated nurses to increase the numbers in their institutional nursing workforce (Davis & Nichols, 2002). Nurses educated in the Philippines, India, Nigeria, Canada, and Poland represented the top five foreign countries from which nurses have been recruited for the national nursing workforce prior to 2000. Various challenges present with the blending of local community nursing staff culture and foreign educated nurses' cultures toward becoming cohesive teams that provide optimum client care. Foreign nurses often provide new insights in care, especially for culturally diverse clients.

Cultural shock (disorientation or being unable to respond cognitively to the new behavior of a group or culture because of strangeness or unfamiliarity; Leininger, 1991) often occurs among nurses recruited from foreign countries. The expanding multicultural workforce also includes new graduates and newly hired nurses arriving to join existing healthcare systems. Travel nurses may not be prepared in transcultural nursing and often become segregated into subcultures because of their differences. As a result, segregated subcultures develop rather than multicultural teams built on promoting supportive and understanding relationships (Pacquiao, 2002). Local nurses may also experience cultural shock as these diverse nursing subcultures work on their teams. Nurse administrators need to provide mentorship and guidance for all these nurses. Administrators are urged to invest in multicultural education and mentorship arrangements for nurses recruited to work in diverse healthcare cultures to help them adjust to the new culture where they live and work, and to guide their practices in providing safe and therapeutic culturally competent care (Bola, Driggers, Dunlap, & Ebersole, 2003; Leininger & McFarland, 2002).

Nurse administrators often make decisions to allocate considerable funds for the recruitment of foreign educated nurses and-or 'travel nurses' to supplement staffing schedules. Many travel nurses have very limited or no knowledge about diverse cultures. Administrators need to allocate funds for transcultural education, mentorship, and supervision of these nurses or culturally destructive care may result. Consequently, culture shock, culture pain, and imposition practices can adversely affect the job performances of the team members. Traditionally, the job orientation has focused on task performance without recognition of nurses' individual cultural knowledge or cultural differences among the recruits and local nurse subcultures, as well as clients. Cultural clashes (major differences between the *emic* [local] and *etic* [outsider] views; Leininger, 1991) frequently occur and lead to dissatisfaction with the work environment, and negatively influence the quality of client care (Leininger, 1997a; Pacqauio, 2002). Nurse administrators need to be more vigilant about these problems to prevent such nontherapeutic outcomes.

An example of a dramatic lack of cultural knowledge and understanding between and among nursing cultures occurred when two foreign educated graduate students were assigned by a college of nursing to precept 20 hours a week with two nurse administrators in the same institution. At the first meeting, the two graduate students identified themselves as being from Iran and Iraq. This preceptorship would be the most indepth time the two nurses would have spent together since starting the program. Initially, there was concern and fear from many in the institution as to how the graduate students would feel towards each other given their political backgrounds. They were also concerned about what they really wanted to learn and whether staff would accept these foreign nurses. The two nurse administrators quickly sought transcultural expertise to help them provide cultural care accommodation in their preceptorship program. The experts also recognized that the nurse managers in their healthcare system needed transcultural knowledge to prevent prejudice, ethnocentricsm, cultural clashes, and cultural pain between and among many cultures and subcultures of nurses in this institution as they would be working closely together for several months. The transcultural nursing orientation focused on the need for *caring as respect* for each other and provided invaluable knowledge to guide the nurses' actions and decisions using the universal and diverse care constructs and findings of the Culture Care Theory.

The Sunrise Enabler with the three modes of decisions and actions guided the team's cohesiveness. The three modes were considered in relation to various cultural beliefs and values. Open discussions were held in meetings, focus groups, and social events. Step one, culture care preservation and-or maintenance, asked: What is important for each foreign nurse, preceptor, and the institution manager involved in the preceptorship? Step two, culture care accommodation and-or negotiation, asked: What can we (foreign nurses, preceptors, and managers) look at to accommodate our diverse and similar cultural views? What is needed for the newly hired nurses' education? What can we negotiate among ourselves and with the preceptors as requirements for their course? Step three, culture care restructuring and-or repatterning, asked: How could this be done differently . . . who would benefit? As a result of transcultural knowledge and use of the Sunrise Enabler, all of the nurse administrators, the more than 20 nurse managers, and the two foreign graduate students found their relationships becoming meaningful, valuable, and trusting. Transcultural holding knowledge as advocated by the theorist (Leininger,

1991, 1997b; Leininger & McFarland, 2002) was greatly expanded within the institutional team and many institution nurses, foreign nurses, preceptors, staff, and clients from many diverse cultures came to cherish their similarities rather than being fearful of their differences.

Cultural Pain Among Teams

Foreign employed nurses may be from cultures where Western behaviors (open and direct questions, confrontational questions, and expectations of assertive behavior) are not valued, and those behaviors from others may result in incidents of cultural pain and even destructive actions. Cultural pain can occur among coworkers who do not understand the beliefs and values, or even communication practices, of others (Leininger, 1995, 1997a). For example, a manager who is unaware of the value of not 'losing face' among Filipinos may openly confront a Filipina nurse, which may inflict cultural pain and loss of self esteem. The nurse manager did not intend to inflict cultural pain, but lacked transcultural mentorship knowledge as a nurse manager and was not able to recognize this important cultural phenomenon and the value of self esteem to the Filipina nurse.

Another example of cultural pain occurred when a Liberian nurse educator came to the Midwest to pursue a master's degree in nursing education. She wanted to work in a hospital as a nursing assistant while waiting to take the Commission on Graduates of Foreign Nursing Schools qualifying exam. Initially, she was not offered any type of mentorship, cultural orientation, or assimilation time. She was faced with unfortunate experiences that led to cultural shock and cultural pain within the hospital unit, in her graduate classes, and her daily lifeway. Although she had been genuinely welcomed, there was no indepth knowledge of her culture held by the school administration, faculty, or the hospital managers and staff. The nurse had no indepth understanding of the culture she was entering or of the administrators' beliefs and values. She needed assistance with verbal and nonverbal communication, hospital routines, medical equipment and supplies, writing skills, eating habits and foods, climate appropriate clothing choices (she had never experienced cold weather), transportation, computer skills, living alone, and homesickness. Many of the people she interacted with were unaware of her cultural values, beliefs, heritage, or the social structural dimensions (active civil war) of the life she had left behind in Liberia. The use of the universal care constructs and the Sunrise Enabler for actions to assist her were crucial for her survival in the USA, and were essential to her success in becoming comfortable and confident in a strange country.

National Travel Nurse Recruitment

Another subculture factor impacting upon local nursing cultures is the quickly growing cadre of nurses who travel nationwide accepting job placements in various healthcare systems (McLinden, 2003). Typically, travel nurses work for an average of 13 weeks before moving on to another assignment. When travel nurses begin an assignment, the other nurses of that particular local nursing culture realize the travelers are *temporary* members of their teams, creating the potential for separate subcultures in the work environment. Nurse managers need to orient travel nurses to the new culture when they arrive, enabling them to become functional team members who can function with multiple nursing team subcultures. Nurses recruited from other parts of the USA may be unfamiliar with the nursing culture in a new region of the country (e.g., a nurse from rural Montana assigned to Atlanta) as well as local cultural values and beliefs in the communities where they will be working. Managers need to include education and mentorship in transcultural nursing concepts, principles, policies, and procedures into the orientation process for travel nurses. Similarly, the travel nurse subculture may bring innovative ideas into local cultures. The Sunrise Enabler with the three modes of decisions and actions can be invaluable for the nurse to discover and expand her knowledge and expertise of the policies and protocols within local nursing cultures. An astute transcultural administrator or manager will recognize the value of transcultural nursing knowledge and mentorship in which they share the knowledge of the universal and diverse care constructs in order to foster positive team outcomes and arrive at culturally congruent client care, as well as providing opportunities for the travel nurse to experience career satisfaction in the employment setting.

Creative Administrative Actions

Nurse administrators and managers are challenged to provide a framework of orientation and education for nurses to work among many cultures. They strive to provide care in collaboration with other nurses and health care providers because ". . . a nurse is assumed to be a nurse and can provide care" (Leininger, 1997b). In the past, many healthcare systems have imposed the traditional Western medical model of care upon clients of various cultures. This cultural imposition (imposing one culture's beliefs, values, and behaviors upon another culture; Leininger, 1991) may lead to negative outcomes for clients. However, nurse administrators and managers with basic transcultural nursing knowledge and skills can greatly facilitate creative programs and policies that can lead to quality cultural care outcomes and result in high levels of client, team, and organizational satisfaction.

An example of a nursing administration creating a unique program to provide culturally congruent care occurred within a Southwestern Catholic healthcare system. Contracts had been acquired from two area Native American tribes for increased services within the system, but the nursing staff questioned how they could provide culturally appropriate care. The system's roots were within the Catholic health care mission and spirituality had been emphasized. A team comprised of a nurse administrator, a nurse from the religious community, and an Apache nurse decided to 'learn from the people's' spiritual leaders about the healing process (*emic* view). The Indian Health Service's national traditional medicine man was Comanche Edgar Monetathchi Jr., and he responded to the nurses' request for knowledge. The cultural sharing evolved to become a series of five- to seven-day experiential conferences, *Traditional Indian Medicine: Spirituality and Healing in Today's Health System*, taught by a faculty of Native American traditional medicine people with over 7000 participants. An evaluation conducted on the value characteristics of the nurses and interdisciplinary team members who were conference participants showed a statistically significant increase in their holistic values, increased self-esteem, and confidence in their ability and willingness to work with and among people of different cultures (Hubbert, 1986). As a result of the popularity of the conferences among the nurses, the health care system's department of nursing revised its mission statement and objectives, and developed new policies to reflect the inclusion of culture care accommodation dimensions. Learning from the people and then applying traditional Indian medicine philosophy to their traditional Western Catholic philosophy led to the recognition of the health care system as a national award winning model of holistic, transcultural nursing care (St. Mary's Second Century Foundation, 1986). The Sunrise Enabler with the three theoretical action and decision care modes were used by the nursing department managers. Mode I, *culture care preservation and-or maintenance*, was initially accomplished by the administrator's decision to create an environment for culturally congruent care of the Native American Indian clients. It included the system's own nursing culture focused on what the clients wanted to preserve of their own values, beliefs, and practices while in the hospital, and what the nurses wanted to preserve of their traditional philosophies and policies. Mode II, *culture care accommodation and-or negotiation*, was accomplished by assessing the client needs thereby gaining an understanding of the clients' and traditional medicine peoples' views (*emic* knowledge) of what the hospital provides. Accommodation was also achieved through the nurses learning from the traditional medicine people's philosophy of the healing process and wellbeing. Mode III, *culture care restructuring and-or repatterning*, was reflected in the development of new policies encouraging traditional (*emic*) care practices in client rooms and hiring native speaking liaisons. These pattern changes also included welcoming traditional medicine people at team meetings, allowing their visits anyplace in the healthcare system, and arranging for nurses to meet with native healthcare councils. Culture care restructuring and-or repatterning also occurred as the nursing department accepted a more holistic mission, objectives, and policies as they learned new philosophical views through participation in the week-long conferences and from working collaboratively with the traditional medicine people.

By restructuring the nursing department's mission, philosophy, and objectives, a newly emerging professional nurse case management (PNCM) program was established to focus on working in partnership with the clients and their families (Stempel, Carlson, & Michaels, 1996). The traditional nursing view regarding the nurse as expert in knowing the care a client needed was identified as a cultural clash (major differences between the professional and people's views, values, and beliefs; Leininger, 1991) between the PNCMs and the clients. However, the program chose to be guided by a holistic nursing model based on the principles learned from the traditional medicine people. The program staff chose to view the client as an expert in her or his own health, and developed a 'working partnership' mutually embracing respect for each person's right and responsibility for personal choice.

Summary

In this chapter several 21st century issues are presented which remain as challenges to transcultural nurse administrators and managers. Transcultural nursing administration is essentially a new area of study. Nurse administrators and nurse managers are increasingly being challenged to become transcultural nurse experts in order to direct, facilitate, and mentor the dominant national and transnational goal of providing culturally congruent care. Cultures and subcultures within nursing, institutional healthcare systems, and all members of the healthcare workforce are challenged to use transcultural nursing theory to provide culturally competent and congruent care. Leininger's Culture Care Theory with the Sunrise Enabler and other enablers can be powerful tools to assist in these endeavors. The Culture Care Theory is an excellent means for nurse administrators and managers to discover transcultural knowledge and to creatively develop care actions and decisions in order to transform health care from unicultural to multicultural perspectives and priorities. Cohesive relationships between and among different multicultural teams are being formed and expanded with the globalization of health care in order to provide culturally congruent care to meet the needs of people of diverse cultures.

References

American Nurses Association. (1991). Cultural diversity in nursing practice. *Position statement from the Council on Cultural Diversity in Nursing Practice*. Retrieved November 10, 2003, from http://www.nursingworld.org/readroom/position/ethics/dtcldv.htm.

Andrews, M. M. & Boyle, J. S. (1999). *Transcultural concepts in nursing care*. (3rd ed.). Philadelphia: Lippincott Williams & Wilkins.

Bola, T. V., Driggers, K., Dunlap, C., & Ebersole, M. (2003). Foreign-educated nurses: Strangers in a strange land? *Nursing Management, 34*(7), 39–42.

Cameron-Traub, E. (2002). Western ethical, moral, and legal dimensions within the culture care theory. In M. Leininger & M. McFarland (Eds.), *Transcultural nursing: Concepts, theories, research, & practice*. (3rd ed.). New York: McGraw-Hill.

Davis, C. R. & Nichols, B. L. (2002). Foreign-educated nurses and the changing U.S. nursing workforce. *Nursing Administration Quarterly, 26*(2), 43–51.

Gardenswartz, L. & Rowe, A. (1998). *Managing diversity in health care*. San Francisco: Jossey-Bass.

Glittenberg, J. (1995). Foreword. In M. Leininger (Ed.), *Transcultural nursing: Concepts, theories, research, and practice* (pp. xi–xii). Columbus, OH: McGraw-Hill College Custom Series.

Hubbert, A. O. (1986). *Effects of a five-day traditional Indian medicine experiential conference on the holistic value characteristics of professional nurses*. Unpublished master's thesis, University of Arizona, Tucson.

Leininger, M. (1988). *Care: The essence of nursing and health*. Detroit, MI: Wayne State University Press.

Leininger, M. (1991). *Culture care diversity and universality: A theory of nursing*. New York: National League for Nursing Press.

Leininger, M. (1995). *Transcultural nursing: Concepts, theories, research, and practice*. Blacklick, OH: McGraw-Hill College Custom Series.

Leininger, M. (1996). Transcultural nursing administration: An imperative worldwide. *Journal of Transcultural Nursing, 8*(1), 28–33.

Leininger, M. (1997a). Understanding cultural pain for improved health care. *Journal of Transcultural Nursing, 9*(1), 32–35.

Leininger, M. (1997b). Transcultural nursing research to transform nursing education and practice: 40 years. *Image: Journal of Nursing Scholarship, 29*(5), 341–347.

Leininger, M. (1998). Dominant culture care (emic) meanings and practice findings from Leininger's theory. *Journal of Transcultural Nursing, 9*(2), 45–48.

Leininger, M. & McFarland, M. R. (2002). *Transcultural nursing: Concepts, theories, research, & practice* (3rd ed.). New York: McGraw-Hill.

Marquis, B. L., & Huston, C. J. (2003). *Leadership roles and management function in nursing theory and application* (4th ed.). Philadelphia: Lippincott Williams & Wilkins.

Mclinden, S. (2003). Going places. *NurseWeek, 4*(17), 16–17.

Nyberg, J. J. (1998). *A caring approach in nursing administration.* Niwot, CO: University Press of Colorado.

Pacquiao, D. F. 2002). Foreign nurse recruitment and workforce diversity. *Journal of Transcultural Nursing, 13*(2), 89.

Stempel, J., Carlson, A., & Michaels, C. (1996). Working in partnership. In E. L. Cohen (Ed.), *Nurse case management in the 21st century.* St. Louis, MO: Mosby.

St. Mary's Second Century Foundation. (1986, Fall). *Traditional Indian medicine conferences: Spiritual focus in healing.* Tucson, AZ: St. Mary's Second Century Foundation.

Uhl Pierce, J. (1999). Managing managed care: The next level for transcultural nurses. *Journal of Transcultural Nursing, 10*(3), 181–182.

United States Department of Health & Human Services, Office of Minority Health. (2001). Revised CLAS standards. Retrieved July 20, 2001, from http://www.omhrc.gov/CLAS/finalcultural1a.htm.

Watson, J. (1994). Watson's philosophy and theory of human caring in nursing. *Conceptual models for nursing practice* (3rd ed.). Norwalk, CT: Appleton and Lange.

Wenger, A. F. (1995). Foreword. In M. Leininger (Ed.). *Transcultural nursing: Concepts, theories, research, and practice* (pp. xi–xii). Columbus, OH: McGraw-Hill College Custom Series.

Wilson, C. K. & Porter-O'Grady, T. (1999). *Leading the revolution in health care: Advancing systems, igniting performance* (2nd ed.). Gaithersburg, MD: Aspen Publishers.

CHAPTER FOURTEEN

Culture Care Theory and Uses in Nursing Administration*
[Revised Reprint]

Madeleine M. Leininger, PhD, LHD, DS, CTN, RN, FAAN, FRCNA

During the past three decades, several theorists, researchers, and scholars in the field of nursing have actively developed and systematically examined nursing's distinct domains of knowledge. A number of conceptual and theoretical perspectives have become evident with different research paradigms to explicate the phenomena of nursing. These developments have been encouraging as nursing delineates what constitutes its distinct focus to guide nursing education and practice. It has been a challenge to explicate nursing knowledge because of the complex and embedded ideas that characterize it, but also because of different theoretical interests and positions taken by nurses of what constitutes nursing's unique perspective as a discipline and profession.

Unquestionably, there is no right or wrong theory of nursing; rather, there are theories that have a lesser or greater potential to explain, describe, interpret, and predict nursing from a local to a worldwide perspective. It is academically and theoretically healthy to see nurses deliberate about different theories and concepts and not close the door on theories that may show some of the greatest potential to explain the universality of nursing and its unique features. It is, therefore, encouraging to see different theories being systematically examined or tested to determine what characterizes the nature and essence of nursing.

It is interesting that some nurses have already been 'fixed on' a few concepts, such as *man* (or *person*), *health*, *environment*, and *nursing* as the central concepts of the metaparadigm of nursing (Fawcett, 1984). But as I have stated earlier, these four concepts must be reconsidered because of their questionable limitations as central, distinct, or unique to nursing (Leininger, 1981, 1984), and for several reasons. First, man as a generic concept is not distinct to nursing, for most humanistic and

*This chapter is a revised and shortened version of the chapter, "Cultural Care Theory and Nursing Administration," as published in *Dimensions of Nursing Administration: Theory, Research, Education, Practice*, by Henry, B., Arndt, C., Di Vincenti, M., and Marriner-Tomey, A. (Eds.), St. Louis, MO: Mosby Publications, 1988, pp. 19–34.
**In this chapter, *nursing administration* refers both to academic education and nursing service administration unless specified otherwise.

scientific fields focus on *generic man*. Some disciplines such as anthropology have been intensively and extensively involved in studying
generic man for more than a century. Second, it is a logical contradiction to declare nursing as a distinct concept and then attempt to explain
the same phenomenon by the same term. Third, while environment and
health are possibilities to help explain nursing, further refinements and
more specificity are needed to show nursing's unique focus in relation
to many other disciplines that claim these concepts as central to their
field. To date, very few nurses have been doctorally prepared in the
environmental sciences, such as ecology, geography, human environments, and other closely related fields, to ensure establishing environment as totally distinct to nursing. Unquestionably, health has been of
historical interest to nurses since the Nightingale era, but only recently
have nurses focused indepth on health *per se*. Health as central to nursing will need more transcultural research to establish it as an epistemo-
logical base unique to nursing. Many disciplines make firm claims to
health as their unique discipline perspective, so it may not be a major
distinct phenomenon to nursing.

From an ethnohistorical and transcultural nursing perspective, *care*
has remained central to nursing, but it has not been studied indepth
and from an epistemic, historical, and ontologic stance until the last
three decades (Leininger, 1976, 1981, 1984, 1990a). Since the 1940s, I
have held that human care and caring are the distinct and unifying features of nursing, and that this perspective will remain well into the
future if nurses are committed to the full discovery and use of care
knowledge. It is of interest that many consumers and society as a collective institution have long viewed nursing as a caring profession, but
as one can see in the above metaparadigm (Fawcett, 1984), *care* is not
mentioned by some nurse leaders. As I have stated in several of my writings, human care and caring acts are, indeed, the essence and the most
promising construct to explain and predict nursing (Leininger, 1970,
1974a/b, 1978, 1981, 1984, 1988, 1990a). Care is the unique, dominant, and unifying focus of nursing. Care is a powerful concept with
which to describe, explain, interpret, and predict nursing outcomes.
Care as a noun is the phenomenon to be explained; *caring* as a gerund
implies the action component of care. And care as a central phenomenon to transcultural nursing has been a major focus since this field was
conceived in the mid-1950s (Leininger, 1967, 1970, 1978).

In this chapter, the theory of Culture Care Diversity and Universality
will be discussed for its importance and usefulness to academic and clinical nursing administrators. The rationale for nurse administrators to use
Culture Care Theory to promote and advance care is presented.

To make humanistic and scientific care an integral and visible part of nursing requires support from nursing administrators. A transcultural comparative cultural perspective is essential and a relatively new area of study and practice for most nurse administrators. It is a major focus for the future of nursing as our world of nursing becomes intensely multicultural. In addition, several research questions will be presented to stimulate nursing administrators to study and use findings generated from the Theory of Culture Care.

Rationale for Culture Care Theory in Nursing Administration

There are a number of reasons for focusing on the theory of Culture Care Diversity and Universality in nursing administration. First, the world of nursing administration with its norms, values, and practices is slowly beginning to shift from largely a unicultural to a multicultural focus. Nursing administration needs to change to a multicultural position to meet diverse consumer needs of clients, students, faculty, and others. Nurse administrators who are culturally alert to transcultural education and service practices realize the importance of understanding and working with people of many different cultures in the management processes, in decision making, and to establish appropriate institutional goals. Accordingly, administrators in their organizational structures, functions, and processes need to reflect these societal and worldwide changes to accommodate cultural diversity factors in their work. For without such knowledge, practices, and commitments a host of cultural conflicts, stresses, and problems will undoubtedly occur.

Nursing administrators as leaders need to make their practices congruent with changing cultural values, beliefs, and lifeways in their local workplace, but they also must reasonably fit with societal and worldwide trends. Healthcare administrators with a unicultural view are challenged by consumers and employees today to make their services responsive to many diverse cultural, individual, and group needs and not treat all consumers alike. Nursing service and education leaders need to become proactive to meet the needs of clients, students, faculty, and staff from diverse cultures. Indeed, far more attention needs to be given to the diverse and universal administrative practices that reflect new and different ways to provide culture care services. Most importantly, nurse administrators need a broad, comprehensive, and culturally based theory in order to expand their worldview and to be sensitive to a global or transcultural view of administrative activities, action modes, and decisions. The theory of Culture Care Diversity and Universality is one of the broadest and most comprehensive theories in nursing to meet some of the major expectations cited above, related to accommodating similarities and differences in educational and service settings. Culture Care Theory can provide a guideline for designing administrative practices based on specific modes of action and decision making from a worldwide perspective (Leininger, 1985a, 1988, 1990a).

A second major reason for using Culture Care Theory is that diverse cultural groups expect or demand that their values and practices be respected as a culture and as individuals. This requires that nurse administrators consider multicultural perspectives and understand different cultures as clients enter and leave administrative systems. There are increasing numbers of clients, staff, faculty, and students from many different cultures in the world who expect that nursing administrators and staff will make decisions and judgments that meet or at least consider their cultural needs as human rights. Cultural minorities in the United States and in foreign countries are not always represented in nursing care services and in nursing schools, and this must change with more minorities having rights to use health and educational services. In schools of nursing in the United States, most students are predominantly Anglo Americans and there are only a few cultural minorities represented (Leininger, 1989). Much more visible administrative efforts are needed to recruit, attract, and retain nursing students from many diverse cultures and subcultures. Nursing administrators need to reexamine their organizational philosophies, structures, values, and recruitment and retention processes to support and nurture multiculturalism.

In nursing care services, it is interesting to observe that service values and practices tend to be focused on one dominant culture, and cultural minority needs, values, and viewpoints may be recognized and addressed in limited fashion only. When the latter occurs, signs of misunderstanding, ineffective communication, cultural shock, cultural imposition, and many kinds of problems or conditions related to cultural negligence or avoidance with minority consumers often appear. The theory of Culture Care can serve as a broad framework to identify and develop nursing administration goals and programs, and as an action theory that will accommodate diverse cultural groups. At the same time, culture care diversity practices can greatly enrich administrative cultural practices and experiences of any environment.

A third reason that nurse administrators need to consider the theory of Culture Care is to develop organizational structures and functions that reflect different cultural values and gender differences in nursing. These dimensions are essential to develop relevant cultural norms and practices in program development, implementation, and evaluation in clinical and educational settings. In clinical settings, for example, one can envision for the immediate future many nurses from diverse and foreign cultures around the world seeking staff positions for client care. Nursing service administrators need to plan now to accommodate and maximize nurses' abilities in many different cultures. Administrators need to develop cultural orientation programs and ways to use the talents and assets of nurses from many different cultures. Nurses from other countries should be respected and understood for the ways they can provide effective, safe, and beneficial care to clients as well as for how they work with multidisciplinary staff. Nurses from diverse cultures have something to contribute to nursing education and service. Transcultural nursing is a two-way process and not a one-way system. As nurses from Egypt, Iraq, Philippines, Mexico, China, Japan, Korea, Eastern Europe, and virtually every place in the world are employed in different clinical settings and schools of nursing, their cultural value differences in gender, role expectations, and life experiences need to be identified and understood. How nursing administrators plan for and respond to these multicultural changes is important, for it is these nurses who will influence nursing care practices and educational systems. Cultural stresses and conflicts between nursing staff and clients will increase unless transcultural nursing education and services prevail that have been grounded in research findings generated from culturally based theory. Thus, nurse administrators need to anticipate worldwide changes and plan to meet multicultural education and service needs in this rapidly changing nursing world. Most importantly, nursing administrators need to maximize and use the knowledge and skills that nurses bring with them, rather than discredit, demean, or misuse nursing talents (Leininger, 1986, 1989).

It also is important to realize that nursing education administrators such as deans, associate and assistant deans, and other staff managers will play a major role in facilitating students and faculty from multicultures. Nursing educators need to support different teaching and learning methods and different ways to help students succeed and function in their career roles within different cultural orientations. Discovering and developing different teaching and learning methods for a new generation of multicultural students will be imperative, for nurses need to succeed and be successful in their career roles in diverse countries. Different teaching methods and a culturally based theory guide administrators and faculty toward that goal. Faculty and student problems and goals related to multicultural value differences are a major factor in student learning, in the recruitment and retention of students, and in educational goal attainment in schools of nursing. Educational administrative structures and policies should be flexible and reflect philosophies and practices that help students and faculty use and learn about multicultural variabilities.

Very few programs exist in nursing service and education that are focused on transcultural organizational structures to support cultural value differences or multicultural human services. Nor have the institutional cultures of nursing education and service been studied to identify and understand current practices that influence values, decision making, and normative practices. In the late 1960s and early 1970s, the theorist described the culture of nursing along with cultural imposition practices, leadership styles, and some changing values and practices in both education and service in the United States (Leininger, 1967, 1970, 1974a, 1978, 1987). The theory of Culture Care Diversity and Universality is a highly appropriate framework to study the culture of nursing and appropriate organizational structures in nursing education and clinical services as the theory includes the worldview, social structure factors, cultural values, environmental context, linguistic aspects, and ethnohistorical considerations. These dimensions are important to design future administrative organizations for nursing service and education systems.

Fourth, the theory of Culture Care has great possibilities to examine different types of professional and academic administrative organizations and their effectiveness or limitations. There is a cultural movement to develop new types of organizations, other than those of the traditional bureaucratic structures, to meet societal and worldwide changes. Culture Care Theory requires a systematic study of worldview, social structures, and cultural values, which would help identify potential patterns for differentiated administrative services. Knowing comparative differences or similarities in nursing service and education with respect to their purposes, goals, and functions is also important to render quality nursing services. What types of organizational structures would be most effective or provide a better linkage between nursing education and service? What criteria should be used to support transcultural programs in nursing education and service? What kinds of nursing organizations would support multiculturalism? What would be the strengths or limitations of different prototypes of nursing organizations for worldwide transcultural nursing education and service? These questions could be explored with Culture Care Theory.

In the United States, nursing faculty generally favor a *collegial type of academic administrative organization* in contrast to the traditional *rational-legal bureaucratic organization* (Henry et al., 1988; Leininger, 1984). *Collegial* type refers to participatory management decisions and actions made in a spirit of collegial respect with participants who are informed on the subject; whereas *rational-legal bureaucratic* type refers to decisions and actions that tend to be coercive, and are mandated from legal or rational stances (Rothschild & Russell, 1986). Some hospitals and clinics tend to espouse bureaucratic-like structures for efficiency and to support the dominant medical-authoritative organizational structure. With democratization growing in the world, one can expect more democratic cultural values and norms being used in institutions. This will be especially evident in nursing schools as nurses move between academic and clinical settings today and experience nondemocratic structures. Many nurses become quite dissatisfied with autocratic structures. Progressive nursing administrators are eager to change existing structures for democratic participatory organizations, and especially in democratized countries.

Professional nurses worldwide are seeking more autonomy and freedom to attain nursing's goals as a discipline and profession. Nurses want to regulate, maintain, and control their professional affairs without undue external pressures and oppressive controls. Tightly controlled bureaucratic organizations and administrative practices in education or service have historically limited nurses to achieve their professional goals. Thus, more collegial rather than legal–bureaucratic organizations are much desired for the new culture of nursing administration, and with a strong caring ethos. Since most Western nursing education schools have moved into institutions of higher learning, several new types of democratic cultures in nursing administration undoubtedly will be developed. However, there will be some nursing education and service administrative organizations that will value what I call the 'cult of efficiency,' the 'cult of compliance,' and the 'cult of pleasing others,' and may, at times, function as highly rational–legal bureaucratic structures. These structures will limit the full development of nursing, reduce multicultural accommodations, and fail to nurture a caring philosophy of administration. These structures tend to show signs of staff dissatisfactions, frustrations, and staff problems. In general, oppressive, controlling, and rigid organizations seldom are supported by nurses because of past oppressive and limiting opportunities with patriarchal systems (Leininger, 1974a). Thus organizational structures that anticipate and accommodate cultural care differences in management, human relationships, decision making, and respect female gender contributions will be in great demand. In addition, nursing education and service organizations will need to interface their organizations closely with local community and multicultural interest groups as well as with the larger society in which nursing functions. Being aware of local and societal perspectives with all their differences and similarities (including folk and professional group systems) will be important for nursing administrators.

An interesting area that merits study today is the growing trend toward the *corporatization of nursing education and health care services*. What are the actual or potential benefits and differences between corporate and noncorporate cultural care nursing systems? How will nursing systems interface and function within large corporate organizations? Comparative studies of corporate nursing systems as independent or interfacing cultures could well lead to some valuable insights about management and their effectiveness. In the future. it is reasonable to predict that corporate structures in institutions of higher education will prevail. Most of these corporate structures will be cloned after business management models rather than transcultural academic and nursing care models. What effect will these business-driven corporate structures have on the quality of nursing education and service where human caring services and a multicultural viewpoint are valued? How might nursing develop its own organizational or corporate care structure to fit with its distinct discipline and professional perspectives? Most assuredly, nursing organizational structures should be culturally congruent with discipline, theoretical, and service perspectives of the nursing profession.

Nursing is entering a new and challenging era with Western and nonWestern nurses coming together. Worldwide administrative organizational structures that support culturally congruent care and multiculturalism will be valued and in demand. Nurse administrators are being challenged to establish organizational structures that reflect these philosophic aspects for a global humanistic care agenda. The theory of Culture Care is an appropriate theory to develop futuristic administrative organizations that can provide culturally congruent care in education and service (Leininger, 1981, 1984, 1988). Most importantly, nursing administrators need futuristic plans that will accommodate rapid value changes and work with nurses from everywhere in the world. These administrators will need to support different configurations of cultures. Working with nurses for short periods of time who are highly mobile will be challenging. The theory of Culture Care provides one means to design future administrative education and service programs with the goals and trends in mind.

Research Areas of Inquiry Related to Culture Care Theory for Nursing Administrators

Since the theory of Culture Care is presented in this book with transcultural care research studies, only research questions for nursing service and education administrators will be discussed in this chapter. These areas of inquiry are offered to stimulate nurse administrators to explore what is universal or diverse about nursing administration worldwide, and to consider ways to get to new knowledge in order to develop administrative organizations and practices. A comparative ethnoadministrative theoretical and research focus is needed to achieve this goal and to obtain fresh perspectives about nursing education and service (Leininger, 1985b, 1990b). Culture Care Theory with the ethnonursing research method is recommended to study ethnoadministrative practices. Other ethnomethods, however, such as ethnography, ethnoscience, life histories, audiovisuals, metaphors, and phenomenology, could be used to discover the often invisible, covert, and little known administrative aspects of human care and other nursing phenomena. The qualitative paradigm offers one of the best means to explicate culture care; however, the ethnonursing method is the method designed specifically for the Culture Care Theory (Leininger, 1985b). The need to discover indepth meanings and comparative cultural data bearing upon a human care and nursing administration within naturalistic and familiar context is important.

Research Questions for Nursing Service Administrators Using Culture Care Theory

1. What are the comparative meanings and interpretive expressions of cultural care to nurse administrators locally and in different countries?
2. In what ways can nurse administrators make human care a clearly visible, coherent, and central focus of nursing services?
3. What attributes and characteristics constitute universal and diverse features of nursing care administration in Western and nonWestern cultures?
4. What alternative types or models of nursing service organization and management practices show the greatest potential to serve people of different cultures?
5. What are the strengths and limitations of a collegial type of organizational structure versus a legalistic–bureaucratic organization for Western and nonWestern nursing service administration?
6. What cultural care stresses and conflicts do clients of diverse cultural backgrounds experience with administrators and staff who espouse cultural values that are clearly different from those of clients or staff nurses?
7. What innovative approaches can nursing service administrators use to accommodate cultural care differences in nursing care practices and provide congruent care practices for clients?
8. In what ways do the worldview, social structure, cultural values, language, history, and environmental context influence nursing education and service practices?

9. What strategies could be used to help nursing administrators shift from the present emphasis on resource reallocation, technological efficiency, and 'bottom line' cost effectiveness to that of quality nursing care services for specific clients of diverse or similar cultures?

10. Given the fact that a number of cultures and minority groups, do not utilize or seek professional nursing and other healthcare services for many cultural reasons, what creative approaches or strategies could be used to attract these cultural groups to use hospital or community-based nursing services when necessary?

11. What are some diverse or universal ethical and clinical problems for nurses when providing care to clients of different cultures, especially those whose values, beliefs, and practices differ considerably from the philosophy, norms, and values of nursing service administration?

12. In what ways could nursing service administrators establish care as the central focus of nursing and with a highly favorable public image of nursing worldwide?

13. How could nursing service managers market the quality of cultural care in a cost-effective, caring way to clients of both diverse and similar cultures?

14. Since Western nursing care values and practices tend to contrast sharply with many nonWestern culture care values, how could nursing service administrators prepare nurses to deal with such differences in order to reduce client stresses, conflicts, and nontherapeutic care practices?

15. Since cultural imposition practices are a serious and prevailing clinical problem (Leininger, 1991a), how might nursing service administrators reduce or change cultural imposition practices?

16. In what ways does the theory of Culture Care contribute to differentiated nursing practices?

17. How can nursing service administrators and staff discover, document, and evaluate culturally congruent care?

18. What are some of the major reasons or factors preventing nurse administrators from focusing on comparative cultural care?

19. What research methods offer the greatest promise to accurately and credibly describe and interpret care phenomena of diverse cultures and their nursing care needs?

20. Given the litigious nature of human beings, what could nurse administrators do today to prevent serious legal suits with multicultural groups and of cultural care negligence?

21. With the future trend for community based home care services, what kinds of nursing service organizations need to be developed to accommodate lifecycle needs and provide culturally congruent home care?

Research Questions for Nursing Education Administrators Using Culture Care Theory

1. What are the universal and diverse meanings and interpretations of cultural care among nursing administrators and faculty in schools of nursing?
2. What universal and diverse administrative care approaches could be used to recruit and retain nursing faculty and students of diverse cultures, and especially cultural minorities that are underrepresented in schools of nursing?
3. What types of organizational structures show the best promise to establish and promote a philosophy of cultural care and concomitant educational practices in schools of nursing?
4. How do the worldview, social structure, cultural values, linguistic expressions, history, and environmental factors influence cultural care education practices in nursing schools?
5. How might nurse administrators and faculty facilitate use of the theory of Culture Care to guide changes in philosophy, organizational structure, and curricula in schools of nursing to accommodate students, faculty, and staff from diverse cultures locally and transnationally?
6. Since so few nurse administrators and faculty have had formal preparation in transcultural nursing and human care, how might the theory of Culture Care help stimulate changes to meet this future emphasis in nursing?
7. In light of the rapid changes and demands for multicultural and transcultural nursing education, what could nurse administrators and nursing service leaders do together to prepare a new generation of nurses to be culturally sensitive, knowledgeable, and skilled in transcultural nursing?
8. What innovative administrative strategies could nursing deans use to support faculty to use a multicultural care approach to teaching, research, and practice?
9. How could Culture Care Theory be used in a collaborative way with nursing service staff in research projects to reinforce and build upon the goal of providing culture congruent care services?
10. How could Culture Care Theory be used to help academic nurse administrators reduce cultural imposition practices with faculty and between nursing service and education?
11. Since cultural conflicts and stresses are anticipated to markedly increase in schools of nursing due to heightened multiculturalism, how might the three modes of actions and decisions in Leininger's (1985a/b, 1988) theory of Culture Care be used to reduce multicultural conflicts and legal suits?

12. What incentives could be used to help nurse educators move from largely a unicultural to a multicultural perspective in administrative services?
13. What accounts for the diverse or similar administrative practices of deans in schools of nursing worldwide?
14. How might the theory of Culture Care be used to generate public policies incorporating transcultural nursing into administrative management practices on university campuses, in local communities, and in public sectors?
15. What is the potential consequence of having 'corporate cultures' in schools of nursing? Will they support humanistic caring ethos with favorable benefits?
16. What might be the predicted outcome if nursing administrators were actively committed to and implemented culturally based humanistic care teaching and administrative practices?
17. What are the universal and nonuniversal ethical care problems that nursing administrators and faculty face when nonsensitive cultural care practices exist? .
18. What universal culture care concepts, principles, and research-based content needs to be taught to students in baccalaureate, master's, doctoral, and postdoctoral nursing degree programs to increase transcultural care knowledge and practices?
19. What are the multicultural public images and interpretation problems related to the current public tagline: "If caring were enough, anyone could be a nurse"? How might this tagline be improved or changed in the future for a more accurate and positive view of nursing?

From the above questions, one can note there are many studies that merit investigation to advance transcultural nursing administration with a care focus. The theory of Culture Care offers good possibilities for its use by nurse administrators in academic and service settings.

Administrators are truly faced with a growing number of diverse cultural and social forces that are influencing nursing education and practice. Many of these critical administrative problems are bearing directly on our rapidly changing society and culture norms. With future demands from clients, nursing students, and faculty to have transcultural care knowledge as an integral part of nursing and a specialization area, nursing administrators must be prepared to meet these needs. No longer can they remain uniculturally oriented or use nursing theories and practices that are ethnocentric or culture-bound. Successful nurse administrators are challenged to be knowledgeable and open to accommodate consumers of multicultural orientations and backgrounds. An open and comprehensive theory such as Culture Care offers a means to discover new insights about administrative practices in nursing service and education.

A number of nursing service and education administrators are using nonnursing theories, ideologies, or philosophies to guide their judgments and actions. Some of these nursing service administrators tend to rely heavily on biomedical disease and symptom alleviation ideologies and practices to guide their administrative decisions rather than nursing care theories and practices. There are some nursing service administrators who borrow, almost wholesale, specific theories and models from economics, public administration, and business to study and guide their administrative practices. In nursing education, there are deans and associate deans who rely on general education theories and practices. Still too few administrators have learned how to use and value nursing theories to generate administrative decisions and actions. It seems ironic to find so many nursing administrators in education and service using only some of the 18 or more major nursing theories to guide their deliberations and for differentiated practices. This is a serious and problematic cultural lag that needs to be recognized if nurses are to advance nursing as a discipline and profession with its distinct perspectives. For without a nursing theoretical perspective, nurses and nurse administrators may be offering questionable client care services.

As nursing moves into the future, I contend that nurse administrators in education and service can benefit from the use of Culture Care Theory or from other similar care theories to help them move soundly into the 21st century. These care theories are needed to provide a worldwide focus to nursing education and services because of future mobility and changing nurses' practices. They need a broad holistic theory as well as an action-oriented specific care theory. Therefore, it is time to prepare nurse administrators for top and middle-level multicultural administrative care practices. These nursing administrators need to reflect nursing's distinct contribution to nursing through the use of current and future transcultural human care knowledge and practices. Nursing administrators as leaders in nursing can make a great difference in changing health care systems, developing new policies and altering public care practices.

Although the future of nursing is promising, nursing administrators, as a key leadership group, must begin to shift from largely a unicultural to a multicultural perspective and use appropriate care theories to guide their judgments and decisions. Nurse administrators will find that the theory of Culture Care with three modes of nursing actions (i.e., cultural care preservation and-or maintenance, cultural care accommodation and-or negotiation, and cultural care repatterning and-or restructuring) should be most helpful to develop new administrative practices in education and service. Unquestionably, the theory is highly relevant and readily available for nurse administrators to use in our rapidly changing multicultural administrative and practice world.

References

Fawcett, J. (1984). The metaparadigm to nursing: Present status and future refinements. *Image: Nurse Scholarship, 16*(3), 84–86.

Henry, B. et al. (1988). *Dimensions of nursing administration: Theory, research, education, practice* (pp. 19–34). St. Louis, MO: Mosby.

Leininger, M. M. (1967). The culture concept and its relevance to nursing. *The Journal of Nursing Education, 6*(2), 27–39.

Leininger, M. M. (1970). The cultural concept and American culture values in nursing. *Nursing and anthropology: Two worlds to blend* (pp. 45–52). New York: John Wiley & Sons.

Leininger, M. M. (1974a). The leadership crises in nursing: A critical problem and challenge. *The Journal of Nursing Administration, 4*(2), 28–34.

Leininger, M. M. (1974b). Towards conceptualization of transcultural health care systems: Concepts and a model. *Human care issues, transcultural health care issues and conditions* (pp. 3–23). Philadelphia: F. A. Davis.

Leininger, M. M. (1976). Caring: The essence and central focus of nursing. American Nurses Foundation. *Nursing Research Report, 12*(1), 2, 14.

Leininger, M. M. (1978). *Transcultural nursing: Concepts, theories, and practices.* New York: John Wiley & Sons.

Leininger, M. M. (1981). *Care: An essential human need.* Thorofare, NJ: Slack.

Leininger, M. M. (1984). Care: The essence of nursing and health. In M. M. Leininger (Ed.), *Care: The essence of nursing and health* (pp. 3–15). Thorofare, NJ: Slack.

Leininger, M. M. (1985a). Transcultural care diversity and universality: A theory of nursing. *Nursing and Health Care, 6*(4), 209–212.

Leininger, M. M. (1985b). *Qualitative research methods in nursing* (pp. 33–73). Orlando, FL: Grune & Stratton.

Leininger, M. M. (1986). Care facilitation and resistance factors. In Z. Wolf (Ed.), *Clinical care in nursing* (pp. 1–24). Gaithersburg, MD: Aspen Publications.

Leininger, M. M. (1987). *Care: Discovery and uses in clinical and community nursing* (pp. 1–30). Detroit, MI: Wayne State University Press.

Leininger, M. M. (1988). Leininger's theory of nursing: Cultural care diversity and universality. *Nursing Science Quarterly, 2*(4), 11–20.

Leininger, M. M. (1989). Transcultural nursing: A worldwide necessity to advance nursing knowledge and practice. In J. McCloskey & H. Grace (Eds.), *Nursing issues.* Boston: Little, Brown.

Leininger, M. M. (1990a). Historic and epistemologic dimensions of care and caring with future directions. In J. Stevenson (Ed.), *Knowledge about care and caring: State of the art and future developments* (pp. 19–31). Kansas City, MO: American Nurses Association Press.

Leininger, M. M. (1990b, Winter). Ethnomethods: The philosophic and epistemic basis to explicate transcultural nursing knowledge. *Journal of Transcultural Nursing, 1*(2), 40–51.

Leininger, M. M. (1991a). Becoming aware of types of health practitioners and cultural imposition. *Journal of Transcultural Nursing, 3*(1).

Leininger, M. M. (1991b). *Current view of the culture of nursing.* Unpublished manuscript.

Rothschild, J., & Russell, R. (1986). Alternatives to bureaucracy: Democratic participation in economy. In R. Turner &. J. Short Jr. (Eds.), *Annual review of sociology* (pp. 12, 307–345). Palo Alto, CA: Annual Reviews.

CHAPTER FIFTEEN

Synposes of Classic Research Studies on Philippine and U.S. Nurses, and the Culture Care of Dying Patients in Hospitals and Hospice

Madeleine M. Leininger, PhD, LHD, DS, CTN, RN, FAAN, FRCNA

In this section, two classic transcultural nursing studies are summarized to show the thoughtful use of the Culture Care Theory with other cultures. Due to space constraints, only a brief summary of each study will be presented. The reader is, however, encouraged to read the full chapter of the research as presented in the First Edition (Leininger, 1991) of the Culture Care Theory book. The authors hold that these two studies are excellent examples of the use of the theory and method with different domains of inquiry to study major American cultures in clinical, hospital, and community contexts.

Culture Care of Philippine and Anglo American Nurses in a Hospital Context

(Zenaida Spangler, RN, PhD)

This transcultural nurse specialist chose as her domain of inquiry to *identify and analyze the similarities and differences in nursing care of Anglo American and Philippine nurses as they cared for clients in a general hospital context* in the United States (USA). Spangler (1991) did an extensive review of the literature and found no studies focused on a comparison of these two nursing cultures. It was the first indepth qualitative study to specifically focus on culture care differences and similarities between caregivers of two different cultures in a hospital setting. The Culture Care Theory was used to explicate the meanings, expressions, and patterns of caregiving by nine key Anglo American nurse informants and 10 Philippine nurse informants. In addition, 13 general Anglo American nurse informants and 16 general Philippine nurse informants were studied. The study was conducted in a 200-bed acute care hospital located in the Northeastern USA. The Leininger Ethnonursing Four Phases of Data Analysis (1991) were used to rigorously and systematically analyze a large amount of rich qualitative data from indepth interviews, direct observations, and participation by the researcher over a considerable time span. The Leininger-Templin-Thompson Ethnonursing software was used to analyze dominant themes related to the domain of inquiry and the theoretical hunches and questions posed by the researcher. Leininger's six criteria for analyzing qualitative research data were used: credibility, conformability, meaning-in-context, recurrent patterning, saturation, and transferability (Leininger & McFarland, 2002, pp. 88–89).

The research findings were significant as they revealed a number of differences between the Anglo American and Philippine nurses in caregiving to hospital clients. Only a few universal themes were discovered, but several differences between the nurses representing the two different cultures were discovered. The first major difference was that Anglo American nurses expressed a strong regard for promoting client independence and self care practices compared with Philippine nurses. Anglo nurses stressed autonomous care and patient education. The promotion of self care and independence with clients fit with Anglo American values for self reliance and independence. These values, however, failed to lead to culturally congruent care with several nonAnglo clients as predicted by Leininger's theory.

Philippine nurses did not discuss and stress self care nor patient education in caring practices. A second major difference was that Philippine nurses included family members in the care of clients. The concept of 'coaxing family' to help clients and to use 'lambing' (which was playful coaxing or cajoling) was used by Philippine nurses. In contrast, Anglo American nurses tried to convince patients to become independent in care practices. Anglo nurses focused less on involving family participation and responsibilities. Most importantly, Anglo American nurses wanted to be in control or to be 'on top of things' in caregiving, especially in the intensive care units. They watched for changes in client behavior and were directive in shaping or influencing situations so they could be and-or were 'in control.'

Third, Philippine nurses had a deep sense of duty and a commitment to function like 'good nurses.' Nursing was a vocation to work and care for patients, and if they did not maintain this attitude 'they felt guilty.' To Philippine nurses, care for clients was a commitment and obligation, and they gave much attention to physical comfort as a major care value. They saw physical caregiving as an important means to develop relationships with patients and spent time making patients comfortable through physical care activities. Interestingly, Anglo American nurses did not view bedmaking and giving baths as care priorities. These comparative care differences between Anglo and Philippine nurses were evident and frequently led to nurse conflicts and misunderstandings with clients and families.

Fourth, the commonly heard universal theme of the 'nurse shortage' in the hospital led to nurse frustrations and to nurses saying they were unable to provide professional nursing care. The nursing shortage was a commonly expressed reason both nursing groups gave for not being able to provide 'total patient care.' It was also a major frustration. The nurses also held that the hospital institutional norms, standards, and values strongly influenced both Anglo and Philippine nursing practices and nurse satisfaction in giving and maintaining quality care.

The study also supported the major tenets of the Culture Care Theory, and the ethnonursing research method was viewed as a critical means to tap rich, informative, and detailed data. These findings were the first detailed documentation available in nursing to show comparisons of nurses from two different cultures as they functioned with their generic and professional care values, beliefs, and practices. Areas of differences and similarities in care were clearly evident. Unquestionably, nurses who had been educated in transcultural nursing used 'holding knowledge' of cultures to provide culturally congruent care. It was clear that to rely on 'encounters' or to learn 'on the spot' with clients was not effective in providing care. Holding knowledge was essential to examine the three modes of care as predicted in Leininger's theory for effective, healthy, and successful outcomes. The researcher discussed how the three modes could or should be used for beneficial health outcomes and to reduce cultural conflicts and care problems. This research study has valuable findings to help nurses provide culturally congruent care for clients.

Culture Care Theory for Study of Dying Patients in Hospital and Hospice Contexts

Marie Gates, RN, PhD

The researcher who conducted this study was a transcultural nurse with considerable experience as a community health nurse. Her domain of inquiry was focused on *discovery of the meanings, experiences, and orientations of caring for dying patients in hospital and in hospice settings*. The researcher was especially interested to learn the meanings and experiences that dying and hospice patients gave to *care* and *cure*.

This researcher was also interested in identifying ways that different sociocultural factors influenced the culture of the patient, the hospital, and hospice, as well as ways holistic care factors influenced the meanings, experiences, and orientation of care and cure with dying patients. She posed several research questions:

1. What are the meanings of *care* and *cure* to persons who are dying?
2. What experiences do persons have with care and cure during the living–dying interval?
3. What characteristics of care and cure orientation exist with dying patients?
4. In what ways does the hospital and hospice setting and the institutional culture influence care and cure meanings, experiences, and the orientations of persons in the dying process?

Unquestionably, this research study was of interest to many health care personnel as the meanings of *care* and *cure* of dying clients had been limitedly studied in a systematic and indepth way. Leininger's theory of Culture Care Diversity and Universality was used along with the ethnonursing research method. The major tenets of the theory were identified with a specific focus on the discovery of linkages between care and wellbeing with dying clients. An explication of such knowledge and the discovery of the influences of the hospital and hospice culture on the dying client were important to advance transcultural knowledge. The researcher examined Leininger's premise: *There can be no curing without caring, but caring can exist with curing.* Thus, care and cure were closely interrelated. Gates (1991) was also interested in exploring evidence of *generic* and *professional* care as practiced by nurses in *the dying and living process* (Martocchio, 1982). Gates used the living–dying interval construct to approach clients, which meant being aware that their illness was likely to lead to death and usually not recovery. These theoretical hunches guided her study with 12 key and 12 general informants in each setting whom she carefully selected for the indepth study. The key informants selected were patients who had an illness designated by the primary physician or nurse that was expected to lead to death within one year. There were 24 key informants who were interviewed and observed over a span of time (approximately 1 year). The age range was from 25 to 84 years and included seven male informants. All informants had a diagnosis of cancer. Two thirds of the informants were Anglo Americans and one third African Americans, all of whom resided in a large urban Midwestern community. The patients varied in marital status. All informants had family members viewed as 'support persons' to help them. All had an identified religion, but two informants no longer practiced their religion.

In contrast with key informants, the general informants were nurses, care providers, family members, volunteers, and visitors. They were interviewed once regarding the domain of inquiry for about 45 minutes. Extensive field notes were kept. Audio taping with the informants' permission was used to document observations, detailed meanings, and experiences. The researcher's observations, reflections, and confirmed observations were all recorded and analyzed. The researcher used Leininger's enabler guides to obtain indepth data and to confirm findings from key and general informants (Leininger & McFarland, 2002). The well known Sunrise Enabler, Participant Observation Enabler, the Researcher's Interview Guide, and the Stranger Friend Enabler were all held as valuable to obtain obscure and subtle data.

There were many very important and revealing findings which the reader is encouraged to read in the full research study (Leininger, 1991, pp. 281–304). New breakthroughs in knowledge were obtained from this study about the hospital and hospice living and dying experiences. A few major findings can be mentioned. First, both diversities and commonalities in themes were discovered. The many detailed descriptions and informant verbatim statements were significant to understand the full meaning and experiences of the dying informants in their specific living–dying contexts. The first major theme and significant recurrent finding was *patients caring for others*. Interestingly, *all* patients were eager to *give care to others without receiving care or something in return*. This finding was evident in both the hospital and hospice care settings. All key informants told of ways they *cared for others*, especially their family members. They gave examples of cooking for family members, giving presence to them, and helping them to organize monthly bills and even to prepare for their anticipated funerals. The informants were grateful for the interval time (before dying) so they could help family members and others prepare for the informant's death. Informants frequently expressed their desire to *give to others*, especially to family, significant others, and friends. They gave something held to be meaningful, important, and valued. They also actively cared for patient–roommates in the hospital by calling for the nurse, writing letters, making phone calls, and offering help in daily activities. The informants' care–caring activities also extended to staff in the hospital and hospice such as bringing them treats, telling jokes (in a caring way), or buying staff members gifts. Some informants spoke of caring for their physicians because some physicians found it 'difficult to care for the dying or to talk about the dying.' They felt caring for others (not self care) helped them to *live* even when they knew they were *dying*. Another finding was that informants *were open to receive care from others,* such as care from family members and professional care providers in each setting. They liked to receive care mostly from their family members. This was held as the greatest value and better than receiving care from professional staff.

In the hospital setting, *care was viewed mainly as doing*, whereas in the hospice setting, *care was largely giving presence* to the client mainly from *family and significant others*. This was a dominant care theme in both settings. Several key informants stressed the importance of receiving care from their physicians in the hospital and hospice setting. Informants valued nonrushing care and to have care by physicians who took time to explain their treatments. In the hospice setting, physicians were often described as 'loved by patients.' In both settings, a major caring value was talking and listening to clients. Most key informants saw physical and psychological care as a priority, but they found differences in giving and receiving care in each setting. Hospital patients valued 'bathing, feeding, control of symptoms and managing their pain and nausea' to be important in caring. In contrast, several hospice clients were not too interested in these caring actions.

Gates (1991) discovered two additional themes. *Hope was the outcome of care while living and dying.* Remaining hopeful was an important care mode. Another theme finding was that *living while dying was manifested in daily living.* Patients often said they were *living while dying* and wanted staff to know and value this idea. The informants were open to talk about their feelings that promoted daily living, dying, and caring for others. Other diverse themes were *reliance on others* and *getting support in the system and from family members.* Physicians needed help from nurses to teach them caring modes especially with dying patients. *Setting limits as caring* was another theme, which meant preventing detrimental acts by caregivers or by clients. *Challenging patients when their behavior was inappropriate while dying* was a diverse finding. It meant 'not getting by with absurd behavior.' The researcher found that while nurses gave care they needed to increase their awareness and knowledge of ways to incorporate cultural, social, and spiritual aspects of care into practices.

Peaceful dying was identified and requested. The need to consciously include culturally congruent care was still an ideal to be attained by the caregivers. The dominant theme of *living while dying* was clearly supported by all informants. The family and significant others were expected to understand this theme in both hospital and hospice contexts. There were many sociocultural factors as depicted in the Sunrise Enabler that influenced care in the living–dying process in both settings. These factors merited full consideration in providing congruent care practices. Additional findings were reported in Gates' chapter (Leininger, 1991).

References

Leininger, M. (1991). *Culture care diversity and universality: A theory of nursing*. New York: National League for Nursing/Jones and Bartlett (Redistributed 1996).

Leininger, M., & McFarland, M. (2002). *Transcultural nursing: Concepts, theories, research and practices*. New York: McGraw-Hill.

Gates, M. (1991). Transcultural comparison of hospital and hospice as caring environments for dying patients. *Journal of Transcultural Nursing, 2*(2), 3–15.

Martocchio, B. C. (1982). *Living while dying*. Bowie, MD: Robert J. Brady.

Spangler, Z. (1991). Nursing care values and caregiving practices of Philippine and Anglo American nurses. In M. M. Leininger (Ed.), *Culture care diversity and universality: A theory of nursing* (pp. 119–146). New York: National League for Nursing Press.

CHAPTER SIXTEEN

Envisioning the Future of Culture Care Theory and Ethnonursing Method

Madeleine M. Leininger, PhD, LHD, DS, CTN, RN, FAAN, FRCNA

Whenever an artist creates anew, undoubtedly a vision into the future comes with one's ideas and new perspectives. In this last chapter, the author will share some of her vision, hopes, and predictions for the future of the theory of Culture Care linking them to the theorist's early ideas about launching the new discipline of transcultural nursing. From its beginning in the 1960s, the theorist was excited about the potential of the theory as nurses learned the theory and the ethnonursing research method. The theorist was optimistic and envisioned that the theory and the method would survive and would be used well into the future. The theory was relevant to a growing multicultural world and filled the critical need for research based culture care knowledge. Most importantly, the theory and the method were highly innovative, challenging to use, and were predicted to have great benefits to consumers. The theorist also believed the findings from the theory would lead to some entirely new ways of knowing, helping, and serving people of diverse cultures. The theory and method were greatly needed as there were no specific nursing theories on cultures and care when the theory was being developed. Furthermore, in the 1960s there was no culturally based nursing care theory that was holistic, and recognized that multiple factors influence people care and lead to wellbeing and health.

Most importantly, a research method was desired by the theorist to fit with the theory instead of using multiple methods borrowed from different disciplines that were not congruent with the theory. At this time in nursing, nurses were heavy borrowers of methods that were narrow in scope and limited to a few variables that would lead to finite measurements. The theorist was concerned how nurses could discover care and caring with people of diverse and complex cultures without reducing their findings to meaningless statements. There were no nursing theories that had a specific method to discover theoretical predictions. Instead, there were narrow hypotheses and a few variables to test with a measurable tool. The theorist had already experienced in nursing and anthropology that many human phenomena about people and cultures could not be reduced and measured for meaningful outcomes. She also knew nursing was holistic and somewhat like anthropology in that one had to enter the people's world and study multiple factors influencing health and wellbeing. Thus, the method had to be holistic for the discovery of complex and subtle aspects of human beings, especially those related to care, health, and cultures. During the past 50 years, this holistic theory and method have been increasingly valued for bringing forth indepth knowledge about care and health. Most encouragingly, other health disciplines have begun to study and value holistic factors influencing the care, health, and wellbeing of diverse cultures.

From the beginning, the theorist envisioned that care and health phenomena were complex and embedded in social and cultural structural factors that needed to be discovered and studied indepth. Astute observations, friendly interviews, trusting relationships, and an appropriate research method that fit with the theory were needed. The theorist also envisioned that obtaining data directly from informants, rather than from secondary sources or by recall, was essential. Obtaining cultural informants' care values, beliefs, meanings, and lifeways was important to obtain new insights about human care and how they contributed to preserving and maintaining health among cultures. No longer could the linguistic use of the word *care* be taken for granted. This important philosophical stance and belief of the theorist led to the use of qualitative research methods to unlock and discover care knowledge. The qualitative approach was predicted to bring forth objective and subjective data related to human beings and their cultural care orientations. The theorist predicted care knowledge would ultimately provide very rich and meaningful data which could profoundly change healthcare services well into the future. Subsequently, these theoretical premises have been studied using the theory and the qualitative ethnonursing method.

This book contains many examples of these theory based discoveries that reveal the ways the theory and method can be used to discover human caring from a transcultural focus. From the work of the authors and that of other transcultural researchers, several major features of the theory and the method are presented. These summary points can be most helpful for the reader to consider while reflecting on the chapters by different authors, and can be helpful to teach and conduct research and to guide students, practitioners, and administrators about providing care services to diverse cultures. The differences and similarities in comparison to other current theories will help to show that quality healthcare services need to be based upon cultural knowledge.

Globalization of health care and the differences and similarities among and between human groups and cultures will continue as a growing imperative. Comparative health knowledge of cultures worldwide will become increasingly important. Discovering the uniqueness of cultures about their health and wellness care patterns will be in demand to provide quality care services, to reduce health costs, and to promote early healing and recovery. Discovering differences and similarities with respect to cultures and subcultures will lead to some new and profound changes in health practices. The old belief to *treat all clients alike* will be eliminated and differentiated care practices will prevail and become essential for use by culture care providers. Comparative care and health research will be one of the greatest contributions to health services for diverse cultures in countries worldwide. Researchers will use the Culture Care Theory for specific human healthcare practices to guide decisions and prevent racial biases. The universals or commonalities of care will be valuable in healing, recovery processes, and to prevent illness as well as disabilities. In keeping with the theory, comparative folk or generic care practices will be more fully discovered in the future and will greatly expand health knowledge for beneficial care practices. The Theory of Culture Care with the ethnonursing method will be used to obtain indepth qualitative and specific data about care expressions and meanings. This will support the goal of the theory, which is *to provide culturally congruent care*—the theorist's goal since the 1960s. This goal will become a transcultural goal worldwide. The universalities or commonalities of care and health will be valued, used, and recognized as the theory helps to open the door to many new discoveries and insights about care and health. These findings will become central for use in healthcare services.

Given that most health disciplines have given limited attention to the role of care to keep people well, to prevent illnesses, or to sustain wellbeing, research guided by the Culture Care Theory will explain and predict wellness, wellbeing, and health. This new focus will be of great importance in the future to reduce health costs and provide safe and therapeutic care. Discovering culture care meanings, symbols, and expressions of care with cultural patterns and benefits in different societies will serve as a powerful guide for nursing actions and decisions. It will be a different theoretical and research approach than in the past. Discovering care patterns and how they can help cultures attain and maintain health and wellbeing will become dominant research and practice foci. Discovering *care* and *caring* patterns that contribute to wellness and health with beneficial outcomes is predicted to be a major new breakthrough in the 21st century and beyond.

The Culture Care Theory has lead to a new paradigm in health care. It moves researchers away from the dominant and narrow focus on medical, pathologic, and symptom focus to a broader perspective of human care behavior. Most assuredly, focusing on cultures has been a new and holistic way to discover health and wellbeing. The theory has led to new emphasis on fully learning about people and their culture care practices. It is an exciting challenge for nurses and others to discover the power of care and wellbeing; it is a different focus for many practitioners and offers some new challenges to the healthcare system. Nurses are becoming very interested in learning about cultures with the goals of discovering human caring symbols, attributes, and care meanings, as well as the ways cultures maintain wellness and prevent illnesses and disabilities throughout the lifecycle. The power and efficacy of care is the new thrust of modern practitioners and researchers.

In the future, as healthcare research becomes focused on generic [emic] derived care and professional [etic] care, some of the greatest changes in health care will occur as these types of care differ from most present day practices. The challenge will be to make generic and professional blend or be safely used together. If they fail to fit, unfavorable outcomes and some destructive or nontherapeutic care will occur. To date, several transcultural nurse researchers have led the way to discover the importance of generic [emic] care and how it contrasts with professional [etic] care of specific cultures. As a consequence, several new ways of knowing, understanding, and helping people have become evident and valued. Generic care needs to be preserved by cultures to prevent cultural imposition practices from clients of diverse cultures. Considerably more research, however, is needed to support generic and professional care to become congruent, safe, and meaningful to diverse cultures. When this occurs, one will find that cultural imposition practices, racial biases, and other negative practices will be markedly reduced or eliminated.

Preventative practices must be research based and examined with cultures using the three action and practice modes explicated in the theory. Discovering ways that these three major care modes fit together requires rigorous study and very thoughtful and creative practices. Several examples are offered by different authors in this book. The theorist holds that *integrative* generic and professional care will prevent cultural imposition and destructive care practices. With integrative care practices, recovery from illnesses will occur more frequently and rapidly. Accordingly, cultures will soon demand or expect that integrative generic and professional care practices be offered by all health professionals. When such practices occur, consumers will be able to function in their work and daily roles more effectively and remain well or healthy.

Consumers of health care will become more active in the decisions about their care. Client resistance and nonadherence will gradually be reduced. Health maintenance and promotion will be based on integrative culture care. Gradually, we will see different outcomes of health services that are culturally congruent with beneficial health outcomes. Challenging health professionals to help clients manage and maintain their wellbeing requires trusting and valuing the culture knowledge with confidence in consumers' decisions. This goal has yet to be realized. Most of all, health professionals must learn to know how to enter the client's cultural world and learn their patterns of care. Health personnel need to gain confidence in clients' ability to manage their own health and care practices.

The theorist envisions that as culture care experts become more dominant, nurses and physicians will act as *healthcare facilitators* to work with clients to transform care services to become culturally based practices. This shift in philosophy and practice, however, will require considerable education and research to develop effective care facilitator roles with cultures. This approach will lead to many positive and enthusiastic responses from clients and families as cultures maintain their own healthcare practices. This trend will require faculty and mentors to be prepared to achieve this goal as nurses and health professionals use the Culture Care Theory and the ethnonursing method. As a consequence, a major transformation in health care will be realized and will lead to institutionalization and globalization of transcultural healthcare services.

But as we move into the future, many more ethical and moral issues will be identified related to culture care practices as individuals, families, and groups assert their rights to preserve their own ethical values and lifeways. A major focus to study ethical and moral concerns of diverse cultures from a holistic perspective will lead to findings that provide the basis for dramatic new policies and ways to serve cultures. Many of these ethical and moral cultural values will be based upon environmental conditions and religious, spiritual, gender, class, and philosophical views. As a consequence, there will be a new appreciation for spiritual healing through caring and a need to reexamine healthcare practices based on spiritual outcomes. Ethical and moral research will be focused on indigenous, theological philosophies, and spiritual care beliefs that will markedly change practices in nursing and medicine. And as many disciplines become involved in ethical and moral arguments, this will lead to new guidelines and policies for health care of diverse cultures, subcultures, and general practices. Several universal as well as markedly diverse ethical and moral principles and issues will be discovered. Transcultural nurse experts and others prepared in transculturalism and direct caregiving will have an important role in codiscovering ethical care research studies with different disciplines. Such interdisciplinary work will lead to a closer linkage of transcultural care and health knowledge and therapeutic outcomes among disciplines in the natural and social sciences.

Based on these predictions, it is anticipated that the theory and method will be used worldwide. It will be used in institutions such as clinics, hospitals, and healthcare centers. It will be used by consultants and international personnel. The theory will be recommended as a guide for institutional accreditation in order to provide quality based culture care practices. Healthcare providers will find the theory and method extremely useful for providing culturally based health care because it is congruent with the way people of diverse cultures expect services. The six enablers of the Culture Care Theory will become major guides for substantiating research findings for culturally congruent and safe care practices. As a consequence, comparative care knowledge among and within cultures in the world will greatly expand and health practitioners will realize they cannot presume to *treat all people and cultures alike* but must culturally individualize their care practices and standards. The theory will be welcomed as a refreshing new approach to traditional ways of discovering and helping cultures, and will lead to many changes in health care including valuing transcultural nursing care and health services. By the end of the 21st century, transcultural health services will be an imperative for most cultures. This approach will be highly rewarding for responsible and sensitive professionals. The real challenge will be to use the research findings from the theory in creative, safe, and appropriate ways.

In summary, the theory of Culture Care Diversity and Universality will grow in demand and use worldwide. The Internet and modern electronic communication systems will facilitate its global usage. The theory and method will be viewed as one of the most comprehensive and holistic means for studying cultures and their healthcare services. Nurses and others prepared in the use of the theory and method will be in great demand. Benefits to Western and nonWestern cultures will be realized along with new insights and care practices. Many new modes of healthcare delivery will occur from universal and diverse research based care and health knowledge. With these developments, transcultural care is predicted to come fully into existence. Transcultural health care will ultimately be heralded as one of the greatest breakthroughs in nursing and many health disciplines in the 21st century. As transcultural care knowledge is used in people care, the consumers will rejoice, for it will be the first time they can rely on culturally based, culturally congruent, safe, and meaningful healthcare practices—a most welcome outcome.

When these predictions become a full reality, then the theorist and many users of the theory and method will experience a universal feeling of reward and satisfaction. The early visions and dreams of the theorist and her followers will be realized and appreciated.

Appendix

Selected Publications with Use of The Culture Care Theory

Ehrmin, J. (2001). Family violence and culture care with African American and Euro American cultures in the United States. In M. M. Leininger & M. R. McFarland (Eds.), *Transcultural nursing: Concepts, theories, research, and practice* (3rd ed.). Columbus, OH: McGraw-Hill College Custom Series.

Finn, J. (1994). Culture care of Euro American women during childbirth: Applying Leininger's theory for transcultural nursing discoveries. *Journal of Transcultural Nursing, 5*(2), 25–31.

George, T. (2000). Defining care in the culture of the chronically mentally ill living in the community. *Journal of Transcultural Nursing, 11*(2), 102–110.

Horn, B. (1995). Transcultural nursing and childbearing of the Muckleshoots. In M. Leininger (Ed.), *Transcultural nursing: Concepts, theories, research, and practice* (2nd ed.).

Leininger, M. M. (1967). The culture care concept and it relevance to nursing. *Journal of Nursing Education, 6*, 27–37.

Leininger, M. M. (1969). Ethnoscience: A promising research approach to improve nursing practice. *Image: Journal of Nursing Scholarship, 3*, 22–28.

Leininger, M. M. (1970). *Nursing and anthropology: Two worlds to blend*. New York: John Wiley & Sons.

Leininger, M. M. (1978). *Transcultural nursing: Concepts, theories, and practices*. New York: John Wiley & Sons.

Leininger, M. M. (1985). Transcultural nursing care diversity and universality: A theory of nursing. *Nursing and Health Care, 6*(4), 202–212.

Leininger, M. M. (1985). *Qualitative research methods in nursing*. Orlando, FL: Grune & Stratton, Inc.

Leininger, M. M. (1988). Leininger's theory of nursing: Culture care diversity and universality. *Nursing Science Quarterly, 2*(4), 11–20.

Leininger, M. M. (1990). Ethnomethods: The philosophic and epistemic basis to explicate transcultural nursing knowledge. *Journal of Transcultural Nursing, 2*(1), 254–257.

Leininger, M. M. (1991). Culture care diversity and universality: A theory of nursing. New York: National League for Nursing Press.

Leininger, M. M. (1993). Culture care theory: The comparative global theory to advance human care nursing knowledge and practice. In D. Gaut (Ed.), *A global agenda for caring*. New York: National League for Nursing Press.

Leininger, M. M. (1993). Culture care theory: The relevant theory to guide functioning in a multicultural world. In M. Parker (Ed.), *Patterns of nursing theories in practice* (pp. 103–122). New York: National League for Nursing Press.

Leininger, M. M. (1993). Gadsup of Papua New Guinea revisited: A three decade view. *Journal of Transcultural Nursing, 5*(1), 21–29.

Leininger, M. M. (1995). *Transcultural nursing: Concepts, theories, research, and practice.* New York: McGraw-Hill College Custom Series.

Leininger, M. M. (1997). Overview and reflection on the theory of culture care and the ethnonursing research method. *Journal of Transcultural Nursing, 8*(2), 32–53.

Leininger, M. M. (1998). Special research report: Dominant culture care (emic) meanings and practice findings from Leininger's theory. *Journal of Transcultural Nursing, 9*(2), 45–56

Luna, L. (1994). Culturally competent health care: A challenge for nurses in Saudi Arabia. *Journal of Transcultural Nursing, 5*(2), 12–20.

MacNeil, J. (1996). Use of the culture care theory with Baganda women as AIDS caregivers. *Journal of Transcultural Nursing, 7*(2), 14–20.

Miller, J. (1996). Politics and care: A study of Czech Americans with Leininger's theory of culture care diversity and universality. *Journal of Transcultural Nursing, 9*(1), 3–13.

McFarland, M.R. (1997). Use of the culture care theory with Anglo and African American elders in a long-term care setting. *Nursing Science Quarterly, 10*(4), 186–192.

Morris, E. (2004). Culture care values, meanings, and experiences of African American adolescent gang members. Unpublished dissertation. Detroit, MI: Wayne State University.

Rosenbaum, J. (1990). Cultural care of older Greek Canadian widows within Leininger's theory of culture care. *Journal of Transcultural Nursing, 2*(1), 37–47.

Stitzlein, D. (1999). The phenomenon of moral care/caring conceptualized within Leininger's theory of culture care diversity and universality. Unpublished dissertation. Detroit, MI: Wayne State University.

Spangler, Z. (1992). Transcultural nursing care values and caregiving practices of Philippine American nurses. *Journal of Transcultural Nursing, 3*(2), 23–38.

Zoucha, R. (1998). The experiences of Mexican Americans receiving professional nursing care: An ethnonursing study. *Journal of Transcultural Nursing, 9*(2), 33–34.

Wenger, A.F. (1995). Cultural context, health and health care decision making. *Journal of Transcultural Nursing, 7*(1), 3–14.

Madeleine M. Leininger

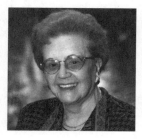

Madeleine M. Leininger, PhD, LHD, DS, CTN, RN, FAAN, FRCNA, is the founder and leader of the academic field of transcultural nursing with focus on comparative human care, theory, and research. She is Professor Emeritus, College of Nursing, Wayne State University, Detroit, Michigan (USA), and adjunct professor, College of Nursing, University of Nebraska Medical Center, Omaha, Nebraska (USA). Dr. Leininger is a well known international nurse lecturer, educator, author, theorist, administrator, researcher, and consultant in nursing and anthropology. She is a fellow and distinguished Living Legend of the American Academy of Nursing and an Emeritus Member of the American Association of Colleges of Nursing. She was first graduate professional nurse prepared with a PhD in cultural anthropology. She initiated the Nurse Scientist and several transcultural nursing programs in the early 1970s and 1980s. She has conducted indepth field studies of 18 Western and nonWestern cultures. Dr. Leininger initiated and was the first Editor of the Journal of Transcultural Nursing and established the Transcultural Nursing Society. She has been a Distinguished Professor and Lecturer in over 100 universities, has given over 1500 invited public addresses throughout the USA and worldwide, and has been the recipient of many honors and awards. Dr. Leininger is author and editor of 30 books and has published over 260 articles. She published the first qualitative nursing research book (1985), an early psychiatric nursing book (1960), and the first Culture Care Diversity and Universality Theory book. Presently, Dr. Leininger resides in Omaha, Nebraska, and remains active as a worldwide nursing consultant, educator, lecturer, and writer.

Marilyn R. McFarland

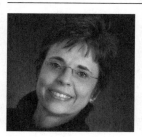

Marilyn R. McFarland, PhD, RN, CTN received her doctorate in nursing with a focus on transcultural nursing under the mentorship of Dr. Madeleine Leininger at Wayne State University, Detroit, Michigan (USA) in 1995. Dr. McFarland has directed her professional work toward the care and study of elders from diverse cultures throughout the USA. She is a Certified Transcultural Nurse, a former editor of the *Journal of Transcultural Nursing*, and is active worldwide in the Transcultural Nursing Society. Dr. McFarland teaches transcultural nursing courses and presents her research findings about the culture care of elders locally, nationally, and worldwide, and is currently pursuing a nurse practitioner certificate with the goal toward integrating transcultural knowledge and caring into advanced practice nursing clinical contexts.

Index

nursing metaparadigm, 6–7, 365–366
nursing organizations, 98
nursing students in baccalaureate
    program (study), 239–252
    economic influences, 244–247
    environmental context, 240, 247
    institutionalization of services, 249
    philosophical and spiritual factors,
        247
    political factors, 241, 247
    research methods and informants,
        242
    social structure, 243–244
nurturance (means of caring), 145,
    147, 150

O

Observation-Participation-Reflection
    Enabler, 26–27, 52, 60–61
    German American elders (study),
        189
    Potawatomi Native Americans
        (study), 215–216
    Southern Sudanese of Africa
        (study), 265
observation, role of, 61
Old Order Amish people (study),
    32–33, 296
openness for discovery, 21, 72–74, 164
    inquiry modes for, 53–54
opportunity for activities (means of
    care), 198
opportunity for cultural knowledge, 165
OPR Enabler, 26–27, 52, 60–61
    German American elders (study),
        189
    Potawatomi Native Americans
        (study), 215–216
    Southern Sudanese of Africa
        (study), 265
orderliness (means of care), 196
organizations, professional, 98
orientational definitions, 12–16. *See
    also individual definitions*
outreach, 166

P

patterns, repeated. *See* recurrent
    patterning
People's Republic of China,
    transcultural nursing in, 90
person, defined, 9
phases of data analysis, 61–64
    German American elders (study),
        190
    Potawatomi Native Americans
        (study), 218
    refugee communities in United
        States (study), 334–335
    Southern Sudanese of Africa
        (study), 273–275
Philippine American values and action
    modes, 292
Philippine and Anglo American nurses
    (study), 381–383
philosophical care influences. *See*
    religious dimensions of care;
    spiritual dimensions of care
philosophical roots of Culture Care
    Theory, 17–18
physical abuse (as noncaring), 227
Polish American values and action
    modes, 297
political dimensions of care
    BSN program (study), 241–242, 247
    Gadsup Akunans (study), 136–137
    refugee communities in United
        States (study), 327–346
        acculturation of refugees,
            327–328
        data analysis, 334–335
        domain of inquiry, 329
        findings, 336–342
        modes of culture care, 342–345
        research methods and
            informants, 331–333
Potawatomi people and family violence
    (study), 207–237
    domain of inquiry, 207–210
    ethnohistory and social structure,
        213–214
    findings, 218–222

W

Z